LEARNING
AND ASSESSMENT
IN CLINICAL PRACTICE

Content Strategist: *Mairi McCubbin*
Content Development Specialist: *Barbara Simmons*
Project Manager: *Vinod Kumar*
Designer/Design Direction: *Miles Hitchen*
Illustration Manager: *Jennifer Rose*

MENTORING, LEARNING AND ASSESSMENT
IN CLINICAL PRACTICE

A guide for nurses, midwives and other health professionals

Third Edition

Ci Ci Stuart BAppSci MED RN RM MTD

City & Guilds Work Based Assessors' Awards D32 & D33

Senior Lecturer in Nursing and Midwifery, Faculty of Health and Wellbeing, Sheffield Hallam University, Sheffield, UK

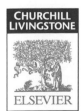

Edinburgh   London   New York   Oxford   Philadelphia   St Louis   Sydney   Toronto   2013

ELSEVIER
CHURCHILL
LIVINGSTONE

© 2013 Elsevier Ltd. All rights reserved.

First edition 2003
Second edition 2007
Third edition 2013

ISBN 978-0-7020-4195-2

British Library Cataloguing in Publication Data
A catalogue record for this book is available from the British Library

Library of Congress Cataloging in Publication Data
A catalog record for this book is available from the Library of Congress

Notices

Knowledge and best practice in this field are constantly changing. As new research and experience broaden our understanding, changes in research methods, professional practices, or medical treatment may become necessary.

Practitioners and researchers must always rely on their own experience and knowledge in evaluating and using any information, methods, compounds, or experiments described herein. In using such information or methods they should be mindful of their own safety and the safety of others, including parties for whom they have a professional responsibility.

With respect to any drug or pharmaceutical products identified, readers are advised to check the most current information provided (i) on procedures featured or (ii) by the manufacturer of each product to be administered, to verify the recommended dose or formula, the method and duration of administration, and contraindications. It is the responsibility of practitioners, relying on their own experience and knowledge of their patients, to make diagnoses, to determine dosages and the best treatment for each individual patient, and to take all appropriate safety precautions.

To the fullest extent of the law, neither the Publisher nor the authors, contributors, or editors, assume any liability for any injury and/or damage to persons or property as a matter of products liability, negligence or otherwise, or from any use or operation of any methods, products, instructions, or ideas contained in the material herein.

ELSEVIER your source for books, journals and multimedia in the health sciences

www.elsevierhealth.com

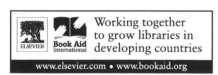

Working together to grow libraries in developing countries

www.elsevier.com • www.bookaid.org

The Publisher's policy is to use paper manufactured from sustainable forests

Printed in the United States of America

Contents

Preface

Having a book published is a 'scary' affair. You never know how it will be received and whether it will be used at all. The writing of the first edition of this book represented my very first attempt at book writing. I made the attempt because I wanted to disseminate my ideas of what I saw are workable strategies to help busy practitioners supervise and assess learners to achieve validity and reliability of assessments conducted; conversations I have had with practitioners who supervise and assess student learning during their clinical placements raised numerous issues about this role. Questions such as 'How do I know I am assessing what I should at the correct level?', 'How do I know how much to allow the student to do?', 'What do I do if a student is not progressing?' were raised frequently. A common comment was 'I simply do not have enough time to give my student as much as I wish to.' The message that was given was 'We want to know how to do it so that we can get on with it.' This informed the approach I took then which was to write a 'how to do it' book. I attempted to provide the 'why' behind the teaching, learning and assessment strategies suggested by referring to the theoretical and evidence base that underpins educational and assessment practice, with particular reference to that body of knowledge on learning and assessment of clinical practice.

On being asked to bring out a third edition, I read through the previous edition and mulled over the solicited comprehensive reviews carried out by a number of professional colleagues. I agreed with them that, since the publication of the second edition, there have been a number of changes in the recommendations, policies and standards made by the Nursing and Midwifery Council (NMC), Health and Care Professions Council and the Department of Health (DoH) about pre-registration programmes and the support of learning and assessment in clinical practice (NMC 2008). The NMC brought out the *Standards* for pre-registration nursing and midwifery education in 2010a and 2009, respectively. These *Standards* replace the *Standards of Proficiency* brought out in 2004. Since 2005 the Health and Care Professions Council has been bringing out *Standards of Proficiency* for the professions it regulates. In all professions there is, again, particular reference to the necessity to train healthcare students for 'fitness to practise'; the crucial contribution of practice learning and assessment to achieve this is again emphasized.

You will not disagree with me when I say that only practitioners who are 'fit to practise' should be allowed on to the professional register. Fitness to practise means having the skills, knowledge, good health and good character to practise safely and effectively (NMC 2010b, HCPC 2010). Therein lies a major problem: there are practitioners on the professional registers whose fitness to practise were questionable prior to initial registration. The issue of 'failure to fail' is a continuing problem in all professions, both nationally and internationally. The section that deals with the management of assessment problems, including the situation where students have to be failed, has been expanded. I have also attempted to provide a synopsis of the key reasons for 'failure to fail' from studies conducted by various professional groups in health care to increase understanding of why assessors give students the benefit of the doubt. To broaden the perspective and discussion around 'fitness to practise', the section on professional behaviours has been expanded.

The complexity and challenges of facilitating learning in the clinical setting remain largely unchanged over time. One of these challenges is supporting students with special needs, including those with dyslexia. The section on how best to support these students has been expanded to include a discussion of strategies to assist the practice educator in meeting the particular learning needs of these students so that they may have successful and fulfilling clinical placement experiences.

In the healthcare professions, competence to perform complex and technical problems only is now increasingly challenged by the public and the professions themselves. There is an expectation that the personal attributes of practitioners are also developed as these are necessary for effective professional practice. It is particularly challenging to assess professional conduct, values and ethics. The assessment of this important aspect of a student's development has been discussed in more detail. There is an inclusion of an assessment tool in Appendix 4 to assess those professional behaviours that reflect the professional conduct, values and ethics expected of health care students.

We carry on having to deal with what Rowntree (1987:ix) refers to as 'the timeless, enduring issues underlying our changing assessment practices'. When working on this edition, I have held on to my views of what I perceive to be workable and sound learning and assessment strategies. Although I have referred to some more educational theory and more recent work on the support of learning and assessment in clinical practice, I have not changed the essence of the clinical learning and assessment strategies used in the previous edition.

In the preface to the first edition I said that clinical settings provide the unique learning experiences and opportunities to assist students to undergo professional socialization positively and develop the competence for professional practice that cannot be readily acquired elsewhere. This means that, during clinical placements, learning needs to be actively facilitated and evaluated; it should not be left to chance. The clinical experience for students should be much more than just learning what to do and how to do it: it should be about the education of students who will one day be our professional peers, colleagues and co-learners. Robertson et al (1997:174) point out that a 'major metamorphosis that must occur in the student clinician is the transformation from dependent, non-skilled, apprenticed technician into an independent, responsible, skilled, self-evaluating professional'. In participating in clinical education, the practitioner who is the practice educator to learners is challenged to empower the learner to reach those goals.

As in the previous editions, I have attempted to keep to an accessible style and used personal overtones. I have chosen the latter approach because I want to convey that in my present role as educator with responsibility for student learning in both theory and practice I engage with those educational processes that I write about. I hope those readers who prefer a more detached style of writing will not feel uncomfortable reading the text. I have kept to the 'how to do it' approach as I still believe that busy practitioners are more likely to look for teaching and learning strategies that are both workable and manageable.

This book is intended for the practice educators of clinical practice in the nursing, midwifery and other healthcare professions who seek to understand, and develop, skills of supporting, supervising, facilitating learning and assessing students to achieve validity and reliability in assessment. Previous editions focused mainly on the education requirements of pre-registration nursing and midwifery students. To make this edition more accessible to registrants from both the NMC and the HCPC, the contents of information and discussion have been broadened to reflect the education requirements of pre-registration students regulated by both statutory bodies.

I hold the rather strong viewpoint that one key capability of a good assessor is that of having the courage to fail students when standards are not achieved. You have the onerous, and crucial, task of ensuring that the clinical practice of students attains fitness for practice at the point of professional registration. In terms of professional functions, this book will be useful for anyone who is trying to understand the complexities of learning and assessing in the clinical setting.

Clinical practice and its assessment are challenging and rewarding professional activities. I hope you enjoy using this book and gain in your expertise as mentor or assessor to the very many students of health care who will pass your way. To the student readers, I hope you are empowered to manage your own learning and professional development.

Sheffield, 2012   Ci Ci Stuart

REFERENCES

Health and Care Professions Council, 2005. Standards of Proficiency. Online. Available: <http://www.hcpc-uk.org/publications/index.asp?action = submit>; (accessed September 2012).

Health and Care Professions Council, 2010. Information for Employers and Managers: The Fitness to Practise Process. HCPC, London, Online. Available: <http://www.hcpc-uk.org/complaints/> (accessed August 2011).

Nursing and Midwifery Council, 2008. Standards to Support Learning and Assessment in Practice, second ed. NMC, London, Online. Available: <http://www.nmc-uk.org/Publications/Standards> (accessed August 2011).

Nursing and Midwifery Council, 2009. Standards of Pre-Registration Midwifery Education. NMC, London, Online. Available: <http://www.nmc-uk.org/Publications/Standards/> (accessed August 2011).

Nursing and Midwifery Council, 2010a. Standards of Pre-Registration Nursing Education. NMC, London, Online. Available: <http://www.nmc-uk.org/Publications/Standards/> (accessed August 2011).

Nursing and Midwifery Council, 2010b. Fitness to Practise: How the Process Works. NMC, London, Online. Available: <http://www.nmc-uk.org/Hearings/How-the-process-works/> (accessed August 2011).

Robertson, S., Rosenthal, J., Dawson, V., 1997. Using assessment to promote student learning. In: McAllister, L., Lincoln, M., McLeod, S. (Eds.), Facilitating Learning in Clinical Settings. Stanley Thornes, Cheltenham, pp. 154–184.

Rowntree, D., 1987. Assessing Students: How Shall We Know Them?, second ed. Kogan Page, London.

Acknowledgements

I wish to say a big thank you to the reviewers for taking the time to carry out the comprehensive reviews for the third edition of this book. Their views and constructive comments have been invaluable in contributing to the revisions made for this edition.

I wish to express a special thank you to the many colleagues, practice educators and students who have continued to contribute to my understanding and thoughts on the assessment, supervision and support of learners during clinical practice.

Introduction

The facilitation and assessment of learning in the practice setting are complex activities and require multifaceted capabilities. My personal experiences of having 'taught', assessed and facilitated learning in both the classroom and clinical settings lead me to say with confidence that these activities are more challenging to conduct well in the clinical setting. Learning situations and settings are more amenable to control in the classroom, but much less so, even impossible to control, in the clinical setting. Teaching and learning have to fit in with the flow of the patient/client care situations; well-developed facilitation skills are required to assist students to extract the learning that each situation has to offer. In this book, strategies are suggested to assist busy practitioners to develop and utilize those skills required for learning and assessing to proceed with success.

This is a practice-centred book. It concerns learning and assessment in clinical practice. There are critical discussions on how supervision, support and valid assessment nurture the development and achievement of competence. As the book has been written with busy practitioners in mind, it has utilized a down-to-earth approach so that the numerous clinical learning and assessment strategies are accessible and workable. For those who wish to delve into the theory and research that underpin the strategies, there is reference to a solid theoretical base that draws on the educational principles and body of knowledge surrounding teaching, learning and assessment, with particular reference to literature applicable to the clinical setting.

The book starts by exploring four broad categories of the purpose of assessment with particular reference to the complex nature of clinical practice and its assessment in the health care professions. There is a critical discussion of how far these purposes are fulfilled, the impact on learners of our assessment procedures and the nature of clinical practice and assessment. The espoused values of these purposes of assessment are challenged. The point is made that, as learning and assessment in clinical practice seem to be rather 'hit and miss affairs', we need to review critically why we assess at all so that we may consider more carefully whether our assessment procedures are justified.

Chapter 2 demonstrates that the very purposes of assessment we set out to achieve may not be fully realized if we do not pause to consider our professional responsibilities and accountability as assessors. What implications are attached to Beaumont's (2004) statement that assessors have a moral responsibility to fail incompetent students, and the requirement of the Nursing and Midwifery Council that its registrants be accountable to their professional statutory body for summative assessment decisions (NMC 2008)? This chapter starts with a consideration of the meaning of the concepts of responsibility and accountability. It then explores the issues of responsibility and accountability surrounding assessment in nursing and midwifery education and other health care professions. It includes an examination of the professional, statutory and institutional regulations governing the assessment of practice and the supervision of students. Regulations for the support of students with learning needs such as dyslexia are examined and strategies are suggested for more effective support of these students to facilitate their development. Attempts are made to answer two key questions surrounding the assessment of clinical practice: 'What are practice educators responsible and accountable for?' and 'Who are practice educators responsible and accountable to?' This latter question is considered in conjunction with the role, responsibilities and accountability of students for learning and assessment. The powerful influence of the practice educator as a role model for learning, and hence raising accountability issues, is considered. Very frequently, a practitioner is mentor as well as assessor to the same student. This may cause dilemmas for this practitioner when assessment decisions are made. The key dilemmas created by the mentor and assessor interface are explored.

In exploring 'What do we assess?' in Chapter 3, there is an investigation of literature that discusses the many challenges that the assessment of competence presents: a notable example is the difficulty in defining the construct and what it means to be clinically competent. Because competence can only be inferred, as it cannot be observed directly, the definition of competence is developed to clarify its components to enable this construct to be assessed with a degree of validity and reliability. The case is made for the use of an integrated competency-based approach for assessing nursing and midwifery practice. Arguments are put forward that a competency-based approach to education and training potentially provides a framework for bringing together professional policies for training and employment requirements to achieve 'fitness to practise'. The competency-based model of assessment is critically evaluated as an assessment tool for assessing professional practice.

Clinical competence is a complex entity and it almost always requires the practitioner to use a combination of attributes simultaneously and adapt practices to different contexts. Equally important will be the requirement to gather sufficient evidence to justify the inference, and, in particular, that a safe inference has been made (Gonczi et al 1993). A 'range of forms of evidence' (Bedford et al 1993) is required to enable assessors to make sound inferences that learners can perform competently in the variety of clinical situations in which they can find themselves. In Chapter 4, the uses and merits, and limitations, of a range of assessment methods that can be used in the competency-based approach for the assessment of clinical practice are explored and debated. The use of the strategy of triangulation to obtain the breadth and depth of assessment evidence to enhance the validity and reliability of assessment is discussed.

Assessment of clinical practice is inevitably based on a sample of the student's performance on assessment tasks perceived to be relevant. An inference of competence is then made from the student's performance on the set of arranged tasks. We rely on assessments to make some quite specific, but also far-ranging, judgements about our students' future behaviour as registered practitioners. A fundamental question we need to ask is this: do our assessments enable us to make such judgements soundly? Deciding whether or not an assessment lives up to this task is not straightforward. In Chapter 5, there is an examination of those issues we need to consider in order to make sound judgements in assessments. Issues surrounding the questions of validity, reliability, feasibility and discriminating powers of assessment are explored. Those factors that can affect validity and reliability are considered, and measures to attain objective assessments and avoid subjective assessments are suggested so that we can begin to work towards assessments that are fairer to all students.

As discussed in Chapters 3 and 4, in a competency-based system, assessment has the key function of obtaining evidence of competence. Chapter 6 discusses the constructive focus of assessment where the aim is to help rather than sentence the individual. Nicklin & Kenworthy (1995) believe that assessments should give students the opportunities to demonstrate the learning that has taken place. In this chapter, the continuous assessment process is explored as the key assessment strategy to facilitate assessment as a learning process. It is suggested that integral to the continuous assessment of clinical practice are the strategies of using learning contracts with its concomitant assessment plan, formative assessment and summative assessment processes. These are examined with respect to the successful management of the continuous assessment of practice in order to realize the positive impact of assessment. Suggestions are made on how to manage constructive feedback.

In Chapter 7, the point is made that monitoring progress, managing feedback and making assessment decisions are interrelated activities that are integral to the continuous assessment of practice. These activities are central to, and essential in, helping students learn through their practice to develop clinical competence. If assessment is to be a learning process as discussed in the last chapter, the student should be an equal partner in these activities; progress is monitored jointly through the formative assessment process set up, and the student participates actively during feedback and assessment decision-making sessions. There is emphasis that assessment is a two-way process between the assessor and student to realize its learning potential. In this chapter, a model comprising four assessment activities is suggested to monitor the progress of learners. This is followed by a discussion of the steps to consider when making formative and summative assessment decisions. Extrapolating from the work of Benner et al (1996) and Glaser (1990), criteria are proposed for the assessment of the development and achievement of competence at the novice, advanced beginner and competent levels. Suggestions are made on how to manage some assessment problems such as students experiencing problems learning during clinical practice with particular reference to the situation when a student has to be failed to avoid the 'failure to fail' scenario.

The clinical experience of students of health care is widely acknowledged as being one of the most important aspects of their educational preparation. The clinical environment is the arena where students from the health care professions learn about care and what clinical practice is all about. The clinical environment must therefore also be an environment where learning can take place, thus becoming an educational environment. This is the ideal setting to promote inter-professional learning and utilize opportunities to enable students to learn and work within the multi-disciplinary team to foster development of the skills of team working.

Marton et al (1984) make the important observation that learning is a function of the relationship between the learner and the environment and is never something determined by one of these elements alone. Learners do not respond merely to tasks assigned; rather, they adapt to and work within the environment taken as an interrelated whole. Chapter 8 examines those human and material factors contributing to a positive clinical learning environment. The centrality of the mentor in supporting learners and facilitating learning is emphasized. Quality assurance processes in place to monitor, maintain and enhance placement experiences for students are described. Criteria for the educational audit of clinical placements are suggested.

The ideal clinical learning environment may not have any fruition if the complexities of learning through experience are not recognized and acknowledged. Chapter 9 provides a systematic account of how competence can be nurtured through the activities of supervision, support and assessment in a clinical practice (Schön 1987). Learning from experience is not a simple rational process: not only do we need to know *what* and *how* to do, we also need to know *what* to think about and *how* to think. Impacting on, and influencing, these psychomotor and cognitive processes are our feelings, values and beliefs. This chapter proposes, and explores, the use of a *model for learning from experience* as the framework to consider experience-based learning, and how learners can be assisted to interact with the clinical environment in order to learn through practice and unearth meaning from experiences. This model emphasizes the centrality and richness of clinical experience as a source of learning. It is also suggested that, as professional knowledge and practices change constantly, the use of this model will enable the practitioner to refine and update knowledge and practices so that professional expertise, and thus practice wisdom (Hull 1998), is continually developing.

The main points of each chapter are provided in the form of 'key points for reflection' at the end of each chapter. This is to provide readers with a quick reference to the contents of the chapter and to give readers a 'checklist' of the main issues of the chapter.

Throughout the book, there are self-directed activities. These are practice-focused as they are intended to assist readers to relate theory to practice, develop the mentoring and assessing roles of the team and also to consider more comprehensively their role as mentor or assessor.

REFERENCES

Beaumont, S., 2004. Stop incompetent nurses. Br. J. Nurs. 13 (11), 663.

Bedford, H., Phillips, T., Robinson, J., et al., 1993. Assessment of Competencies in Nursing and Midwifery Education and Training. The English National Board for Nursing, Midwifery and Health Visiting, London.

Benner, P., Tanner, C.A., Chesla, C.A., 1996. Expertise in Nursing Practice. Springer, New York.

Glaser, R., 1990. Toward new models for assessment. Int. J. Educ. Res. 14 (5), 475–483.

Gonczi, A., Hager, P., Athanasou, J., 1993. The Development of Competency-Based Assessment Strategies for the Professions. Australian Government Publishing Service, Canberra, National Office of Overseas Skills Recognition. Research Paper No. 8.

Hull, C., 1998. Open learning and professional development. In: Quinn, F.M. (Ed.), Continuing Professional Development in Nursing. Stanley Thornes, Cheltenham, pp. 182–204.

Marton, F., Hounsell, D., Entwistle, N., 1984. The Experience of Learning. Scottish Academic Press, Edinburgh.

Nicklin, P.J., Kenworthy, N., 1995. Teaching and Assessing in Clinical Practice, second ed. Baillière Tindall, London.

Nursing and Midwifery Council, 2008. Standards to Support Learning and Assessment in Practice, second ed. NMC, London, Online. Available: <http://www.nmc-uk.org/Publications/Standards> (accessed August 2011).

Schön, D.A., 1987. Educating the Reflective Practitioner. Jossey-Bass, San Francisco.

Terminology

MENTOR

In Greek mythology, Mentor was the wise and faithful advisor to Odysseus. Today the term 'mentor' is generally used to describe a friend, role model, an able advisor and a person who supports in many different ways.

The term *mentor* is used in this book to describe the clinical practitioner who supports, guides, supervises and facilitates student learning during clinical practice, who participates in the formative assessment of competence only.

PRACTICE EDUCATOR

The term *practice educator* is used in this book to describe the identified clinical practitioner who supports, guides, supervises and facilitates student learning during clinical practice, who also has responsibility for the formative and summative assessment of competence. The practice educator is very likely to assume the role of mentor as well.

Throughout the literature, the identified practitioner who supports, supervises and facilitates student learning during clinical practice generally also has responsibility for the formative and summative assessment of competence. These practitioners may be referred to as the mentor, assessor, preceptor, work-based supervisor, field work teacher, practice learning facilitator, practice educator, clinical tutor or trainer. These terms are likely to have different connotations for different readers. With the potential for confusion that may arise from the use of so many terms to describe this role, the decision was made to use the term practice educator in this text to describe this role for several reasons.

The principle that underpins much of the discussion in this book is that assessment should seek to facilitate learning through the use of formative and summative assessment processes. Generally, among other activities, the activities of supporting, supervising and facilitating learning take place during formative assessment. During summative assessment the crucial decision to pass or fail the student is generally made on the basis of evidence generated from formative assessment activities. The term practice educator therefore reflects most closely the role of the practitioner who engages in the use of formative and summative assessment processes to assess competence.

In the context of the assessment of clinical practice in the health care professions in the UK, the practice educator is a qualified practitioner whose name is on the statutory professional register that confers the right for a person to practise in that professional capacity. The practice educator would normally work alongside students while guiding, supervising and assessing their practice. Assessments conducted would be both formative and summative. These students would normally be undergoing the pre-registration educational programme to obtain the same professional qualification as the practice educator.

In the case of nurses and midwives, the practitioner who fulfils the role outline of the practice educator as described above is referred to as the mentor; this is not to be confused with the use of the term mentor in this book.

Chapter | 1 |

The purposes and nature of assessment and clinical assessment

INTRODUCTION

In this chapter, I shall consider why we assess at all in the health care professions. These supposedly educational and professional purposes of assessment will be explored in conjunction with their potential for causing short- and long-term negative consequences for the students on whom we have passed 'judgement'. Mindful of the context of assessment being discussed in this book, this chapter will also take a look at the complexities of clinical assessment. The phrase 'complexities of clinical assessment' is used with intent: it is used on the assumption that, for many readers of this book, the nature of learning and assessing in the clinical setting will be close to their hearts as a direct result of significant and meaningful personal experiences of having been a learner and been assessed, and having worked and been an assessor, in that setting.

In this chapter, 'assessment' is used as a global term incorporating tests and examinations of coursework (whether oral or written), the judgement of performance during clinical practice, and any other ways of measuring professional learning. The term 'assessor' is used to encompass all clinical practitioners who support and assess students during practice, or lecturers from higher education institutions who assess academic work and/or clinical practice.

THE NATURE OF ASSESSMENT

We all are keenly aware of the importance of assessment and the influence it has on our lives. As Rowntree (1987:xii), in perhaps one of his philosophical moments, points out:

> *Assessment will remain with us from the cradle to beyond the grave. Scarcely have we taken our first breath before we have a label fastened to our wrists, giving weight at, and method of, birth, and, somewhere, our first file (medical) has already been opened. And even in death we cannot escape the assessors – obituary-writers for the famous; just family, workmates and friends for the rest of us.*

And don't Rowntree's sentiments strike a strong chord! Consciously or subconsciously, we are assessing most of the time, be it at work, at home or even when out walking in the countryside. And as Broadfoot (1996:3) noted, 'assessment is a central feature of social life'.

Passing judgement on people, on events, on ideas, on things and on values is part of the process of making sense of the world around us and where we stand in any given situation. Sometimes we judge to reassure ourselves – *I am glad I am not as selfish as she is* – (and we might be rather lacking in self-awareness)! We are all assessors; even very young children are capable of making assessments – ask a young child whether she or he likes her/his new school and, of course, the response will be either a 'yes' or a 'no'. The ability to respond implies that the child has activated the mental processes involving a mental review of perhaps the teachers, the other children, the events and the activities that she or he likes or dislikes and has applied more or less conscious criteria to what would constitute, for instance, a like or dislike of the teacher. In social settings and during social interactions we may not be asked to justify our judgements and, indeed, may be most taken aback and even feel embarrassed if asked to do so. However, in educational and professional settings, such justification is frequently required as the process of assessment is overt, formalized and controlled. The criteria we use are often subject to scrutiny and we are required to make our assessment decisions on the basis of available evidence.

Much has been written about educational assessment as it is a legitimate concern of practitioners, learners, teachers and those responsible for the development and accreditation of courses. Rightly or wrongly, assessment is assumed to be the nexus of learning. It might seem to be common sense and, indeed, it is the 'custom and practice' today that students undertaking an educational programme should be assessed. It is easy to polarize to the position of unquestioning acceptance of the necessity for assessment as we have all been subject to some form of educational assessment ourselves, such as sitting a timed, invigilated written examination or a multiple-choice paper, carrying out a practical procedure or enduring the agonies of an oral examination. Assessment can reduce us to experience extremes of emotions.

As a student of health care, you would have been observed, tested and questioned in the clinical setting: e.g. while giving patient/client care and performing procedures in conjunction with care delivery, and carrying out tasks such as preparing a trolley or cleaning a piece of equipment. A comprehensive list will be long. Many of you may also recall that, on your 'good' days, after completion of a span of duty you leave the clinical area feeling glad to have been on duty as you have had a positive and productive day – you have learnt from feedback from your assessors. Conversely, on your 'bad' days, you may have cried and threatened to hand in your notice! Staff had been too busy to help and supervise what you were doing – you made errors, and staff and patients complained about your work. You became emotionally and physically drained, and were also thoroughly demoralized. You perceived that time had been wasted as you had not learnt on those types of days.

The scenario of 'bad' days as painted appears to be an ongoing one and remains a problem. In 1989, Watts reported that, after an initial period of supervision, student nurses on a first clinical placement were left to practise independently. If they sought supervision and

feedback, it was given. Students who were unaware of incorrect practice would continue to practise incorrectly without seeking help. The assumption made was that, if no help was required, 'all was well'. Even assessment was carried out by inference; trained staff would assume safe and competent practice from students' expressions of confidence. Assessors of pre-registration nursing and midwifery students in the studies by Bedford et al (1993) and Phillips et al (2000) reported experiencing role strain and role conflict, and teaching and assessing students became an additional burden. Later studies by Henderson et al (2006) and Hurley & Snowden (2008) found that assessors could not attend to students' needs fully when demands of patient care overrode teaching duties. Consequently, students' learning and assessing needs were marginalized and placed in opposition to client care needs, with students having to fend for themselves.

Learning and assessment in clinical practice seem to be rather 'hit and miss affairs'. Why then do we bother to assess students in clinical practice, and during their educational programme in general? What are the purposes of assessment? It is perhaps appropriate to explore these at this point. You may wish to try Activity 1.1 before you proceed.

ACTIVITY 1.1

Ask yourself the following questions: Why do I assess students? What justifications can I give that these purposes are realized by my assessment procedures and processes?

THE PURPOSES OF ASSESSMENT

The nursing, midwifery and medical professions have required their 'trainees' to be examined since the 19th century. The medical profession was the first profession to institute qualifying examinations in order to determine competence (Broadfoot 1979). This commenced in 1815. In 1872, the London Obstetrical Society took the initiative to set up its own examination board to examine women between the ages of 21 and 30 who wanted to be certified as a 'skilled Midwife, competent to attend natural labours' (Donnison 1988:85). This examination comprised a written and oral examination (Sweet & Tiran 1997). In the case of nurses, the first examination was held with the establishment of a School of Nursing at the London Hospital in 1880 (Seymer 1949). Students had to sit an examination consisting of a paper, a viva voce and a practical test in the wards, at the end of their first and second years of training (Bendall & Raybould 1969). Certificates were awarded on successful completion of the 2-year course.

With the passing of The Midwives Act in 1902 it became a statutory requirement to be registered on the Midwives Roll in order to practise as a midwife. Likewise, with the passing of The Nurses Registration Act in 1919, nurses were required to register on the Nurses Register. Statutory registration was instituted to raise standards of care. In the early years of the Acts, one route to registration was to fulfil the prescribed conditions of practice and pass state examinations. In the case of health professionals regulated by the Health and Care Professions Council (HCPC), the Health Professions Order of 2001 requires these practitioners to register with the HCPC following successful attainment of assessments. Professionally, then, nurses, midwives and registrants on the HCPC register have been impressed with the necessity to be assessed and most are likely to have internalized this value.

To accept the necessity for assessment unthinkingly denies a complex debate concerning the purposes of assessments. The effects of the assessment on the learner as an individual, and its impact on the curriculum, teaching and learning, may also be overlooked. Rowntree (1987:xii) pointed out that even though educational assessment is confined to a fairly small proportion of our lifespan it can have a disproportionate negative effect on the rest of our lives. The 'evidence' from these assessments can make or break us in life as it can tell other people (and ourselves) what to think and feel about us – life's doors may either be open or shut for us as a result of being so judged. Critically reviewing 'why' we assess may make us consider more carefully whether our assessments are reasonable and just. As professionals, we like to think that we know why we are doing what we are doing most, if not all, of the time. However, Foucault (1982:182) has this to say: 'People know what they do; they frequently know why they do what they do; but what they don't know is what what they do does'.

Klug (1975) acknowledged that one of the many difficulties of discussing the theme of assessment lies in the tangle of issues involved: even its explicit and acknowledged functions are multifarious and conflicting. In an earlier publication Klug (Klug 1974 in Rowntree 1987) gathered 32 reasons for formal assessment. Here, I shall concentrate on what I see are the four main reasons commonly advanced for assessment in professional health care education.

Assessment for entry into the profession

Selection for training

Assessment for entry into a profession starts at the point of application for training. Candidates are screened for the required 'academic' qualifications, their ability to complete the course and the potential qualities of being a professional of the profession applied for. For the purpose of illustrating whether it is possible to carry out this aspect of 'assessment' with some semblance of reliability and validity, some findings from the pre-registration nursing and midwifery programmes in the UK are used as a case study.

In the UK, the typical academic qualifications (with some variations between the requirements of different Higher Education Institutions) required for entry to pre-registration nursing and midwifery programmes include three GCE 'A' levels, grade C or above; or five GCSE/GCE 'O' levels, grade C or above; or the General National Vocational Qualification (GNVQ) Advanced level or an Access course for Higher Education. Candidates have to prove that their ability to contribute to the profession is greater than that of others. One of the assumptions implicit in this selection procedure is that only those who are deemed capable of successfully completing the training are funded for the education programme. Disappointingly, the correlation between fulfilment of selection criteria and successful completion of training is low. Levels of discontinuation from pre-registration nursing and midwifery courses are a source of concern. In earlier years, statistics published by the English National Board (ENB 2002) for the period 1996–2001 show that the non-completion rate of all pre-registration student nurses and student midwives was between 15 and 18%. Later statistics show that the situation has worsened. Statistics from the Higher Education Statistics Agency in the UK show that, for the period 2002/03 to 2003/04, just 68% of nursing students stayed the course (Waters 2006). In 2006 in the UK, the Department of Health (2006) declared that nursing student attrition rates of more than 15% are unacceptable. In the intervening period to 2010, despite various policy initiatives, the attrition rate has risen to almost double that target in England. It hit 30 per cent in Scotland (Scott 2010). Scott went on to say that the admissions process cannot be working effectively if applicants accepted on courses discover after a matter of weeks that nursing is not for them. Table 1.1 show the attrition rates for the UK for the years 2006, 2008 and 2010 (Waters 2010). The statistics clearly show a high 'casualty' rate.

Table 1.1 Attrition rates for pre-registration nursing students in the UK: 2006, 2008, 2010

	2006	2008	2010 (estimate)
England	30	27	20
Scotland	29	27	28
Wales	17	25	13
Northern Ireland	9	23	16

(From Waters A 2010 The question for universities: how can they win the war on attrition? Nursing Standard 24(24):12–15.)

Internationally, the scale of the problem is difficult to quantify from the literature, partly because of differences in definition and partly because of incomplete and non-comparable data. Ehrenfeld et al (1997) gave a figure of 23.5% over a 5-year period for their own institution in Israel. Mashaba & Mhlongo (1995) from South Africa reported an attrition rate of 31.2% over a 5-year period for the institution under investigation. This compared with 64% over the same 5-year period for eight institutions (including the study institution) offering the same course.

Reasons for discontinuation are many and varied. There is no intention here to explore these but to refer only to those that, by our stringent selection criteria, we seek to prevent from occurring. These reasons are listed in

Table 1.2 for ease of reference. Readers are directed to the work of Urwin et al (2009) where a comprehensive critical review and analysis of 123 records to identify factors contributing to student nurse attrition found that individual student factors, institutional issues and broader political, professional and societal issues were the key reasons for the attrition.

The non-completion rate is similar in occupational therapy (Ilott 1993, in Ilott & Murphy 1999). Ilott reports that, for the period 1987–1990, the collective rate for three intakes of students was 14.6%. The most common reason was academic failure, which was defined as an inability to cope with the course, and/or to learn by failure on internal or professional assessment.

Table 1.2 Reasons for discontinuation of training			
Author	**Year**	**Country**	**Reasons**
Waters	2010	UK	Financial pressures Academic failure Wrong career choice
Urwin et al	2009	UK	Academic failure Wrong career choice Personal problems Financial pressures Dissatisfaction with the course and clinical placements
White et al	1999	UK	Academic failure –39% Personal problems Wrong career choice
Ehrenfeld et al	1997	Israel	Academic failure –39% Inappropriate professional behaviour –16% Personal problems
Richardson	1996	UK	Academic failure –20% Misconduct
Mashaba & Mhlongo	1995	South Africa	Dissatisfaction with the course Negative attitude of lecturers Exploited in clinical areas
MacKeith	1994	UK	Academic failure –21%
Braithwaite et al	1994	UK	Academic failure Disciplinary proceedings Personal problems Disillusionment
Hutt	1988	UK	Academic failure Disciplinary proceedings Unsuitable for the training
Lindop	1987	UK	Unsatisfactory performance Not suited to nursing Personality disorders

Salvatori (2001) reviewed 83 articles from the disciplines of medicine, nursing, midwifery, physiotherapy, occupational therapy, respiratory care and medical imaging for the reliability and validity of both cognitive and non-cognitive measures used to select students to health care programmes. The conclusion drawn was that an admissions process that provides a 'thorough, fair, reliable, valid and cost-effective assessment of applicants remains an elusive goal for health profession education programs'.

Our selection procedure invests us with the power to reject those whom we perceive do not fulfil our selection criteria. Prior academic achievement may be seen as one criterion that is an objective measure for selection for entry to health care education, and ultimately the health care profession. Even the relevance and usefulness of this perceived 'objective measure' has serious shortcomings. As can be seen in Table 1.2, academic failure is cited as a key reason for discontinuation of nurse education in all studies. This certainly casts great doubt over the assumption that those who perform best in current examinations are those who would become most capable as a result of further educational investment. Perhaps such factors as maturity, personality and motivation are also important in determining success in nursing and midwifery education. Readers are directed to discussions of these latter issues in the papers by Deary et al (2003) and Glossop (2001).

Thomas Love Peacock (1860 in MacLeod 1982:7) railed against the preponderance of examinations that would 'infallibly have excluded Marlborough from the Army and Nelson from the Navy'! Of the candidates we reject, we will never know how many would have become the sensitive and caring nurse or midwife or physiotherapist or doctor – their potential may never be realized. The academic high-flyer may not be the better practitioner if she/he does not possess qualities such as compassion and empathy.

Students in training

Statutory regulation of health professionals is well established. The primary purpose of statutory regulation is to protect the public. In the UK, medical practitioners have been subject to state registration since 1858 with the passing of the Medical Act; midwives since 1902 with the Midwives Act, and nurses since 1919 with the Nurses Registration Act. Regulation of the professions supplementary to medicine (chiropodists and podiatrists, dieticians, medical laboratory scientific officers, occupational therapists, orthoptists, physiotherapists and radiographers, both diagnostic and therapeutic) followed in 1960 with the passing of the Professions Supplementary Act 1960. This was extended in 1997 to include prosthetists and orthotists and arts therapists (Department of Health 2000). With the passing of The Health Professions Order 2001, the Health

Professions Council was created and currently regulates 16 professions: arts therapists, biomedical scientists, chiropodists/podiatrists, clinical scientists, dietitians, hearing aid dispensers, occupational therapists, operating department practitioners, orthoptists, paramedics, physiotherapists, practitioner psychologists, prosthetists/orthotists, radiographers, social workers in England and speech and language therapists (Health and Care Professions Council 2012). With statutory regulation, Parliament grants a profession the right to self-regulation. This means that a profession is given the right to maintain professional discipline, standards of conduct and entry into the profession. Standards of professional behaviour and for employment have to be observed by those who are registered with a statutory body. These standards are upheld through the key functions of education, registration and discipline.

The standards of conduct, performance and ethics of the Nursing and Midwifery Council (NMC, 2008a) and the Health and Care Professions Council (2008) are concerned with maintaining a standard of practice such that high-quality care is provided to the recipients of health care at all times. As discussed earlier, the issue of a 'licence' to practise by a professional statutory body offers some measure of public protection. The public has a fundamental right to expect competence from the qualified professional in health care, and protection against unsafe, unscrupulous or sick practice. The mechanism of statutory registration is designed to ensure that those legally entitled to call themselves 'midwife', 'nurse', 'physiotherapist', 'occupational therapist', 'operating department practitioner' and so on possess the outcomes and competencies described in statute. For nurses and midwives and those professions regulated by the HCPC, the rules and standards of proficiency for pre-registration programmes leading to registration on the NMC and HCPC registers are currently set out in the Nursing and Midwifery Council (Education, Registration and Registration Appeals) rules 2004 (NMC, 2004a) and in The Health Professions Order 2001 (Education and Training rules).

More recently, the NMC (2009, 2010a) mandated that pre-registration nursing and midwifery programmes must be designed to prepare the student to provide the nursing and midwifery care that patients/clients require, safely and competently, and to be able to assume the responsibilities and accountabilities necessary for public protection. The HCPC (2009a) mandated that all pre-registration programmes must prepare the student to have the knowledge, skills and experience to practise safely and effectively in a way that meets the standards of the HCPC, and no danger is posed to the public or the self.

The educational and professional outcome of pre-registration education is a competent practitioner who is fit to practise. Both the NMC (2008a) and the HCPC (2008) make it clear that fitness to practise is a registrant's suitability to be on the register without restrictions. This means that, prior to being admitted to the professional registers, there must be evidence that the student is able to uphold the standards of conduct, performance and ethics expected of registrants set out in the respective professional's codes of practice. It is incumbent upon practitioners to facilitate the learning and development of students so that evidence of fitness to practise is generated and provided through assessment processes. This evidence needs to be valid and reliable to provide the objective data upon which assessment decisions of fitness to practise can then be made. We may need to remind ourselves that the NMC and HCPC are reliant on this assessment decision for conferring professional registration upon the nurse or midwife, or orthoptist, radiographer or paramedic and so on.

Take a few moments to consider Activity 1.2.

ACTIVITY 1.2

How well are we preparing health care practitioners to be competent so that they are fit for practice as required by the NMC and the HCPC? Be objective in your considerations.

If it is accepted that one of the purposes of assessment is to prepare practitioners who are fit for practice, the answer to the question posed in Activity 1.2 is that this purpose is not fully realized (Cleland et al 2008, Luhanga et al 2008, Duffy 2004, Bradshaw 2000, Glen & Clark 1999, Runciman et al 1998). The following point was made by the UKCC Education Commission on nursing and midwifery education (UKCC 1999a):

> ... there is concern that newly-qualified nurses, and to a certain extent midwives, do not possess the practice skills expected of them by employers, and public perceptions about levels of preparedness for practice are sometimes negative.

Similar concerns were expressed by the NMC (2005a). Reasons for this are wide ranging (Cleland et al 2008, Luhanga et al 2008, Glen & Clark 1999). Among the most notable is the confusion in the terminology of 'competence' – thereby contributing to difficulties experienced by assessors when required to assess competent practice (Watson et al 2002, Bradshaw 2000, Fraser et al 1997, Bedford et al 1993). Other studies reported assessors' lack of skills, knowledge and confidence to assess and report underperformance in order to take the necessary remedial action (Cleland et al 2008, Luhanga et al 2008, Dudek et al 2005).

If the purpose of assessing students for entry into the profession is to be achieved with validity, there needs to be a more careful examination of how pre-registration health care education, including the assessment of

clinical practice, can be managed better, so that when students qualify they can meet service needs and requirements – that is, they are 'fit for practice' and 'fit for purpose'. Within this framework more concerted efforts are required to make valid and reliable assessments of students' clinical practice.

Assessment as a form of quality control

Students in training

Closely related to the purpose of assessing for entry into the profession is this second purpose. In industry such as manufacturing, quality control of production enables those items below the required standard to be rejected. With the purpose of assessment as a form of quality control for the health care professions, assessors should be able to identify those students who have not achieved the educational standards, and therefore, make a 'fail' decision so that the names of those who are not 'competent' are not entered into the professional register. Among other roles, assessors need to be the 'gatekeepers' of their profession to achieve the quality control function of assessment. A crucial question to ask is 'How adequately, or how well, is this "gatekeeping" role being performed?' Again, the sobering answer is that this purpose of assessment is not fully realized as the 'gatekeeping' is inadequate. There is a 'failure to fail' students with grave consequences for the public that we serve: their health and well-being are supposed to be protected by the registrants on the professional register. In fairly recent times, the case of Beverley Allitt (Clothier et al 1994) is perhaps a tragic example of how the nursing profession has let the public down. Beverley Allitt was an enrolled nurse who was convicted of murdering four children and harming nine others, some of who have been left severely brain damaged. In 1990 when she was still a student she took 94 days of sick leave, which delayed her qualification. As a student, she had a history of inflicting injuries on herself and others. How did she pass her training, or, why was she not failed? Allitt's fitness to practise was impaired but she achieved professional registration. The points of *fitness to practise* and *fitness for practice* will be developed in Chapter 3.

This complex problem of 'failure to fail' is not new and appears to be a continuing challenge for assessors of students on pre-registration professional courses. In the health care professions, the issue of 'failure to fail' is reported in literature relating to assessment in the fields of social work (Brandon & Davis 1979), medicine (Cleland et al 2008, Green 1991), nursing and midwifery (Luhanga et al 2008, Duffy 2004, Fraser et al 1997, Bedford et al 1993, Lankshear 1990) and occupational therapy (Ilott & Murphy 1999). References are made to assessors giving students the benefit of the doubt in marginal situations instead of awarding a fail when it was clearly warranted.

To determine whether pre-registration students have achieved the threshold standards or competence, assessors must make the crucial 'pass/fail' assessment decision. Higher-education institutions have to make decisions of impairment of fitness to practise. These vital decisions protect the public from unsafe, incompetent or unscrupulous practitioners. This is crucial for quality control and, as one of the purposes of assessment, it also serves to safeguard the standards of the profession. The complex situation of 'failure to fail' will be explored further in Chapter 7.

Qualified professionals

Professional conduct The quality control purpose of assessment for qualified professionals serves to maintain the standards of the profession through the regulation of the education, training and conduct of its registrants. In the case of nurses and midwives and those professions regulated by the HCPC, both the NMC and HCPC maintain a register of practitioners who have met the standards for entry to the professions. This is central to the Councils' role in protecting the public. Being on the NMC and HCPC registers demonstrates to the public that practitioners have accepted the responsibilities and accountability that go along with registration, and that they will abide by the professional standards set by the NMC and the HCPC. This is done through professional self-regulation. Professional self-regulation means that, in exercising professional accountability, professional knowledge, judgement and skill are used to interpret and apply professional standards in practice. Although the NMC and the HCPC administer the system of professional self-regulation, it is through its practitioners who are accountable for their own practice that professional standards are maintained in the workplace.

The Standards of conduct, performance and ethics of the NMC and the HCPC (NMC 2008, HCPC 2009a) are the basis of the regulatory framework. Practitioners are required to monitor and maintain not only their own professional standards but also those of their colleagues. In exercising individual professional responsibility and accountability, the *Standards* require practitioners to report to an appropriate person or authority any circumstances that may put patients and clients at risk. The position of the NMC and the HCPC on this is explicit. Two of the clauses in the NMC standards above state that:

> *You must act without delay if you believe that you, a colleague or anyone else may be putting someone at risk ... You must inform someone in authority if you experience problems that prevent you working within this Code or other nationally agreed standards.*

The HCPC standards are equally explicit in stating that:

> *You must not do anything, or allow someone else to do anything, that you have good reason to believe will put the health or safety of a service user in danger. This includes both your own actions and those of other people ... You must protect service users if you believe that any situation puts them in danger. This includes the conduct, performance or health of a colleague. The safety of service users must come before any personal or professional loyalties at all times. As soon as you become aware of a situation that puts a service user in danger, you should discuss the matter with a senior colleague or another appropriate person.*

In 2004, the NMC published guidelines for employers and managers for reporting unfitness to practise (NMC 2004b) and reporting lack of competence (2004c); later guidelines (2010b) gave information on the four broad areas of misconduct, lack of competence, character issues and poor health when allegations are investigated. Likewise, guidelines published by the HCPC in 2007 gave similar guidance for reporting allegations against its practitioners.

The guidance provided by these publications reinforces the quality control purpose of assessment of practitioners, which in turn supports the primary mandate of the NMC and the HCPC: to safeguard the health and well-being of the general public. Between 2010 and 2011, the NMC received 4211 allegations (0.7% of registrants, compared with 2988 the previous year) against its registrants for their fitness to practise (NMC 2011), and the HCPC received 759 allegations (0.35% of registrants, compared with 772 the previous year) (HCPC 2011). The allegations of fitness to practise against these practitioners indicate that the quality control purpose of assessment of practitioners is necessary.

Education and training *The Post-Registration Education and Practice* (PREP) standard of the NMC (2008) and the HCPC standards (HCPC 2010) for continuing professional development (CPD) are professional standards that practitioners must meet to demonstrate that their professional knowledge and competence are maintained and continue to be developed. Practitioners must undertake and record their CPD in a personal professional profile in order to renew their registration prior to renewal of their registration in a personal professional profile. The NMC will audit compliance with the PREP (Practice and CPD) standard (NMC 2008b). The NMC will assess directly whether practitioners have maintained this standard by monitoring a sample of registrants who will be asked to provide the NMC with evidence of their learning activity and the relevance of this learning to their work. In the case of the HCPC, whenever a profession renews its registration there will be a random audit of the CPD of a proportion of health professionals from that profession. The health professionals randomly chosen have to send in evidence to show how their CPD meets the standards.

There is a general recognition across the health care professions that CPD is a planned process by which

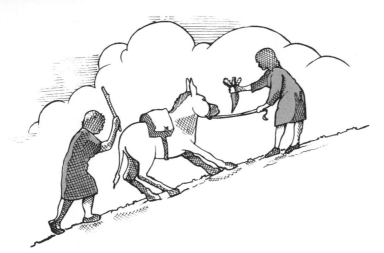

Figure 1.1 Assessments – the carrot or the stick?

individuals both maintain and update their current individual skills and knowledge portfolios but, at the same time, is an opportunity to develop new skills and extend the knowledge base. The Department of Health (2004) publication titled *The NHS Knowledge and Skills Framework (NHS KSF) and the Development Review Process* attempted to provide a more consistent national structure for post-registration development for the CPD of health care professionals. It facilitated the process of defining criteria for demonstrating continuing levels of competence throughout a professional career by establishing formal standards for recognition of post-registration development. The quality control of practice was thus made more consistent.

In its paper titled *A First Class Service* (Department of Health 1998), the government stated that clinical governance would provide a framework through which National Health Service (NHS) organizations would be accountable for continuously improving the quality of their services and safeguarding high standards of care by creating an environment in which excellence in clinical care would flourish. For the first time, NHS organizations and individuals have a statutory duty to achieve quality improvement. NHS organizations are required to develop processes for monitoring and improving clinical quality.

Like professional self-regulation, clinical governance is all about promoting high standards of care in order to protect the public. The government sees clinical governance as the main vehicle for continuously improving the quality of patient care and developing the capacity of the NHS to maintain high standards, including dealing with poor professional performance. The established professional self-regulation of nursing and midwifery and the professions regulated by the HCPC can thus make a major contribution to clinical governance.

For qualified practitioners, the quality control purpose of assessment starts at the point of entry into the profession and terminates on exiting the profession. Assessment is a means of answering the demands of public accountability. Assessment for qualified professionals takes the forms of self-assessment through professional self-regulation and clinical governance as systems of monitoring clinical quality are developed through this framework.

Assessment for the motivation of students

Assessments serve as a powerful motivating force for students – were it not for the carrot of success or stick of failure created by summative assessments, many students, it is claimed, would lack any real incentive to work (Figure 1.1). With motivation, assessment is used to encourage the student to learn. From this standpoint, assessments are seen as a form of positive help to students. Rowntree (1987:23), however, reminds us in no uncertain terms that 'assessment can be used as an instrument of coercion, as a means of getting students to do something they might not otherwise be inclined to do – especially if unfavourable assessments can have unpleasant consequences'. He goes on to say that the line between coercion and encouragement is hard to draw. Let us take the case of professional health care education – one key aim of these programmes of education must be to prepare practitioners who are safe and competent. Of necessity, then, students are assessed for their achievement of statutory standards of proficiency. How else can we measure such learning? Failure to pass these standards of proficiency results in being discontinued from the course. The reader may wish to decide whether assessments in this instance are used to coerce or encourage the student!

It is important not to take too simplistic a view of motivation and assessment, as motivation is a complex concept. A high level of motivation is not a sufficient condition, but is a necessary one for learning (Gipps 1994). The importance of motivational factors influencing learning was succinctly stated by Howe (1987:142):

> *I have a strong feeling that motivational factors are crucial whenever a person achieves anything of significance as a result of learning and thought, and I cannot think of exceptions to this statement. That is not to claim that a high level of motivation can ever be a sufficient condition for human achievements, but is undoubtedly a necessary one. And, conversely, negative motivational influences, such as fear of failure, feelings of helplessness, lack of confidence, and having the experience that one's fate is largely controlled by external factors rather than by oneself, almost certainly have effects that restrict a person's learned achievements.*

In an extensive review of the impact of classroom evaluation on students, Crooks (1988) found that research repeatedly demonstrated that the responses of individual students to educational experiences and tasks are complex functions of their abilities and personalities, their past educational experiences, their current attitudes, self-perception and motivational states, together with the nature of their current experiences and tasks. Crooks' review also revealed just how important assessment is in defining the attitude students take towards their work, their sense of ownership and control of their own learning, the strategies they employ in learning and their confidence and self-esteem – all of which impact profoundly on the quality of learning achieved. The significant effects of assessment on motivation for learning (Crooks 1988) and their implications for assessment in health care education are discussed below.

Student self-efficacy

Self-efficacy refers to students' perceptions of their capability to perform certain tasks. Perceptions of self-efficacy have a strong influence on effort and persistence with difficult tasks, or after experiences of failure: under such circumstances, students high in self-efficacy usually redouble their efforts, whereas students low in self-efficacy tend to make minimal efforts or avoid such tasks. Self-efficacy can be developed if repeated success is experienced. Conversely, repeated failures lead to lowered self-efficacy. Success at tasks perceived to be difficult or challenging is more influential than success on easier tasks.

Self-efficacy is best enhanced if longer-term goals are supported by a carefully sequenced series of sub-goals with clear criteria that students find attainable. In addition, standards must be clearly specified. The setting of clear and attainable goals has significant implications for strategies used by clinical assessors in relation to the level and type of work that is aimed at individual students. These important points are discussed further in Chapters 6 and 7.

Intrinsic motivation and continuing motivation

Intrinsic motivation to learn (defined as a self-sustaining desire to learn) and continuing motivation (defined as a tendency to return to and continue working on tasks away from the instructional context in which they were initially confronted) are highly related concepts. Both, in turn, are closely related to interest in the material that is being studied. Where students initially lack intrinsic motivation in a particular subject area, a carefully planned programme of positive educational experiences accompanied by extrinsic motivation can lead to the development of interest in the area, and thus to intrinsic motivation. On the other hand, where students are initially intrinsically motivated, attempting to stimulate learning through extrinsic motivation usually leads to decreased intrinsic motivation, especially on challenging tasks.

These findings have obvious implications for teachers and assessors when designing learning experiences for students. Crooks' statement below of what effective education should be (Crooks 1988:460) may help us focus more carefully on how, through our educational endeavours, which include assessment strategies we use, we can help our students develop and/or maintain intrinsic and continuing motivation:

> *Effective education requires the fusing of 'skill and will', and intrinsic interest and continuing motivation to learn are educational outcomes that should be regarded as at least as important as cognitive outcomes.*

This aspect of learning and assessment is explored in Chapter 6.

Assessment anxiety

The fact that clinical experience is overwhelming and stressful for many students is well documented (see, for example, James and Chapman (2009–2010), Lincoln et al 2004, Deary et al 2003, Phillips et al 2000, Smith 1992, Williams 1993, Kleehammer et al 1990, Parkes 1985). These authors also reported that anxiety can contribute to decreased learning. To be subject to assessment in the face of this negative emotion can only compound the situation. Crooks (1988) found that the debilitating effects for high-anxiety students are greater when the student perceives good performance to be particularly important, when the test is expected to be difficult and when the testing conditions are particularly intrusive (e.g. rigid timing). Although extrapolations must be made with caution, it seems possible to draw parallels between these findings and the circumstances faced by health care students during clinical practice. The performance of students in the clinical setting must meet the required standards within the time frame of the clinical placement. The achievement of some aspects of care can be difficult, such as being able to perform cardiopulmonary resuscitation, communicating with the very ill/dying client/patient and managing the care of a group of clients/patients. For some students, experiences of assessment may then be rather dispiriting and demotivating.

As can be seen from this presentation of the possible impact of assessment on motivation, there are many factors to be considered to realize this purpose of assessment. A comprehensive review of the motivational aspects relating to assessment can be found in Crooks (1988).

Assessment to support teaching and learning

Knowledge of performance in an assessment exercise, such as during clinical practice or a written assignment, will help students benefit educationally from assessors' response to work that has been done. The importance of this type of feedback is probably captured by Rowntree (1987:24) when he stated that 'feedback, or "knowledge of results", is the life-blood of learning'. Student nurses and student midwives work at getting helpful feedback (Bedford et al 1993, O'Neill and McCall (1996), Spouse 1996). In O'Neill & McCall's study, student nurses found face-to-face feedback a very positive aspect of their learning, helping them to identify strengths and weaknesses so that they improved where they were weak and built upon what they did best. Likewise, students' skills of self-assessment and motivation for self-directed learning improved when feedback on practice-based learning was linked to constructive feedback on performance (Embo et al 2010, Srinivasan et al 2007, White 2007).

For feedback of this nature to be effective, assessment needs to be used as a 'diagnostic aid' to learning throughout the course so that it becomes an integral part of the educational process, continually providing both 'feedback' and 'feedforward' (Torrance 1993:334) for both students and assessors. This formative element of the assessment process will then have a positive impact on learning, particularly if it focuses on helping the student to achieve short-term goals and provides specific and detailed feedback on progress. A comprehensive discussion of unhelpful forms of feedback, such as the award of marks, grades, a pass or fail, can be found in Rowntree (1987). In summary, being awarded just a mark or a pass or a fail does not indicate to the student how well or badly he may have performed in aspects of the assessment exercise. Such grades are meted out by the teacher at the end of a term or a course. Students may therefore not know how to improve future performance. Rowntree (1987) believes that such feedback can begin to be useful only when it includes verbal comments.

Insofar as assessment evidence reveals the quality and quantity of learning, the assessor may be able to identify what has been taught well, what has not been so well explained and therefore may have confused the issue for the student, what further experiences are required, and so on. In the clinical setting, such information will further enable the assessor to plan those clinical experiences and teaching sessions the student will require in order to achieve learning outcomes. The use of the formative assessment process is explored in Chapter 6, where the process of the continuous assessment of clinical practice is discussed.

Torrance & Pryor (1998:10) contend that 'all assessment practices have an impact on [student] learning'. As revealed by Crooks' review of 1988, teaching arrangements, notably the assessment approaches used, is particularly potent in influencing how students go about studying and learning. Marton & Säljö (1984) reported that students' approaches to learning tasks could be categorized into two broad categories that they labelled as *deep* or *surface* approaches. Deep approaches involve an active search for meaning in order to understand material for oneself. The content is interacted with vigorously and critically. Organizing principles are used to integrate ideas. Surface approaches, in contrast, rely primarily on attempts to memorize course material, treating the material as if different facts and topics were unrelated.

Assessment strategies should encourage deep learning, higher-order thinking and self-monitoring, alongside the acquisition of knowledge, from the earliest stages of professional education to develop the practitioner who is 'fit for practice' (HCPC 2007, NMC 2010b). Higher-order learning is retained longer and encourages the development of intrinsic motivation and positive attitudes to continued learning (Gipps 1994). The health care professions can only stand to benefit given the professions' aim of developing and fostering the attitude of lifelong learning in its practitioners in order to strive constantly to improve standards and quality of client/patient care (Department of Health 1999, 2001, HCPC 2010, NMC 2008b).

ASSESSMENT IN CLINICAL PRACTICE

The nature of clinical assessment

You may be able to recall your experiences of being assessed when you were a student. Some of these memories may no doubt be rather vivid! Not only were you required to sit written tests and be subjected to oral and practical examinations, but also you were assessed while you were 'working'. In the classroom, your teacher gave you feedback on your test papers and assignments. In the clinical area, your assessor gave you feedback, thus implying that some form of assessment of your practice had taken place. At a personal level, you were either pleased or dissatisfied with your performance – you had therefore assessed yourself. Colleagues may have indicated to you how they thought you were doing on a surgical ward – they had assessed you. Patients gave you feedback on the care you had given them – you were subject to yet further assessment!

All in all, you may have frequently felt quite overwhelmed as you knew that what you said or did or the way you behaved, or even the way you dressed, was under scrutiny. If we reflect on our experiences of being assessed as a health care student, some of us may even begin to say that we experienced assessment as though we had experienced a 'phenomenon'. What is the nature of this *phenomenon*? Pause for a moment to consider the questions posed in Activity 1.3.

ACTIVITY 1.3

From the above sketch of assessment, what inferences can be drawn about the nature of assessment in general, and about assessment in the clinical setting? How were you affected by the many occasions when you were assessed?

In most of the instances in the sketch, feedback you received about your performance and abilities or otherwise was based on another person's inferences and estimations of your actions and behaviours. In other words, you had been judged by someone else. Rowntree (1987:4) states that, when we assess, we enter into human encounters whereby we make attempts to know that person. He explains further:

> … *assessment in education can be thought of as occurring whenever one person, in some kind of interaction, direct or indirect, with another, is conscious of obtaining and interpreting information about the knowledge and understanding, or abilities and attitudes of that other person.*

Assessors of students in the clinical setting make judgements about, for example, how students are integrating into the ward team, how they are developing as practitioners, what they are learning and what they have accomplished. Assessments may reveal the positive changes in the student's knowledge and understanding, abilities and attitudes as a result of supervision and guidance given, the practical experiences, influences and effects of the clinical milieu on the student. The nature of clinical practice, and the clinical milieu itself, places multiple demands on the skills of the practitioner as mentor, assessor and teacher. The dynamic clinical setting is ever changing and unstructured. It provides a range of clients whose conditions are varied and changeable. Learning experiences for students are therefore not consistent. Each of these situations has to be dealt with in a different way. Real people in the real world of practice do not see things

in a uniform way. Bedford et al (1993) make the point that assessors are individuals who are not automatons, but people who interpret and make sense of what they encounter in terms of their own experience. Our own values will also influence the interpretations we make of situations. The subjectiveness of the clinical world will inevitably mean that assessments we make are likely to be influenced by our own personal and professional experiences and perceptions of the situation.

The diversity of context and the differing demands of each context also mean that the student's knowledge, understanding, abilities and attitudes can be assessed only within those contexts that the student has encountered. In Rowntree's terms then, assessments of students during clinical practice are truly *only attempts* to know our students. We may have worked with the student for the maximum number of shifts possible within the student's allocation, but will have been able to form such opinions of the student's learning only on the basis of what was observed of the student's performance. While we are observing, we cannot be sure that we have picked up every aspect of performance – there may have been some aspect of care or nuance that has been missed, or the interpretation of ability to perform or otherwise may have been made based on our personal biases for, or against, the student. During clinical placements then, finding out about a student's abilities to perform is done mainly through informal processes and as opportunities arise. As assessments are likely to be based on these 'snapshots' of practice (Bradshaw 1989), there is a need to question how well we truly know the student. Knowledge of the student's achievements is of course important when assessment decisions are made, be they formative or summative.

As the student works alongside us, we hope that they are learning through observation of our practices. Throughout the student's placement, their learning is facilitated through instruction, guidance and supervision as they participate in care delivery. While they are adjusting to clients, staff and other personnel and also learning to perform care, students are being assessed and given feedback on their performance. This means that while the student is learning he/she is being assessed. Wood (1982) says that this situation is less than ideal and it would be better to separate learning and assessment. Working in the demanding clinical setting may prevent practitioners from carrying out their roles of mentor and assessor as effectively as they would wish to. At the grass roots, the first responsibility of health care practitioners is to care for clients (Whiting 1997, Bedford et al 1993). Consequently, even the extremely important activity of teaching and assessing students comes second to this.

Fretwell's study in 1980 showed that student nurses were taught and supervised for 11.6–36.9% of the time. In a lengthy and detailed study of all aspects of student nurses' clinical experience, Jacka & Lewin (1987) reported that learners spent more than 50% of their time, with some spending more than 75% of their time, working alone. The results of these studies indicate that teaching and assessing activities were left to chance. The situation today appears to be similar; the study by Allan et al (2011) reported that busy staff left students unsupervised with an allocated workload. There were also instances when students were not allocated work and mentors. If this is the case, how then can we be sure that students are learning what they should in order to achieve professional competence? Strategies to facilitate more effective learning and assessment are made in Chapters 7 and 9.

The complexities of clinical assessment

From the discussion above, it can be seen that the nature of clinical assessment is complex. There is much in the literature that says the assessment of students in clinical practice is a continuing problem (Fitzgerald et al 2010, Cleland et al 2008, Duffy 2004, Ilott & Murphy 1999, Fraser et al 1997, While 1991, Wood 1982, Woolley 1977, Wood 1972), and one that 'will not go away' (Chambers 1998:201). The basic issues complicating clinical assessments discussed by Wood in 1982 are as real today. Try Activity 1.4.

ACTIVITY 1.4

Think of the clinical experiences in the different placements you experienced, either as a student or as an assessor. From these experiences, identity the problems that arose as you attempted to learn to care for clients/patients or when assessing students.

From your experience both as student and assessor, the problems you most commonly identified are likely to be similar and could also be shared by your colleagues. Problems you experienced might be as follows:

- Clinical assessment is based predominantly on direct observation of practice. Human observation inevitably possesses inherent biases and subjectivity and is therefore a subjective process. Interpretations of standards of performance are hence very likely to be inconsistent, leading to unreliable assessments.
- Unreliable assessments are also contributed to by the considerable amount of official assessments that occurred at different points in the clinical experience schedule for different students (Phillips et al 2000). The number of times that different students were assessed was also different.
- Over the course of a pre-registration programme, students have to adapt to new and differing clinical areas on a regular basis, with some clinical placements lasting for only a short duration. During each placement, students have to adjust and adapt to a multitude of personalities. They have to interact with each other, nurses and midwives, doctors and other health professionals such as the physiotherapist and dietician who are also attending the client/patient. Students also have to adjust to, and learn to care for, a range of clients/patients with their differing illnesses and needs, possibly attempting to apply what has been learnt in the classroom to the real-life situation of the clinical world. As already mentioned earlier, students are assessed while adapting, coping and trying to learn and achieve the competencies of being a health care professional. It is therefore important to remember that students are assessed in their capacity as students at the pre-specified level. This point is discussed in more detail in Chapter 7.
- The attainment of behavioural skills forms one essential element of learning in the clinical environment (Department of Health 1999, While 1991). The unpredictability of the clinical learning environment means that there can be little educational control over clinical learning experiences for students. Patient turnover and changes in patient dependency mitigate against consistency of experience. There is a variation in the quality and quantity of practical experience on apparently similar wards. The diverse experiences mean that the demonstration of behavioural skills may vary from occasion to occasion (Boreham 1978). Boreham cited the example of explaining a procedure to an articulate English-speaking patient as compared with achieving the same level of understanding in an anxious non-English-speaking patient. The second student was assessed on her ability to communicate with an anxious non-English-speaking patient. Should this student be judged to be more skilful than the first student? Given the multicultural society of Great Britain, should all students be expected to be able to communicate likewise? And can clinical experiences be provided to enable the development of these skills? If the second student is unable to achieve the same level of understanding in her patient, should she be given a fail grade?
- The Department of Health (1999) requires nurses and midwives to be trained to 'broadly the same standards and have the same skills' wherever they are trained. Is this an 'order' that is achievable? Likewise, the NMC (2009, 2010a) and the HCPC (2009a) require pre-registration students to achieve mandatory standards of proficiency. The reality of being able to achieve the requirements of pre-registration education uniformly, and to the same standard, is perhaps summed up in the following statement by Young (1994:47):

Even for students following the same course, the variations in clinical experience ensure that no two people's trainings, and therefore learning outcomes, are ever identical. For example, a student may not be involved in cardiac resuscitation at all during a three-year training, while a colleague on the same course may have assisted with resuscitation on a number of occasions. This means that even with detailed training criteria, it is impossible to specify precisely in what skills a registered nurse will be competent.

- The issues of uniformity, consistency and fairness of clinical assessment have remained contentious over the years (Fitzgerald et al 2010, Dolan 2003, Phillips et al 2000, Chambers 1998, Bedford et al 1993, Girot 1993, While 1991, Wood 1982). These issues are addressed in more detail in Chapters 4 and 5, where strategies to try to achieve fairness of assessment are discussed.
- Clinical areas are under pressure to accommodate large numbers of students for increasing periods of the year. The total assessment demands within many placement areas are thus increased. Large student intakes and staff shortages mean that even the most committed practitioners, and these are the majority, are hard pressed to support and supervise students adequately (Allan et al 2011, Eraut 2003a). Many practitioners are involved in assessing a range of health care students. This may result in an assessor supervising several students simultaneously, resulting in 'mentor overload' (Hallin & Danielson 2009, Hurley & Snowden 2008). The assessment of an individual student's performance is likely to be based on a sample of the student's total experience, as it would be impossible to achieve a constant 1:1 supervision and observation of the student. The potential for making inaccurate assessment decisions based on 'snapshots' of practice is high.
- In a study by White et al., (1994:103), students cited examples where assessments of their practice were made in the absence of any witness of it! One student blatantly said that it was virtually impossible to fail the practical part of the course and there would always be ways of getting round a weak area of practice. Herein lies a grave concern – if it is accepted that one of the purposes of assessment is to ensure that the student has achieved professional competencies prior to professional registration, this way of making assessment decisions clearly indicates that this purpose is not fulfilled. Further evidence that this purpose of assessment is not fulfilled comes from literature around 'failure to fail' (see above).
- There is much rhetoric on the theory–practice gap in nursing. Few people would doubt its existence, and supporting evidence is available from many studies and official reports (see, for example, Wellman 2010, and McCaugherty 1991 for a review). Patients and clients are individuals with individual needs. Thus health care practice cannot be an exact science: there needs to be more than one way of meeting patient and client needs. In attempts to describe health care, the unique psychological and social dimension of each patient and client cannot be captured. Theory gleaned can paint only incomplete and generalized pictures of the realities of practice. However good classroom and textbook theory may be, clinical practice may not always correlate, making it difficult for the student to apply theory to practice. From the student's viewpoint, clinical practice can appear quite different from theory learnt during lectures and from books (Michau et al 2009, Corlett 2000, McCaugherty 1991).
- The student has to learn to integrate knowledge learned in a context away from the world of practice with the real world of clinical practice. Many students will find this very difficult, as cognitive processes indicate that there is an intimate connection between the acquisition of knowledge and the context in which it is used (Gipps 1994). Educationally, this suggests that we cannot teach theory in one setting and expect it to be applied automatically in another. Studies in educational research confirm that facts cannot be learned in isolation and then used in any context, as skills and knowledge acquisition are now understood to be dependent on the context in which they are learned (Eraut 2003b, Gipps 1994).
- Clinical assessors are frequently not party to theoretical instruction in the classroom. This may militate against the ability to assist students in successfully integrating theory with practice, which many struggle with (Moriaty et al., 2010). If students encounter such difficulties in relating theory to practice, they will not be as likely to develop the clinical competencies required of them. In these circumstances, we need to question the validity of our assessment processes.
- Accurate feedback on professional values and behaviours to facilitate professional development was frequently not given (Fitzgerald et al 2010, Miller 2010).

In the face of the complexities of learning and assessment in the clinical setting, it would appear that it is difficult to realize fully the purposes of assessment of clinical practice in the health care professions. Perhaps this is not surprising. In pre-registration health care education in the UK, students have been set the onerous task of becoming 'fit for practice' in what I would suggest is a short period of 2–3 years – short, because the nature of health care education and practice today is making increased demands on students. Students now also have to achieve the academic demands of study at an institution of higher education. Other factors, to name but a few, such as the dynamic health care setting with its changing patient/client needs, the reduced number of clinical areas to attain clinical experiences, the constantly changing and increased demands made on the health care practitioner, an increasing number of specialties, technological innovations and an ever-increasing knowledge base, stretch students' resources much more today. If the support that many students require is not readily available, many may fall by the wayside. Without an adequate level of support and supervision of students during clinical practice, the very purposes of assessment we set out to achieve will not be fully realized.

CONCLUSION

Four broad categories of purpose in nursing and midwifery education have been outlined. These are not entirely without overlap and conflict. In our role as assessors of learners in the health care professions, we need to consider carefully the learning that must be achieved and balance this against the needs of the learner as an individual, which on occasions may conflict. Our personal philosophy of what teaching and learning in clinical practice is about is powerful in determining our attitudes

to the assessment of clinical practice, which in turn influences our use of any assessment system, tools and procedures. As we examine the nature of clinical assessment, we might begin to analyse the reasons underpinning our attitudes towards learning and assessment in clinical practice.

Reilly (1980:2–3) posed the following questions of us as accountable self-regulating professionals:

> *Do our educational offerings stand the test of accountability? Can we demonstrate that the [health care practitioners] sent into the health care system have made a difference for the better in the quality of health care provided in proportion to the scope of their educational preparation?*

Who is responsible and accountable? After you have examined the issues of responsibility and accountability surrounding assessment in health care education and professional practice in the next chapter, you may be in a better position to contribute to the wider debate surrounding the achievement of the purposes of assessment in the health care professions.

KEY POINTS FOR REFLECTION

1. To accept the necessity for assessment unthinkingly denies a complex debate around the purposes of assessments. It may also make us overlook the effects of the assessment on the learner as an individual, and its impact on the curriculum, teaching and learning. Critically reviewing 'why' we assess may make us consider more carefully whether our assessments are reasonable and just. Four key purposes of assessment in professional education put forward are:

To regulate entry into the profession through:

   ◆ Selection for training where only those who we perceive fulfil our selection criteria are admitted. These are those who are supposed to be the 'best' and who will complete the course successfully. Non-completion and discontinuation rates tell us that our 'stringent' selection criteria may not be so valid and reliable.

   ◆ Assessment of pre-registration students so that they achieve 'fitness for practice'. Concern about the competence (and by implication the 'fitness for practice') of newly qualified nurses and midwives has a long history. In 1999, the UKCC stated that: 'there is concern that newly-qualified nurses, and to a certain extent midwives, do not possess the practice skills expected of them by employers, and public perceptions about levels of preparedness for practice are sometimes negative' (UKCC 1999). More recently the same concern has been raised by Clark & Holmes (2007) and Snow & Harrison (2008).

To use assessment as a quality control mechanism for the profession through:

   ◆ Assessment of students in training so that only those who are safe and competent are allowed to register. There is overwhelming evidence that there is a 'failure to fail' marginal students, and therefore, there are practitioners on professional registers who are not safe and competent.

   ◆ The quality control purpose of assessment for qualified professionals serves to maintain the standards of the profession through the regulation of the education, training and the continuing 'fitness to practise' of its registrants. Regulations are in place for the reporting of 'fitness to practise' and to ensure the continuing professional development of practitioners.

To motivate students:

   ◆ Assessments can encourage or discourage students to learn. They define the attitude students take towards their work, their sense of ownership and control of their own learning, the strategies they employ in learning and their confidence and self-esteem, all of which impact profoundly on the quality of learning achieved.

To support teaching and learning:

   ◆ 'Feedback, or "knowledge of results", is the life-blood of learning' (Rowntree 1987:24). Feedback needs to become an integral part of the educational process, continually providing both 'feedback' and 'feedforward' (Torrance 1993:334) for both students and assessors, so that strengths and weaknesses in student learning and teaching by the practitioner can be identified. Specific and detailed feedback is required to enable students to progress.

2. Teaching and assessing activities in clinical areas are frequently left to chance. As assessments of competence are frequently based on 'snapshots' of practice, the validity and reliability of assessment decisions are questionable. Reliability is compromised further by the subjective nature of clinical assessments.

3. The dynamic nature of clinical practice militates against consistency of experience and learning. This is likely to lead to variations in fitness to practise at the point of registration.

REFERENCES

Allan, H.T., Smith, P., O'Driscoll, M., 2011. Experiences of supernumerary status and the hidden curriculum in nursing: a new twist in the theory-practice gap? J. Clin. Nurs. 20, 847–855.

Bedford, H., Phillips, T., Robinson, J., et al., 1993. Assessment of Competencies in Nursing and Midwifery Education and Training. The English National Board for Nursing, Midwifery and Health Visiting, London.

Bendall, E.R.D., Raybould, E., 1969. A History of the General Nursing Council for England and Wales: 1919-1969. Lewis & Co., London: H.K.

Boreham, N.C., 1978. Test-skill interaction errors in the assessment of nurses' clinical proficiency. J. Occup. Psychol. 51, 249–258.

Bradshaw, A., 2000. [Editorial.] J. Clin. Nurs. 9, 319–320.

Bradshaw, P.L. (Ed.), 1989. Teaching and Assessing in Clinical Nursing Prentice Hall, Hemel Hempstead.

Braithwaite, D.N., Elzubeir, M., Stark, S., 1994. Project 2000 student wastage: a case study. Nurse Educ. Today 14, 15–21.

Brandon, J., Davis, M., 1979. The limits of competence in social work: the assessment of marginal students in social work education. Br. J. Soc. Work. 9 (3), 295–347.

Broadfoot, P., 1979. Assessment, Schools and Society. Methuen, London.

Broadfoot, P.M., 1996. Education, Assessment and Society. Open University Press, Buckingham.

Chambers, M.A., 1998. Some issues in the assessment of clinical practice: a review of the literature. J. Clin. Nurs. 7 (3), 201–208.

Clark, T., Holmes, S., 2007. Fit for practice? An exploration of the development of newly qualified nurses using focus groups. Int. J. Nurs. Stud. 44, 1210–1220.

Cleland, J.A., Knight, L.V., Rees, C.E., 2008. Is it me or is it them? Factors that influence the passing of underperforming students. Medical Education 42, 800–809.

Clothier, C., Macdonald, C.A., Shaw, D.A., 1994. The Allitt Inquiry. HMSO, London.

Corlett, J., 2000. The perceptions of nurse teachers, student nurses and preceptors of the theory–practice gap in nurse education. Nurse Educ. Today 20, 499–505.

Crooks, T.J., 1988. The impact of classroom evaluation practices on students. Rev. Educ. Res. 58 (4), 438–481.

Deary, I.J., Watson, R., Hogston, R., 2003. A longitudinal study of burnout and attrition in nursing students. Journal of Advanced Nursing 43 (1), 71–81.

Department of Health, 1998. A First Class Service, Quality in the New NHS. Department of Health, London.

Department of Health, 1999. Making a Difference. Department of Health, London.

Department of Health, 2000. Health Service Circular: Professions Supplementary to Medicine (HSC 2000/006). Department of Health, London.

Department of Health, 2001. Working together, Learning together: A Framework for Lifelong Learning in the NHS. Department of Health, London, Online. Available: <http://www.dh.gov.uk/

publicationsandstatistics> (accessed May 2006).

Department of Health, 2004. The NHS Knowledge and Skills Framework (NHS KSF) and the Development Review Process. Department of Health, London, Online. Available: <http://www.dh.gov.uk/PublicationsAndStatistics/Publications/PublicationsPolicyAndGuidance/fs/en> (accessed December 2005).

Department of Health, 2004. The NHS Knowledge and Skills Framework (NHS KSF) and the Development Review Process. Department of Health, London.

Department of Health, 2006. Managing Attrition Rates for Student Nurses and Midwives. Department of Health, London.

Dolan, G., 2003. Assessing student nurse clinical competency: will we ever get it right? Journal of Clinical Nursing 12, 132–141.

Donnison, J., 1988. Midwives and Medical Men, second ed. Historical Publications, London.

Dudek, N.L., Marks, M.B., Regehr, G., 2005. Failure to fail: the perspectives of clinical supervisors. Academic Medicine 80 (10), S84–S87.

Duffy, K., 2004. Failing Students Report. Nursing and Midwifery Council, London.

Earnshaw, G.J., 1995. Mentorship: the students' views. Nurse Educ. Today 15, 274–279.

Ehrenfeld, M., Rotenberg, A., Sharon, R., et al., 1997. Reasons for attrition on nursing courses: a study. Nursing Standard 36 (8), 393–396.

Embo, M.P.C., Driessen, E.W., Valcke, M., et al., 2010. Assessment and feedback to facilitate self-directed learning in clinical practice of midwifery students. Medical Teacher 3, e263–e269.

English National Board, 2002. Student Statistics Report: 1996/97–2000/2001, third ed. English National Board for Nursing, Midwifery and Health Visiting, London.

Eraut, M., 2003a. Editorial: assessment in a wider context. Learning in Health and Social Care 2 (4), 177–180.

Eraut M. 2003b Transfer of knowledge between education and the workplace. Paper presented at the Conference of the Professorship in Educational Technology. Netherlands. January 2003. Available at: <http://www.ou.nl/otecre-search/publications/oratie%20Els%20Boshuizen/deel3.pdf> (accessed April 2005).

Fitzgerald, M., Gibson, F., Gunn, K., 2010. Contemporary issues relating to assessments. Nurse Education in Practice 10, 158–163.

Foucault M. (1982) Letter quoted in Dreyfus HL, Rainbow P (Eds.) Michael Foucault: Beyond Structuralism and Hermeneutics, Harvester, Brighton.

Fraser, D., Murphy, R., Worth-Butler, M., 1997. An Outcome Evaluation of the Effectiveness of Pre-registration Midwifery Programmes of Education. English National Board for Nursing, Midwifery and Health Visiting, London.

Fretwell, J.E., 1980. An inquiry into the ward learning environment. Nursing Times 76 (16), 69–75.

Gipps, C.V., 1994. Beyond Testing: Towards a Theory of Educational Assessment. The Falmer Press, London.

Girot, E., 1993. Assessment of competence in clinical practice: a review of the literature. Nurse Educ. Today 13, s83–s90.

Glen, S., Clark, A., 1999. Nurse education: a skill mix for the future. Nurse Educ. Today 19, 12–19.

Glossop, C., 2001. Student nurse attrition from pre-registration courses: investigating methodological issues. Nurse Educ. Today 21, 170–180.

Green C. 1991 Identification of the responsibilities and perceptions of the training task held by workforce supervisors of those training within the caring professions. Project 551 prepared for the Further Education Unit, Anglia Polytechnic.

Hallin, K., Danielson, E., 2009. Being a personal preceptor for nursing students: registered nurses experiences before and after introduction of a preceptor model. Journal of Advanced Nursing 65 (1), 161–174.

Health and Care Professions Council, 2007. Managing Fitness to Practise: A Guide for Employers and Registrants. HCPC, London, Online. Available: <http://www.hcpc-uk.org/assets/documents/10001344Managingfitnesstopractise.pdf> (accessed July 2011).

Health and Care Professions Council, 2008. Standards of Conduct, Performance and Ethics. HCPC, London, Online. Available: <http://www.hcpc-uk.org/assets/documents/10002367FINALcopyofSCPEJuly2008.pdf> (accessed July 2011).

Health and Care Professions Council, 2009a. Standards of Education and Training. HCPC, London, Online. Available: <http://www.hcpc-uk.org/assets/documents/10002C0EHCPCStandardsofeducation(A5)(final).pdf> (accessed July 2011).

Health and Care Professions Council, 2009b. Guidance on Conduct and Ethics for Students. HCPC, London, Online. Available: <http://www.hcpc-uk.org/publications/brochures/index.asp?id=219> (accessed July 2011).

Health and Care Professions Council, 2010. Continuing Professional Development and your Registration. HCPC, London, Online. Available: <http://www.hcpc-uk.org/assets/documents/10001314CPD_and_your_registration.pdf> (accessed July 2011).

Health and Care Professions Council, 2011. Fitness to Practise Annual Report 2011. HCPC, London, Online. Available: <http://www.hcpc-uk.org/publications/index.asp?startrow=11&sCategory=0&sKeyword=fitness> to practise reports (accessed February 2012.

Health and Care Professions Council, 2012. About Us. HCPC, London, Online. Available: <http://www.hcpc-uk.org/aboutus/> (accessed September 2012).

Henderson, A., Fox, R., Malko-Nyhan, K., 2006. An evaluation of preceptors perceptions of educational preparation and organizational support for their role. Journal of Continuing Education in Nursing 37 (3), 130–136.

Howe, M.J.A., 1987. Using cognitive psychology to help students learn how to learn. In: Richardson, T.E., Eysenck, M.W., Piper, D.W. (Eds.), Student Learning: Research in Education and Cognitive Psychology Open University Press and Society for Research into Higher Education, Milton Keynes., 135–46.

Hurley, C., Snowden, S., 2008. Mentoring in times of change. Nursing in Critical Care 13 (5), 269–275.

Hutt, R., 1988. Lasting the course, Part IV: findings and conclusions. Senior Nurse 10 (3), 4–8.

Ilott, I., Murphy, R., 1999. Success and Failure in Professional Education: Assessing the Evidence. Whurr, London.

Jacka, K., Lewin, D., 1987. The Clinical Learning of Student Nurses. NERU Report No. 6, Dept of Nursing Studies. King`s College, London.

James, A., Chapman, Y., 2009–2010. Preceptors and patients – the power of two: nursing student experiences on their first acute clinical placement. Contemporary Nurse 34 (1), 34–47.

Kleehammer, K., Hart, A.L., Keck, J.F., 1990. Nursing students` perceptions of anxiety producing situations in the clinical setting. Journal of Nursing Education 29 (40), 183–187.

Klug, B. (Ed.), 1975. A Report by the Group for Research and Innovation in Higher education The Nuffield Foundation, London.

Lankshear, A., 1990. Failure to fail: the teacher`s dilemma. Nursing Standard 4 (20), 35–37.

Lincoln, M., Adamson, B., Covic, T., 2004. Perceptions of stress, time management and coping strategies of speech pathology students on clinical placement. Advances in Speech–Language Pathology 2 (6), 91–99.

Lindop, E., 1987. Factors associated with student and pupil nurse wastage. Journal of Advanced Nursing 12, 751–756.

Luhanga, F., Olive, J., Yonge, O.J., et al., 2008. Failure to assign failing grades: issues with grading the unsafe student. International Journal of

Nursing Education Scholarship 5 (1) article 8.

MacKeith, N., 1994. A study of students who leave pre-registration midwifery. Nursing Times 90 (39), 40–41.

MacLeod, R., 1982. Science and examination in Victorian England. In: MacLeod, R. (Ed.), Days of Judgement. Driffield, N. Nafferton Books, Humberside, pp. 2–24.

Marton, F., Säljö, R., 1984. Approaches to learning. In: Marton, F., Hounsell, D., Entwistle, N. (Eds.), The Experience of Learning Scottish Academic Press, Edinburgh, pp. 36–55.

Mashaba, G., Mhlongo, T., 1995. Student nurse wastage: a case study of the profile and perceptions of students of an institution. Journal of Advanced Nursing 22, 364–373.

McCaugherty, D., 1991. The theory–practice gap in nurse education: its causes and possible solutions. Findings from an action research study. Journal of Advanced Nursing 16, 1055–1061.

Michau, R., Roberts, S., Williams, B., et al., 2009. An investigation of theory-practice gap in undergraduate paramedic education. BMC Medical Education 9 (23) doi: 10.1186/1472-6920-9-23 Online. Available: <http://www.biomedcentral.com/content/pdf/1472-6920-9-23.pdf> (accessed July 2011).

Miller, C., 2010. Improving and enhancing performance in the affective domain of nursing students: insights from the literature for clinical educators. Contemporary Nurse 35 (1), 2–17.

Moriaty, J., MacIntyre, G., Manthorpe, J., et al., 2010. My expectations remain the same. The student has to be competent to practise: practice assessor perspectives on the new social work degree qualification in England. British Journal of Social Work 40, 583–601.

Nursing and Midwifery Council, 2002. The PREP Handbook. Nursing and Midwifery Council, London.

Nursing and Midwifery Council, 2004a. Nursing and Midwifery Council (Education, Registration and Registration Appeals) Rules 2004. Statutory Instrument 2004/1767. The Stationery Office, Norwich, Online. Available: <www.hmso.gov.uk> (accessed December 2005).

Nursing and Midwifery Council, 2004b. Reporting Unfitness to Practise: A Guide for Employers and Managers. Nursing and Midwifery Council, London.

Nursing and Midwifery Council, 2004c. Reporting Lack of Competence: A Guide for Employers and Managers. Nursing and Midwifery Council, London.

Nursing and Midwifery Council, 2005a. Fitness to Practise Annual Report 2004–2005. NMC, London, Online. Available: <http://www.nmc-uk.org> (accessed December 2005).

Nursing and Midwifery Council, 2005b. Consultation on Proposals Arising from a Review of Fitness for Practice at the Point of Registration. NMC, London, Online. Available: <http://www.nmc-uk.org> (accessed December 2005).

Nursing and Midwifery Council, 2006. Standard to Support Learning and Assessment in Practice. NMC, London, Online. Available: <http://www.nmc-uk.org> (accessed 2006).

Nursing and Midwifery Council, 2008a. The Code: Standards of conduct, performance and ethics for nurses and midwives. NMC, London, Online. Available: <http://www.nmc-uk.org/Documents/Standards/The-code-A4-20100406.pdf> (accessed July 2011).

Nursing and Midwifery Council, 2008b. The PREP Handbook. Nursing and Midwifery Council, London, Online. Available: <http://www.nmc-uk.org/Documents/Standards/nmcPrepHandbook.pdf> (accessed July 2011).

Nursing and Midwifery Council, 2009. Standards for Pre-registration Midwifery Education. NMC, London, Online. Available: <http://www.nmc-uk.org/Documents/Standards/nmcStandardsforPre_RegistrationMidwiferyEducation.pdf> (accessed July 2011).

Nursing and Midwifery Council, 2010a. Standards for Pre-registration Nursing Education. NMC, London, Online. Available: <http://www.nmc-uk.org/Publications/Standards> (accessed July 2011).

Nursing and Midwifery Council, 2010b. Fitness to Practise. NMC, London, Online. Available: <http://www.nmc-uk.org/Employers-and-managers/Fitness-to-practise> (accessed July 2011).

Nursing and Midwifery Council, 2010c. Guidance on Professional Conduct for Nursing and Midwifery Students. NMC, London, Online. Available: <http://www.nmc-uk.org/Documents/Guidance/NMC-Guidance-on-professional-conduct-for-nursing-and-midwifery-students.PDF> (accessed July 2011).

Nursing and Midwifery Council, 2011. Fitness to Practise Annual Report: 2010–2011. Nursing and Midwifery Council, London, Online. Available: <http://www.nmc-uk.org/About-us/Statistics/Statistics-about-fitness-to-practise-hearings/> (accessed August 2011.

O`Neill, A., McCall, J., 1996. Objectively assessing nursing practitioners: a curricular development. Nurse Educ. Today 16, 121–126.

Parkes, R., 1985. Stressful episodes reported by first year student nurses: a descriptive account. Social Science and Medicine 2 (9), 945–953.

Phillips, T., Schostak, J., Tyler, J., 2000. Practice and Assessment in Nursing and Midwifery: Doing it for Real. The English National Board for Nursing, Midwifery and Health Visiting, London.

Reilly, D.E., 1980. Behavioural Objectives – Evaluation in Nursing, second ed. Appleton-Century-Crofts, Norwalk.

Richardson, J., 1996. Why won't you stay? Nursing Times 92 (32), 28–30.

Rowntree, D., 1987. Assessing Students: How Shall We Know Them?, second ed. Kogan Page, London.

Runciman, P., Dewar, B., Goulbourne, A., 1998. Employers` Needs and The Skills of Newly Qualified Project 2000 Students. National Board for Nursing, Midwifery and Health Visiting for Scotland, Edinburgh.

Salvatori, P., 2001. Reliability and validity of admissions tools used to select students for the health professions. Adv. Health. Sci. Educ. 6, 159–175.

Scott, G., 2010. Time to address attrition. Nursing Standard 24 (24), 1.

Seymer, L.R., 1949. A General History of Nursing, second ed. Faber and Faber, London.

Smith, P., 1992. The Emotional Labour of Nursing: How Nurses Care. Macmillan Education, London.

Snow, T., Harrison, S., 2008. Carter to raise nurse education concerns with University heads. Nursing Standard 22, 8.

Spouse, J., 1996. The effective mentor: a model for student-centred learning in clinical practice. Nursing Times Research 1 (2), 120–133.

Sweet, B.R., Tiran, D., 1997. History and development of the midwifery profession. In: Sweet, B.R., Tiran, D. (Eds.), Mayes` Midwifery: A Textbook for Midwives, twelfth ed. Baillière Tindall, London, pp. 1005–1010.

The Health Professions Order, 2001. Consolidated Text Incorporating Repeals and Amendments made up to 1st April 2010. HCPC, London, Online. Available: <http://www.hcpc-uk.org/Assets/documents/10002D20HPORDER-2010CONSOLIDATION.pdf> (accessed July 2011).

Torrance, H., 1993. Formative assessment: some theoretical problems and empirical questions. Cambridge Journal of Education 23 (3), 333–343.

Torrance, H., Pryor, J., 1998. Investigating Formative Assessment. Open University Press, Buckingham.

UKCC, 1986. Project 2000, UKCC: A New Preparation for Practice. United Kingdom Central Council for Nursing, Midwifery and Health Visiting, London.

UKCC, 1990. The Report of the Post-registration Education and Practice Project. United Kingdom Central Council for Nursing, Midwifery and Health Visiting, London.

UKCC, 1999a. Fitness for Practice. United Kingdom Central Council for Nursing, Midwifery and Health Visiting, London.

UKCC, 1999b. Register, Spring 1999, No. 27. United Kingdom Central Council for Nursing, Midwifery and Health Visiting, London.

UKCC, 2000a. Requirements for pre-registration nursing programmes. United Kingdom Central Council for Nursing, Midwifery and Health Visiting, London.

UKCC, 2000b. Requirements for Pre-registration Midwifery Programmes. United Kingdom Central Council for Nursing, Midwifery and Health Visiting, London.

Urwin, S., Stanley, R., Jones, M., et al., 2009. Understanding student nurse attrition: learning from the literature. Nurse Educ. Today 30, 202–207.

Water, A., 2006. What a waste. Nursing Standard 20 (23), 14–17.

Waters, A., 2010. The question for universities: how can they win the war on attrition? Nursing Standard 24 (24), 12–15.

Watson, R., Stimpson, A., Topping, A., et al., 2002. Clinical competence assessment in nursing: a systematic review of the literature. Journal of Advanced Nursing 39, 421–431.

Watts, G., 1989. Students` feedback from practical learning. Nursing Times 85 (18), 63.

Wellman, D., 2010. Mind the gap: philosophy, theory, and practice. Nursing Philosophy 11, 85–87.

While, A.E., 1991. The problem of clinical evaluation – a review. Nurse Educ. Today 11, 448–453.

White, E., Riley, E., Davies, S., et al., 1994. A Detailed Study of the Relationship between Teaching, Support, Supervision and Role Modelling in Clinical Areas within the Context of the Project 2000 Courses. The English National Board for Nursing, Midwifery and Health Visiting, London.

White, J., Williams, W.R., Green, B.F., 1999. Discontinuation, leaving reasons and course evaluation comments of students on the common foundation programme. Nurse Educ. Today 19, 142–150.

Whiting, L., 1997. Clinical assessment of student nurses. J. Child. Health. 1 (1), 33–37.

Williams, R.P., 1993. The concerns of beginning nursing students. Nursing and Health Care 14 (4), 178–184.

Wood, V., 1972. Evaluation of student nurse clinical performance: a problem that won't go away. Int. Nurs. Rev. 19 (4), 336–343.

Wood, V., 1982. Evaluation of student nurse clinical performance – a continuing problem. Int. Nurs. Rev. 29 (1), 11–18.

Woolley, A.S., 1977. The long and tortured history of clinical evaluation. Nursing Outlook 25 (5), 308–315.

Young, A.P., 1994. Law and Professional Conduct in Nursing, second ed. Scutari Press, London.

Chapter | 2 |

Responsibility and accountability surrounding clinical assessment

CHAPTER CONTENTS

health care education and professional practice. There is a discussion of the meanings and implications of the concepts of responsibility and accountability in professional practice. This is followed by an exploration of two key questions surrounding the assessment of clinical practice:

- What are practice educators responsible and accountable for?
- Who are practice educators responsible and accountable to?

This latter question is considered in conjunction with the role, responsibilities and accountability for student learning and assessment. Very frequently, a practitioner who is the mentor to a student is also required to assess the student (Health and Care Professions Council (HCPC) 2009a, Nursing and Midwifery Council (NMC) 2008a). Some of the dilemmas of this dual role are also explored.

INTRODUCTION

For the many busy nursing and midwifery practitioners, having the additional role of practice educator to students adds to the role strain (Allan et al 2011, Dolan 2003, Phillips et al 1993, 2000). Teaching and assessing are add-on activities and the adjuncts that are attended to when time permits. Practitioners who are in this unenviable position frequently feel unhappy that the supervision and support of students cannot be made more of a priority. What students learn may be left to chance. Positive assessment decisions about performance may have been made without the concrete evidence of having observed the student in action (White et al 1994). Practitioners may, or may not, be aware of the many legal and ethical ramifications of making assessment decisions in this manner, and for providing an insufficient level of supervision and support for learners.

This chapter explores the issues of responsibility and accountability surrounding assessment in pre-registration

ACCOUNTABILITY AND PROFESSIONALISM

As the nursing and midwifery professions and the professions regulated by the Health and Care Professions Council strive for professional status and self-regulation, the term 'accountability' has assumed increasing importance (Allen & Dennis 2010, Ormerod 1993, Emerton 1992, Bergman 1981).

Accountability as an integral part of health care practice in the UK has been high on the agenda of the NMC and the HCPC. The position taken by the NMC and the HCPC will be discussed later. Health care professionals are required to consider and observe – often simultaneously – ethical, psychological, ethnic and human rights aspects in the discharge of their duties. Society places a high value on the health care professions. The confidence and trust in which health care professionals are held are measures of the special relationship between them and the vulnerable patients and clients in their care.

In the UK, the NMC was established under the Nurses and Midwives Order 2001 (NMC 2001, SI 2002 No. 253) and came into being in April 2002. This Act set out the constitution, establishment and functions of the NMC. The responsibility for the regulation of nursing, midwifery and specialist community public health nurses is vested with the NMC. The HCPC was established under the Health Professions Order 2001 (HCPC 2001, SI 2002 No. 254) and came into force in February 2002. The primary mandate of the NMC and the HCPC is to safeguard the health and well-being of the general public. This is done by keeping a register of all their registrants and ensuring they are fit to practise. The NMC and HCPC also set the standards for the education, training and conduct of those on the register. In all their work, the NMC and HCPC act in collaboration with others, including statutory and professional bodies, education providers, employers and education commissioners.

In 2002, the NMC published its first code of professional conduct. This is now called The Code: Standards of conduct, performance and ethics for nurses and midwives (NMC 2008b). Likewise, the HCPC published standards of conduct, performance and ethics for its registrants in 2003 when their register opened that year. An updated edition was published in 2008 (HCPC 2008). In addition to safeguarding standards and principles of practice for patients and clients, the *Standards* are intended to assist individual practitioners by an expression of the components of acceptable professional practice and related ethical considerations. The *Standards* set out the responsibilities and accountability of the registered practitioner and are the basis of the regulatory framework. They stress the personal accountability of each practitioner for her/his own practice, and that accountability may not be delegated or transferred to another person.

The *Standards* expressly require that the interests of patients and clients should take precedence over all other considerations. Accountability becomes strikingly real when set in the context of clinical situations where professional knowledge and competence are exercised when caring for the diverse range of patients and clients. It is evident that professional accountability in the health care professions is a complex matter. It includes 'ethical, societal and public duty and protective elements for patients and clients' (Royal College of Nursing (RCN) 1990:4).

ACCOUNTABILITY AND RESPONSIBILITY

There are many questions that can be asked about accountability in general. You may wish to carry out Activity 2.1 before progressing with an exploration of the concept of accountability.

ACTIVITY 2.1

What is meant by accountability? What is the relationship between responsibility and accountability?

It is not possible to enter into an extensive philosophical discussion of the concepts of accountability and responsibility. The discussion is therefore limited to aspects of what I see is relevant to the educational role of practitioners as practice educators. Responsibility is linked inextricably with accountability. The focus of responsibility is on the task and not on accounting for it (Cornock 2011). We talk of a 'responsible person' as one who accepts and executes an undertaking so long as it is within her/his capabilities (Champion 1991). To be responsible implies being answerable to either another or oneself for some act – it implies a moral accountability for one's actions as one is capable of rational conduct and fulfilling obligations for vested trust (Brykczynska 1995). Brykczynska goes on to point out that a responsible person is reliable and can justify a trust. Bergman (1981) believes that responsibility is the key component of accountability. However, it is only a part of accountability, as accountability is more inclusive than responsibility. Cornock (2011) suggests that accountability is a higher-level activity than responsibility because the person is not only responsible for an action undertaken but is also required to give an account, reason or explanation for the action. The necessity for this account is not only in instances when something has gone wrong. For instance, it may be required as part of a monitoring system or because things are going right. As an example, in the case of nurses and midwives who assess the clinical practice of pre-registration nursing and midwifery students in the UK, the NMC states that they are accountable for confirming that students have met, or not met, the NMC competencies in practice (NMC 2008a).

Before one can be accountable, several preconditions have to be present. These preconditions (Figure. 2.1) are shown in the model used by Bergman (1981:55). The basic precondition is to have the ability (knowledge, skills, values) to decide and act on a specific issue to be able to act autonomously. Next, one must be given, or take, the responsibility to carry out that action. One also needs the autonomy to carry out the action as there is a link between accountability and autonomy (Cornock 2011). Without the autonomy to make decisions freely about the form of action required to be taken, the practitioner is unable to be accountable. If a health professional is instructed to undertake an action, and also the manner in which it should be undertaken, then the health professional is not accountable but responsible. Champion (1991) describes two forms of autonomy: personal and structural autonomy. Personal autonomy

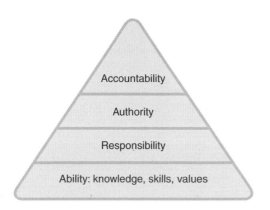

Figure 2.1 Model of the preconditions leading to accountability.
(From Bergman, R., 1981. Accountability – definition and dimensions. Int Nurs Rev, *28 (2): 53-59. Reproduced with permission from Blackwell Science Publishers.)*

refers to the expertise, knowledge and skills related to the defined area of work, the understanding of personal limits of competence and the willingness to take responsibility. Structural autonomy is the 'authority to act' given by the organization. To be accountable, one needs the authority to be able to decide whether to act and how to act. A practitioner cannot be accountable if told how to carry out an action and is not able to make the decision on the way the action is to be performed or even whether the action should be carried out at all. When these preconditions are present, one can then be held accountable for the actions one takes. It can thus be expected that 'an accountable person does not undertake an action merely because someone in authority says to do so. Instead, the accountable person examines a situation, explores the various options available, demonstrates a knowledgeable understanding of the possible consequences of options and makes a decision for action which can be justified from a knowledge base' (Marks-Maran 1993, in Cornock 2011).

Professional accountability involves accepting responsibility for professional decisions. Stated more simply, practitioners are 'entrusted with, answerable for, take the credit and blame for and can be judged within legal and moral boundaries' (Castledine 1991). The RCN (1990:4) suggests the following working definition of professional accountability for nurses:

It is that obligation on the practitioner that binds her [sic] to a code of conduct, based on the expectations of society that she will use her discretion and skill to safeguard her patients and act in every way to uphold professional standards. This obligation, and the values of the profession provide a framework for professional and ethical behaviour within which nurses must personally and professionally conduct themselves and within which the primacy and vulnerability of those served is observed and protected.

In view of the substantial clinical role of practitioners, the *Standards of conduct, performance and ethics* for registrants (HCPC 2008, NMC 2008b) appropriately focuses on professional accountability to patients and clients. Generally, practitioners are in little doubt about their professional accountability towards their patients and clients. Professional accountability for nursing and midwifery education has not received the same attention and interest (Marks-Maran 1995, Harding & Greig 1994). It was not until the publication of the NMC *Standards to support learning and assessment in practice* (NMC 2008a, 2006) that accountability for student learning and assessment in clinical practice started to receive due attention.

There can be few health care practitioners who are not in some way involved in the training and supervision of others. These roles are frequently part of the contract of employment. NMC registrants who support pre-registration nursing or midwifery students and make summative assessment decisions are termed *mentors*. The educational role of nurses and midwives in clinical practice is formalized by the NMC in the *Standards to support learning and assessment in practice* (NMC 2008a). These standards specify the responsibility and accountability of NMC registrants who are mentors to pre-registration nursing and midwifery students. Mentors are required to support and make summative assessment decisions of students' fitness to practise, i.e. determine that students have met the relevant standards of proficiency for entry to the register or for a qualification that is recordable on the register. Those registrants on the NMC register who make summative assessment decisions that determine whether students have met the relevant standards of proficiency for entry to the register must be on the same part or sub-part of the register as that which the student is intending to enter (NMC 2008a). Also, they must hold professional qualifications equal to, or at a higher level than, the students they are supporting and assessing. Additionally, the designation of *sign-off mentor* has been introduced to sign-off proficiency for all nursing students at the end of the programme. All midwifery mentors are sign-off mentors (NMC 2010a, circular 05/2010). In addition to the possession of the other criteria of a sign-off mentor, a sign-off mentor must have clinical currency and capability in their field of practice and an in-depth understanding of their accountability to the NMC for the decision to pass or fail a student (NMC 2008a, section 2.1.3).

In the case of registrants on the HCPC register, practice placement educators will normally be registered with the HCPC in the relevant profession. However, the HCPC recognizes that there are other appropriate practice placement educators whose backgrounds do not match the specific profession that the student is studying. For example, occupational therapists may supervise physiotherapy students in areas such as hand therapy, and nurses may supervise radiographers in aseptic techniques (HCPC 2009a:48). Whilst the *Standards of education and training* of the HCPC (HCPC 2009a) state that practice placement educators involved in formative and summative assessment must undertake appropriate practice placement educator training, the HCPC does not specify any precise standards to guide the practice of HCPC registrants who assess students' clinical practice.

The requirements for training, supervision and support of pre-registration health care students, and the concomitant assessment of learning, mean that more and more practitioners must take on these roles. Dimond (1994:272) says that 'for the most part this is unlikely to give rise to many legal issues'. However, an awareness of the potential pitfalls and problems associated with these roles may prevent grief from arising. The rest of the chapter therefore examines accountability issues surrounding the assessment of clinical practice; there is an exploration of the moral and legal obligations that practice educators have to fulfil. The rights of learners and why they have legal means of redress will be explained.

Due to the differences in terminology used by the NMC and the HCPC for the educational role of registrants to pre-registration students in clinical practice, in all health care practitioners who support and supervise pre-registration students and conduct their summative assessments during clinical practice are referred to as 'practice educators' in the rest of this book.

ACCOUNTABILITY FOR THE ASSESSMENT OF CLINICAL PRACTICE

Before going on to explore this section, consider the questions posed in Activity 2.2.

ACTIVITY 2.2

What are practice educators responsible and accountable for?

Who are practice educators responsible and accountable to?

In its document *Making a Difference* (Department of Health 1999:24), the government made it clear that it wants practitioners who are fit for purpose, with excellent skills and the knowledge and ability to provide the best care possible in a modern National Health Service (NHS). The point was made that every practitioner shares responsibility to support and teach the next generation

of health care professionals. Both the NMC (2008b) and the HCPC (2009a) expect that students who complete pre-registration programmes must have met the standards of proficiency. Prior to entry to the NMC and HCPC professional registers, students must also meet the standards of conduct, performance and ethics, and the health and character requirements of registration (HCPC 2009a, NMC 2010b). To enable the fulfilment of these professional requirements, practice educators need to be cognizant of their responsibility and accountability for the supervision and assessment of clinical practice.

The following section examines WHAT the practice educator is responsible and accountable for when supervising and assessing learners.

Responsibility and accountability FOR WHAT?

For nurses and midwives, direct reference is made to professional accountability for the support and supervision of learners, and, by inference, the assessment of standards of practice, in the NMC *Standards of conduct, performance and ethics* (NMC 2008b). The Standards state:

> *You must facilitate students and others to develop their competence.*

For nurses and midwives and registrants on the HCPC register, your respective *Standards of conduct, performance and ethics* (HCPC 2008, NMC 2008b) make it clear that no one else can answer for you and it will be no defence to say that you were acting on someone else's orders. The NMC states:

> *As a professional, you are personally accountable for actions and omission in your practice and must always be able to justify your decisions.*

Whilst the HCPC is not as explicit as the NMC in its statement about accountable practice, it states that:

> *As an autonomous and accountable professional, you need to make informed and reasonable decisions about your practice to make sure that you meet the standards that are relevant to your practice. … You are responsible for your professional conduct, any care or advice you provide, and any failure to act.*

Both sets of *Standards* also make it clear that, if you delegate work to someone, your responsibility and accountability is to make sure that the person who does the work is able to carry out your instructions safely and effectively and that proper supervision and support are provided. The NMC further state that nurses and midwives must also confirm that the outcome of any delegated tasks meets required standards.

When these requirements for professional practice are applied to assessment, it can be seen that the practitioner has professional responsibility and accountability to fulfil in her/his role as a practice educator. It is suggested here that the practice educator can be answerable for standards of personal professional practice, with its inevitable impact on learning, and the following aspects of supervision and assessment:

- standards of personal professional practice
- standards of care delivery by learners
- what is taught, learned and assessed
- standards of teaching and assessing
- professional judgements about student performance.

Personal professional standards of practice

It is discussed in Chapter 1 that one purpose of assessment in pre-registration health care education is as a form of quality control for the outcome of the educational process. The educational and professional outcome is a nurse or midwife or physiotherapist or social worker, and so on, who is able to apply knowledge, understanding and skills to perform to the standards required in employment. This professional must have met the standards of proficiency, and prior to entry to the NMC and HCPC professional registers; students must also meet the standards of conduct, performance and ethics, and the health and character requirements of registration. The full realization of this outcome is dependent on the successful achievement of both theoretical and clinical learning and professional development measured by assessment. Assessment is an integral part of professional health care programmes. The processes of clinical teaching, learning and assessment are complex. The committed input of practice educators is required to plan and implement these processes if learning outcomes are to be achieved successfully. I would suggest that this commitment starts with the individual practitioner's competence and standard of practice. Eraut et al (1995) state that, if aspects of clinicians' practice are ill-defined, lack quality or make insufficient use of scientific knowledge, the next generation of practitioners will suffer.

Much of the learning that takes place in professional education does so in the practice setting (Baskett & Marsick 1992, Schön 1983). Role modelling is an important (Fowler 2008, Pollard 2008, Spouse 1998, Wood 1987), and an almost inevitable, learning strategy in this environment. Within social learning theory, Bandura (1977) suggests that, in role modelling, one person sets a pattern of behaviour that is then copied by another. Learning takes place constantly from observing role models deliver care – these practices are subsequently emulated (Charters 2000). Davies' (1993) study of role modelling showed that major aspects of nursing were learnt by students when they observed role models providing direct patient care. Students who worked alongside knowledgeable and respected practitioners developed an enthusiasm and commitment to their professional development that was unparalleled by any other learning experience (Spouse 1998). As stated succinctly by McAllister et al (2007:305), 'students are a product of their schooling'. It is therefore important for the practice educator to adhere to high standards of professional practice so that students learn this high standard of care and are assessed against these professional practices. A high standard of care from students cannot be expected if this is not role modelled. Without modelling high standards of practice one aspect of professional and moral accountability will not be fulfilled.

Nicklin & Kenworthy (1995:72) say that 'assessment inevitably takes place in a role-relationship'. The usual relationship that exists between a student and a practice educator is hierarchical in nature. Neary (2000) pointed out that many practice educators take for granted their position of power in the assessment relationship. Her study in 1996 (in Neary 2000) showed the extent to which this 'taken-for-granted' power imbalance became explicit at early stages of the relationship when practice educators quickly confirmed their expertise and established the subordination of their students. In a review of the literature on how practice educators influence practice, Armstrong (2010) found that a student's actual experience is one of control and coercion. Students felt powerless in challenging practice owing to their lack of status and the fear of jeopardizing their clinical assessment and securing a job.

Within this hierarchical situation, one assumption made of the practitioner as practice educator is that she/he possesses the requisite professional qualities and can recognize these in the learner (Harding & Greig 1994). This assumption is of course open to debate. Hepworth (1991:46) expressed her disagreement when she said that:

> *the assessor of a student's clinical nursing skills can only assess the student in the light of her own perceptions of the nursing situation, and her own nursing expertise.*

Our assessments, then, are likely to be based on our own standards of practice and perceptions of the situation. Therefore, as practitioners who are also practice educators, there is the responsibility for maintaining competent practice so that assessments are made against these standards. Furthermore, in exercising professional accountability, the NMC (2008b) and the HCPC (2008) require their practitioners on the professional registers to maintain and improve professional knowledge and competence. One point arising from debates on competence is the requirement for the practitioner to keep up to date in order to claim that practice is competent (Hager & Gonczi 1996, McGaghie 1991). Notwithstanding professional requirements, the bottom line in the argument for keeping up to date must be the legal requirement that professional health care practitioners can exercise contemporary professional practices as the law expects current practice to be the accepted practice (Dimond 2011, Young 2009, 1994). There is an expectation that practitioners will employ evidence-based practice and, generally speaking, judges will take a dim view of practitioners who fail to follow the latest clinical guidelines (Young 2009). The duty of care to patients requires practitioners to keep their knowledge and practice up to date (Griffith & Tengnah 2010).

Young (1994) states that the legal implication of omitting certain information, or of giving wrong information, is potential negligence on the part of the instructor. This potential exists whenever a failure in instruction jeopardizes the safety of the learner being instructed, or of the patient in her care. I would also suggest that, unless a practice educator is also a competent practitioner, training requirements may not be fulfilled owing to the inability to teach what constitutes competent practice. The practice educator thus has a legal duty, as well as moral and professional accountability to fulfil, in terms of keeping up to date and maintaining competent practice. If it could be established that a patient/client suffered harm as a consequence of negligent instruction (e.g. incorrect information to a student), the patient/client could instigate legal action against the instructor.

Standards of care delivery by learners

The practice educator has a dual responsibility: to the patient/client and to the student. A major aspect of the concept of professional negligence in clinical practice is that practice educators have a 'specific duty or responsibility to foresee or anticipate the possible adverse outcomes of their actions' (Gunby 2008:414). This applies to both client care and supervision of students. Practice educators must meet a standard of care with respect to the patient/client and a standard of conduct with respect to the student. Practice educators must ensure that students have the necessary clinical experiences and supervision to develop professional competencies in such a way that the patient/client is not harmed in any way while the student is giving the care. The NMC (2008b) and the HCPC (2008) state that patient safety must always take precedence above all else. The NMC and HCPC *Standards of conduct, performance and ethics* (HCPC 2008, NMC 2008b) make sure that practitioners put the interests of patients, clients and the public before their own interests and those of professional colleagues: i.e. accountability to the patient is always more important than to the student.

The Bolam Test (see later discussion) applies to delegation (Dimond 2011). In the eyes of the law, the student's performance must be equal to that of a registered practitioner. The law is quite clear that a lack of experience or knowledge is never an excuse for incompetent

care (Griffith & Tengnah 2010, Young 1994). Students of health care are thus required to provide care equivalent to that of the registered practitioner. One judge (in Young 1994:56) adopted the following view:

The law requires the trainee or learner to be judged by the same standard as his more experienced colleagues. If it did not, inexperience would frequently be urged as a defence to an action for professional negligence.

Another judge linked the expected standard of care to that of the post rather than to the status of the person performing the care, saying:

To my mind the notion of a duty tailored to the actor, rather than to the act which he elects to perform, has no place in the law of tort.

Therefore, in a highly specialized clinical setting, the standard must be 'not just that of the averagely competent and well-informed [nurse] but of such a person who fills a post in a unit offering a highly specialized service' (Wilsher v Essex AHA 1988, in Young 1994).

For students to deliver care to a standard equivalent to that of a registered practitioner, that care to be given must be within the student's capabilities. So far as the NMC and HCPC (HCPC 2008, NMC 2008a) are concerned, it is the registered practitioner working with the student who is professionally responsible for the consequences of the actions and omissions of that student. A pre-registration student, or any other unqualified staff, who is not on the professional register cannot be called to account for her/his actions or omissions as registered practitioners are accountable for care given whether directly or through delegation. It is the personal and professional responsibility of the practitioner who delegates an activity to make sure that the person carrying out the activity is trained, competent and has the necessary experience to undertake the activity safely (Dimond 2011). The delegating professional must also make sure that the appropriate level of supervision is provided. The provision of appropriate levels of supervision is developed in Chapter 7.

A number of cases of qualified staff were reported to the then United Kingdom Central Council for Nursing, Midwifery and Health Visiting (UKCC 1996) for inappropriate delegation of responsibilities. One case, which was closed by the Preliminary Proceedings Committee (PPC) of the UKCC, concerned the delegation, by a nurse to a care assistant, of the task of administering an insulin injection. The case was reported on the basis that such administration by a care assistant was prima facie wrong. The issue considered by the PPC was not that the care assistant could not give the injection, but whether the person to whom the responsibility was being delegated was competent to carry out the task. The UKCC concluded that the issue was about supervision, the appropriateness of the delegation and the instruction of unqualified staff, and not about the rigid demarcation of work into tasks to be done by one group or another.

It is therefore important to know *when* and to *whom* it is safe to delegate. In order to delegate safely and to avoid negligent delegation, the practitioner must be satisfied that the person performing the delegated task is competent to carry it out (Dimond 2011, Young 1994). Making the following two checks may help you to decide when it is safe to delegate. Assess:

- The extent of the person's knowledge and understanding of the task – this requires skilful questioning of the person. This point is developed in Chapter 4.
- How skilful the person is in the task delegated – this may require observation and close supervision of the person initially. It is important to provide ongoing supervision. The amount and extent of the supervision will vary from person to person. However, Wood (1987) holds that students must be under strict supervision at all times. This point on supervision of students will be developed in Chapter 6 when management of the continuous assessment process is discussed.

The learning and assessment programme for the student must therefore be planned so that the patient/client is protected from harm while the student is enabled to develop and achieve the professional standards of proficiency required.

The NMC (2008c) has issued detailed guidance on delegation that is available on its website. The guidance considers the principles of delegation by nurses and midwives, the responsibility and accountability of the practitioner who delegates and the documentation required.

What is taught, learned and assessed

The practice educator has the responsibility for ensuring that the learning environment is conducive to learning. A wide range of high-quality learning opportunities should be arranged and provided to enable the student to achieve learning outcomes and competencies. The Nursing and Midwifery Order 2001 (NMC 2001) and the Health Professions Order 2001 require the NMC and HCPC to determine the standard, kind and content of training to be undertaken with a view to registration. The standards of proficiency and standards of education required for all pre-registration health care education regulated by the NMC and the HCPC are set out in the Registration Rules (NMC 2004) and Standards of Education and Training under Article 15(1)-(9) of the Health Professions Order, 2001, respectively.

Pre-registration nursing and midwifery programmes in the UK now require students to achieve national NMC standards of proficiency (NMC 2010c, 2009). In the case of professions regulated by the HCPC, each profession

has defined its own standards of proficiency with varied dates of implementation (HCPC 2011a).

It is a requirement that pre-registration programmes must be designed to enable students to apply knowledge, understanding and skills when performing to the standards required in employment and to provide the care that patients/clients require, safely and competently, in order to assume, on registration, the responsibilities and accountability necessary for public protection. Both the NMC and HCPC make it clear that these standards of proficiency are achieved under the direction of the practice educator. In accepting the roles of practice educator as defined by the NMC and the HCPC (HCPC 2009a, NMC 2008a), the practitioner is responsible for ensuring that teaching and learning activities, including clinical experiences, assist the student in achieving these standards of proficiency. This requires practitioners to have a sound knowledge and understanding of the learning outcomes to be achieved, expectations of professional conduct and assessment procedures including the implications of, and any action to be taken in the case of, failure to progress. This will enable the practice educator to identify and plan appropriate teaching and learning activities and clinical experiences.

As in any practice discipline, it is not enough just to have 'knowledge of' – one also needs to know what to do with that knowledge. This leads into the next 'what for' aspect of accountability of the practice educator: namely that of facilitating and measuring that learning.

Standards of teaching and assessing

The student is entitled to the best instruction available (Young 1994, Wood 1987). Failure to instruct properly could be construed as a negligent act (Dimond 2011, Goclowski 1985). The standard of teaching and learning that an academic institution is expected to provide is generally stated in the educational institution's 'student charter'. Service providers for patient/client care enter into contracts with higher education institutions to provide clinical experience for students. Within such contracts is an agreement to provide a standard of teaching and learning in the clinical setting commensurate with that set by the educational institution. To achieve the required standards of the teaching and assessment of clinical practice, practice educators need to attain and maintain competent practice in these roles (HCPC 2009a, NMC 2008a). It is recognized that clinical staff exercise a major influence on the quality of pre-registration programmes (Allan et al 2011, Eraut et al 1995). They do much of the teaching, supervision and assessment of students, and as it is likely that this will continue, it is imperative that they are capable of fulfilling these roles. Activities that practice educators are expected to provide will include planning learning opportunities for and with students to enable them to achieve their individual learning needs;

facilitating and supporting the learning process; assessing learning; and providing feedback to students on their performance (NMC 2008a, Neary 2000, Eraut et al 1995). To support these educational processes in the clinical setting, higher education institutions include a policy for the management of the assessment of clinical practice in its curriculum document. Generally, the practice educator is required to carry out an initial interview with the student to negotiate and formulate a learning contract/plan to facilitate the achievement of learning outcomes and standards of proficiency. Subsequently, an intermediate interview should take place half way through the placement to review the student's progress and achievement, and formal feedback given and documented. A final interview allows the practice educator to make a summative assessment of whether the student has achieved the learning outcomes of the placement.

Practice educators must be aware of, and be careful that, any policy regulating the assessment of practice is followed, as any deviation from such regulations could give rise to students appealing against any unfavourable assessment decision on the grounds of not having received the supervision, guidance and support to which they are entitled. Cases of students suing nursing institutions in the courts using the above grounds as educational malpractice are well documented in the North American literature (see, for example, Johnson & Halstead 2005, Goudreau & Chasens 2002, Graveley & Stanley 1993, Goclowski 1985, Spink 1983). Courts have recognized that, by virtue of their training, practice educators are uniquely qualified to observe and judge all aspects of their students' performance. Court decision ruling in favour of the student has been on the basis of practice educators not following established guidelines for the supervision of the student.

Practice educators require adequate preparation to enable them to manage the educational activities to support learning and assessment. Subsequently, regular updates are important to keep abreast of developments and/or changes in the curriculum, the assessment process and new local and national policies influencing health care education. In the case of nurses and midwives and registrants with the HCPC, the NMC and HCPC require practice educators to update regularly (HCPC 2009a, NMC 2008a). The practices of mentoring and assessing can be enhanced if these 'update' sessions are also used as opportunities to discuss assessment problems and how these had been dealt with by individuals.

Unfortunately, there is current unease about the expertise of practice educators. Research shows that the initial preparation and continuing development of practice educators are inadequate, particularly with respect to knowledge of programmes and assessment of practice (Luhanga et al 2008, Duffy 2004). Whereas practice educators are personally accountable for their practice of the supervision and assessment of students (HCPC 2009a, NMC 2008b), service providers and higher education institutions have the joint responsibility for ensuring that training, support and updating opportunities are provided for practitioners to develop their role as practice educator (HCPC 2009a, NMC 2008a, Department of Health 1999).

Professional judgements about student performance

By virtue of their role, practice educators have the right to make, and are indeed vested with the onerous responsibility and accountability for making, professional judgements about the performance of students (HCPC 2009a, NMC 2008a, 2005). These professional judgements require the practice educator to make and report on two important professional decisions: first, they are reporting on the degree to which a student has met the programme learning outcomes and standard; secondly, they are reporting on the ability of the student to provide professionally competent and safe care to the public. Practice educators to students on NMC-approved programmes leading to registration, or a qualification that is recordable on the register, are **accountable** to the NMC for their assessment decisions about *fitness to practise* of students to enter the register, and whether they have the necessary knowledge, skills and competence to take on the role of registered nurse, midwife or specialist community public health nurse (NMC 2008a, 2005). Whilst the HCPC does not make a direct reference to accountability for summative assessment decisions, it may be inferred from the *Standards of conduct, performance and ethics* (HCPC 2008) that HCPC registrants who are practice educators are also accountable, thus:

> *As an accountable health professional, you will be responsible for the decisions you make and you may also be asked to justify them (p. 16).*

It is important for the practice educator to remember that professional judgements not only assess the student's current competence but also provide a prediction of the student's potential ability to practise as a professional nurse or midwife, or physiotherapist, or social worker and so on. Therefore, the conclusion about a student's performance should attempt to elicit reliability and predictive validity. These important criteria of sound assessments are discussed in Chapter 5.

Literature on the assessment of clinical practice abounds with discussions about the subjective nature of this process. Ashworth & Morrison (1991:260) stated that:

> *… assessing involves the perception of evidence about performance by an assessor, and the arrival at a decision concerning the level of performance of the person being assessed. Here there is enormous, unavoidable scope*

for subjectivity especially when the competencies being assessed are relatively intangible ones.

Assessments about a student's performance frequently reflect the practice educator's personal perception of what performance constitutes professional practice. Such an assessment is based on both objective and subjective criteria. There is, therefore, a danger that some decisions about student performance may be biased and unfair. Practice educators should be aware that many factors, some of which they are unaware of, can interfere with fair and equitable professional judgements, resulting in the student being treated unfairly.

As noted earlier, students have the right to expect that they will be notified of any deficiencies in their performance. The practice educator is behaving unfairly and unethically if the student is not informed about unsatisfactory performance (Orchard 1994). Furthermore, practice educators who fail to evaluate a student's unsatisfactory performance accurately, either through reluctance to expose the student to the experience of failure or through a fear of potential redress by the student, are guilty of misleading the student, potentially jeopardizing patient/client care and placing the higher education institution in a difficult situation. It is much fairer to students to inform them of unsatisfactory performance as soon as such performance is identified. Informing students of deficiencies in a caring and constructive way allows students the opportunity to improve their performance, not to inform them denies them this opportunity and right (Killam et al 2010, Johnson & Halstead 2005).

Practice educators have a moral responsibility to fail incompetent students (Gopee 2008, Beaumont 2004, Ilott & Murphy 1999). Beaumont's call came after Duffy (2004) reported that practice educators were 'failing to fail' nursing students. Being 'kind' to students by not failing them is not in the best interest of the student, especially when there is a delay to fail until late into the programme, such as in the final year. Having to inform family and friends that one will now not be able to graduate owing to failure, after having been on the programme for two years, can do untold damage to the self-esteem of that student. Failing to fail students is also not in the best interest of the profession for obvious reasons. An awareness of those factors that contribute to 'failure to fail' may be a first step to understanding why difficulties are experienced when dealing with a failing student, and may assist the practice educator in not passing a student when a fail is clearly warranted. It is suggested here that the responsibility for seeking assistance and/or support to make valid summative assessment decisions rests with the individual practice educator. The issues of the unsafe student and 'failure to fail' will be explored further in Chapter 7.

I have put forward what I see are the main aspects that practice educators are responsible and accountable for

when they supervise and assess learners. The next section examines the 'TO WHOM?' aspects.

Responsibility and accountability TO WHOM?

As discussed earlier, one position that the RCN takes in relationship to professional accountability is that it comprises ethical, societal and public duty and protective elements for patients and clients. These elements of professional accountability may also be applied to the supervision and assessment of learners. With professional registration, each practitioner is vested with personal autonomy. A contract of employment gives the structural autonomy for the authority to act in the best interests of patients and clients. This contract frequently also requires the practitioner to take on the role of practice educator – this gives the practice educator the authority to act in the best interests of the learner.

Based on the above context of accountability, and extrapolating from the work of mainstream education, practice educators responsible for the supervision and assessment of clinical practice can be seen to assume the three aspects of educational accountability described by Becher et al (1981):

- professional accountability: responsibility to self, colleagues and the profession
- contractual accountability: accountability to the employer or someone in authority
- moral accountability: answerability to students.

Teachers are accountable for their professional conduct, such as the selection and implementation of appropriate forms of practice. Contractually, they are under an obligation to report to, and be partly directed by, a specific person or group of persons. A teacher in mainstream education is contractually accountable to the head teacher. Moral accountability is of special importance in education as it pervades the teacher–pupil relationship. These aspects of accountability will now be used to examine the

ACTIVITY 2.3

Make a list of the individuals and bodies that you consider you are responsible and accountable to when you supervise and assess students. Why do you think you are responsible and accountable to them?

to whom aspects of responsibility and accountability when supervising and assessing the clinical practice of students. Before you proceed, you may wish to try Activity 2.3.

These individuals and bodies are listed in Figure 2.2. In acknowledgement of professional responsibility and accountability required of the practitioner by the NMC

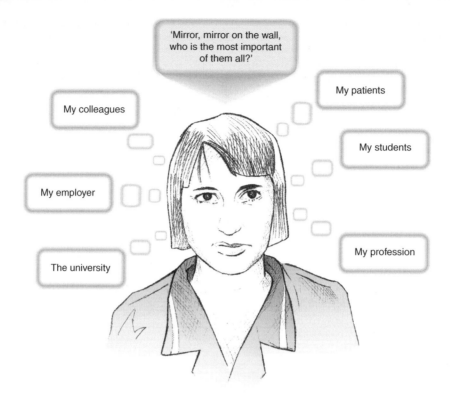

Figure 2.2 Juggling responsibilities?

and HCPC, the most important individual would be the patient/client.

Each of the above individuals and bodies shown in Figure 2.2 will now be considered in an examination of why you might be responsible and accountable to them. This will be developed in four sections, namely that of responsibility and accountability to:

- the patient/client
- the student
- the trust/employing authority and the higher education institution
- yourself, colleagues and your profession.

The patient/client

The practitioner on the NMC or HCPC professional register has both a legal and a professional duty of care to patients and clients. In law, the courts could find a registered practitioner negligent if a person suffers harm because the practitioner has failed to provide proper care to that person. Professionally, the NMC's and HCPC's Conduct and Competence Committee could find a registered practitioner guilty of misconduct and remove the practitioner from the register if there has been failure to

provide adequate care for patients/clients (HCPC 2010a, NMC 2010b). The practitioner's accountability and duty of care to the patient/client when supervising students has been discussed at some length in the previous section (see responsibility and accountability for standards of care delivery by learners). It will be reiterated here that the pre-registration student cannot be called to account by the NMC or HCPC for any actions and omissions. It is the registered practitioner with whom the student is working who is professionally responsible and accountable for the consequences of the student's actions and omissions. In law, the practitioner could also be found to be negligent for the actions and omissions of the student (Goudreau & Chasens 2002). These authors reported the case of a patient in North America who was injured while under the care of a medical student who had been left to make inappropriate decisions. The courts determined that the supervisor was negligent in his duty due to lack of adequate supervision of the student.

When making arrangements for students to care for patients and clients, the wishes of patients and clients should be respected at all times. Under the *Patient's Charter*, patients/clients have the right to choose whether or not to take part in medical research or student training

(Department of Health 1995). This right should be made clear to them when they are first given information about care they will receive from students. Their rights as patients or clients supersede at all times the student's rights to knowledge and experience (NMC 2010b, HCPC 2009b).

The student

Students have rights; practice educators need to respect these, while maintaining professional standards and expectations of their performance at the same time. Students also have obligations and responsibilities to fulfil. It is important for the practice educator to recognize what these rights, obligations and responsibilities are so that the student may be assisted in the most appropriate ways to succeed during clinical practice. The practice educator also needs to recognize that there are legal, professional and moral obligations towards students under supervision.

Student rights, obligations, responsibilities and accountability

Student rights

Higher education institutions have the right to set academic standards for students. They have the responsibility to communicate those standards to students. Institutions have written policies that govern student progression, grading and discipline. These policies are typically made available to students through the student handbook, which serves as a contract between the student and the institution (Johnson & Halstead 2005). Policies made within a programme of study regarding progression, grading and dismissal of students must be in agreement with the institution's policies. Any student who has enrolled in a course has implicitly agreed to abide by the policies of the course and those of the higher education institution. Within assessment regulations (Johnson & Halstead 2005) students have the following rights:

- to know the professional conduct and competencies that are expected of them in order to pass the clinical placement successfully
- to receive timely feedback about their performance and conduct, and the opportunity and support to correct unsatisfactory performance and conduct
- to be made aware that their performance is not meeting the criteria that have been set for satisfactory performance before being failed
- to work under the supervision of a qualified practitioner who has been appropriately trained to be a practice educator. The NMC (2008a) stipulates that, whilst giving direct care in the practice setting, at least 40% of the student's time must be spent being supervised (directly or indirectly) by a practice educator.

Within any scheme of the continuous assessment of practice, there must be formalized meetings between the student and the practice educator to guide student learning, which will also enable these rights to be met. Assessment regulations relating to the continuous assessment of practice generally require practice educators to conduct a minimum of three documented formal interviews with student nurses and student midwives. Failure to do so could give rise to grounds for student appeal against an unfavourable assessment decision.

All higher education institutions have established policies for hearing student grievances and appeals. These policies exist to protect students' rights and to provide student recourse to appeal assessment decisions previously made (Johnson & Halstead 2005). The grievance and student appeal process provides the opportunity for the original assessment decision to be reassessed. Generally, the assessment grade and/or summative assessment decision cannot be altered, but it is likely to be declared null and void if those educational processes that were in place to support student learning and progression had been violated.

Student obligations and responsibility

As stated above, any student who has enrolled in a course has agreed to abide by the policies of the course and those of the higher education institution. Higher education institutions generally have regulations governing the progress and discipline of students. Practice educators have the responsibility of assisting higher education institutions to uphold these regulations. These regulations serve to safeguard standards of training and conduct. Failure to fulfil and/or comply with these regulations could result in the student being dismissed from the course. Students are thus directly accountable to their higher-education institution. I have known students to be disciplined by the higher education institution for falsifying their practice educators' signatures in the assessment of practice records. This misconduct has resulted in those students being dismissed from their course.

Several responsibilities are conferred on the student. Higher education institutions can expect students:

- to fulfil regulations governing the progress of students
- not to behave in ways that can be alleged as misconduct.

Additionally, nursing and midwifery students need to abide by the guidance set out in the NMC document *Guidance on professional conduct for nursing and midwifery students* (NMC 2010b). Students studying for a profession regulated by the HCPC need to abide by the guidance set out in the HCPC document *Guidance on conduct and ethics for students* (HCPC 2009b).

The NMC (2010b) and HCPC (2009b) and higher education institutions make it clear to students that they must always work under the supervision of a registered practitioner. Furthermore, students should not participate in any procedure for which they have not been fully prepared or in which they are not adequately supervised (NMC 2010b,

HCPC 2009b). Students must learn when to ask for help and not to allow themselves to be placed in situations where practice becomes unsafe. Working in collaboration with their practice educator, students must learn to appraise for themselves whether they are personally willing to take any risks that may be involved in any care-giving situations (Goudreau & Chasens 2002). In general, students should be allowed to practise only to the level of competence consistent with course requirements. When it becomes unclear whether engagement in an aspect of care delivery could be beyond the student's usual scope of practice, it becomes incumbent upon the student, and the practice educator, to seek guidance from the educational institution.

Student accountability

The student can also be called to account by the law for the consequences of actions or omissions as a pre-registration student (NMC 2010b, HCPC 2009b). The student must behave in a reasonable way (Castledine 2000). What is reasonable? The case of Bolam v Friern Hospital Management Committee produced the 'Bolam Test' of what is reasonable (Dimond 1994, 2011, UKCC 1996). The test derives from a case heard in 1957 where a psychiatric patient was given electroconvulsive therapy without any relaxant drugs or restraint. He suffered several fractures and claimed compensation. The judge, in deciding how to determine the standard that should have been followed, said:

> *When you get a situation that involved the use of some special skill or competence, then the test as to whether there has been negligence or not is the standard of the ordinary skilled man exercising and professing to have that special skill. A man need not possess the highest expert skill; it is well established that it is sufficient if he exercises the ordinary skill of an ordinary competent man exercising that particular art.*
>
> *He is not guilty of negligence if he has acted in accordance with a practice accepted as proper by a responsible body of medical men skilled in that particular art (in Dimond 1994:115).*

Although the case concerned a doctor, the Bolam Test can be used to examine the actions of any professional person. Thus the negligence of a professional (e.g. a nurse) is to be determined by the standard of the ordinary skilled nurse exercising and professing to have the skills of a nurse. The case of Wilsher v Essex AHA (1986, in Dimond 2011:66, 419) sets the standard of reasonable care to be expected of students and junior staff. The case involved a premature baby in the special care baby unit who required oxygen therapy. The junior doctor inadvertently inserted the catheter to monitor blood levels of oxygen into a vein rather than an artery. He had asked the senior registrar to check the position of the catheter following the procedure. The registrar failed to see the mistake.

This resulted in incorrect oxygen levels being monitored with the consequent administration of too much oxygen. The outcome was that the baby developed near blindness due to incurable damage to the retina. The Bolam Test was applied. The court ruled that the standard of care required was that of the ordinary skilled person, but that standard was to be determined in the context of the particular posts in the unit rather than according to the general rank or status of the post holder. The duty ought to be tailored to the act performed rather than to the doctor himself. Therefore, inexperience is no defence to an action for negligence. The judges held that the junior doctor had not been negligent and had upheld the relevant standard of care by consulting his superior. As students have to practise under supervision (direct or indirect) at all times, they can be held liable for what they chose to do or failed to do under their own volition, and will be judged according to the standards expected of a student.

Good health and good character The requirement for *good health and good character* to enter the professional Registers and renewing registration are laid down in legislation. The Nursing and Midwifery Order (the Order, NMC 2001) and the Health Professions Order 2001 state that these regulatory bodies must prescribe the requirements to be met as to the evidence of good health and good character to satisfy the NMC and HCPC Registrars that an applicant is capable of safe and effective practice without supervision: that is, the registrant is fit to practise. The requirement for evidence of good health and good character was introduced into the Order to enhance protection of the public, following a number of high-profile cases involving the health and character of doctors and nurses; see, for example, the cases that involved the nurse Beverly Allitt (Clothier 1994), and the doctor Harold Shipman (Baker 2001).

For the purposes of the NMC's and HCPC's legislation, the term 'good health' is a relative concept. The NMC (2010e:8) defines good health as the capability of 'safe and effective practice without supervision. It does not mean the absence of any disability or health condition. Many disabled people and those with health conditions are able to practise with or without adjustments to support their practice'. A registrant may have a disability, such as impaired hearing, or a health condition, such as depression, epilepsy, diabetes or heart disease, and yet be perfectly capable of safe and effective practice. However, there are some conditions that would be likely to affect a practitioner's ability to practise safely and effectively. These include alcoholism or other substance abuse. The type of issues raised in cases considered by Health Committee panels of the NMC in 2010-2011 (NMC 2011a) includes substance abuse (27%) and mental or physical health (39%). In 2009-2010, Health

Committee panels of the HCPC considered 256 allegations of registrants' fitness to practise was impaired by reason of their physical and/or mental health (HCPC 2010b). The panels made the decision that 70% of these cases were founded.

Good character is central to the Standards of conduct, performance and ethics in that practitioners must be honest and trustworthy. The NMC (2010e:8) states that 'good character is based on an individual's conduct, behaviour and attitude. It also takes into account any convictions, cautions and pending charges that are likely to be incompatible with professional registration. A person's character must be sufficiently good for them to be capable of safe and effective practice without supervision'. Both the NMC and HCPC state that an important determinant of good character is the individual's commitment to compliance with the Standards of conduct, performance and ethics (HCPC 2011b, NMC 2011b, NMC 2010d). Examples of the nature of the allegations made in cases considered by panels of the Conduct and Competence Committee during 2010-2011 (NMC 2011a) include dishonesty (e.g. theft or obtaining goods by deception), inappropriate conduct with patients (e.g. verbal/physical/sexual abuse of a patient or inappropriate relationships with patient), convictions and theft of drugs. In 2010, the HCPC considered similar cases where there were allegations of attending work under the influence of alcohol, engaging in sexual relations with a service user, fraudulent claims for paid sick leave and self-administration of medication (HCPC 2011c).

Prior to being admitted to a pre-registration health programme, good health will normally be checked and assessed by a local occupational health department. This includes the completion of a health questionnaire. Additionally, students are required to declare their good health annually during the programme. Good character will normally be assessed by taking up character references from reliable referees. Programme providers are also required by the NMC and HCPC to carry out an enhanced criminal conviction check through the Criminal Records Bureau or Disclosure Scotland or Access Northern Ireland and request confirmation that the person is not barred from working with children or vulnerable adults.

Students are required to maintain good health and good character throughout the educational programme. Students must inform the programme provider immediately if they have any charges, convictions or cautions during the programme.

Programme providers are required by the NMC and HCPC to set up processes to monitor good health and good character throughout the programme to deal with any new issues that arise. A local 'fitness to practise' process and panel must be in place to consider any health or character issues to ensure that public protection is maintained. Concerns include those relating to a student's health, behaviour or attitude which may affect the student's fitness to practise in the relevant profession. These concerns may be brought to the attention of the university by any person or organization. Generally, within assessment structures and processes, practice educators contribute evidence to enable the higher education institution to judge whether the student is suitable to remain on the educational programme and, ultimately, to enter the NMC and HCPC professional registers. If you suspect, or are aware, that a student's good health and/or good character may be in question, you must inform the university. This is normally done via the university lecturer who liaises with your clinical area.

A student must be of 'good health' and 'good character' before being admitted to the NMC and HCPC professional registers (NMC 2010b, HCPC 2009b). Students are required to make a self-declaration of good health and good character to their regulatory body when applying for registration. In the case of nurses and midwives, good health and good character must be confirmed by the designated registered nurse or midwife at the university (see Appendix 1). For nurses, this is the NMC registrant responsible for directing the pre-registration nursing programme. For midwifery programmes, this should be the lead midwife for education. This confirmation of good health and good character does not happen as a matter of course – there are occasions where directors of educational programmes do not support the declaration because of gross misconduct or criminal convictions during the training (Castledine 2000). In the case of students applying for registration with the HCPC, confirmation of good health and good character by the university is not required. Instead, a character reference and a health reference from referees outside the university are accepted by the HCPC. In the case of nurses on the Overseas Nurses Programme, the designated NMC registrant responsible for directing the programme confirms competence, good health and good character to the NMC. In the case of midwives on the Overseas Midwives Programme, the lead midwife for education in the relevant approved educational institution or her designated registered midwife substitute confirms competence, good health and good character to the NMC.

Professional and legal responsibility and accountability to the student Professional accountability to the student requires the practitioner to respect and uphold student rights and the higher education institution's regulations as discussed above. It also requires the practitioner to be aware of those aspects of accountability when supervising and assessing students. These have been discussed in the section Responsibility and accountability FOR WHAT?

The practitioner has a legal duty of care not only for patients/clients but also for others under her/his care, such as students (HCPC 2008, NMC 2008b,c). In law, the courts could find a registered practitioner negligent if a person suffers harm because she or he failed to care for that person properly. Lord Atkin (House of Lords 1932) defined the duty of care when he gave judgement in the case of Donoghue v Stephenson:

You must take reasonable care to avoid acts or omissions that you can reasonably foresee would be likely to injure your neighbour. Who, then, in the law is my neighbour? The answer seems to be persons who are so closely and directly affected by my act that I ought to have them in contemplations as being so affected when I am directing my mind to the acts or omissions that are called in question.

This means that a practitioner has a duty in relation to colleagues to ensure that they are reasonably safe from her/his actions (Dimond 1994). This important duty to safeguard the health and safety of other persons who may be affected by the practitioner's acts or omissions also comes under Health and Safety at Work regulations (Young 1994). For example, if work is delegated, a failure to supervise can lead to the practitioner who delegates being sued for negligence by the less experienced person if she/he (rather than the patient) suffers harm (Young 1994:58). In addition, under the Health and Safety at Work Act 1974, a practitioner could be prosecuted for any such acts or omissions. Giving students verbal instructions only about safety is not enough, as the level and amount of care and supervision required are generally commensurate with the level and amount of danger of a situation (Goudreau & Chasens 2002).

Under health and safety at work regulations, the employer has a statutory duty to keep employees informed, as well as provide training, on topics that are likely to affect health and safety (Young 1994). Examples of training are the provision of information on particular diseases that have health implications to the practitioner, such as HIV infection and AIDS, and treatments that carry risks to those administering them, such as the toxic effects of certain drugs. Practitioners working in some areas will often face particular risks. For example, the community nurse will need specialist training to enable her/him to move and handle clients safely in their homes and the nurse in the psychiatric or learning disability areas may need a greater input on preventing and dealing with aggression and violence. Careful record keeping of any training is important under the Health and Safety at Work Act for the protection of both the employer and employee.

Training needs to be given to both qualified and unqualified personnel. This means that students must also receive such training. The higher education institution must ensure that a student receives sufficient training on health and safety prior to the start of clinical placement. This is to protect the student as well as patients and others. Areas of particular concern are moving and handling, the handling of aggression and violence, firefighting regulations and safety, and the control of infection. Subsequently, when the student starts the clinical placement, it is the joint responsibility of the practice educator and the student to ensure that the following training takes place on the student's first working day:

- the student understands her/his responsibilities in the event of a fire, cardiac arrest and any other emergency
- the student has been shown the layout of the clinical area, including fire exits and fire and resuscitation equipment
- the student knows her/his responsibilities regarding health and safety at work
- the student has been instructed in moving and handling patients/clients in the clinical area
- the student knows his/her responsibilities in respect of data protection and confidentiality.

The training should be documented in the student's records. This is to protect the student, the service provider and the higher education institution in case of any later legal action for negligence.

Students with special needs

Anti-discrimination law In the United Kingdom, the Equality Act 2010 became law in October 2010. It consolidates and replaces the numerous arrays of Acts and Regulations that formed the basis of anti-discrimination law. These were, primarily, the Equal Pay Act 1970, the Sex Discrimination Act 1975, the Race Relations Act 1976, the Disability Discrimination Act 1995, much of the Equality Act 2006, the Employment Equality (Religion or Belief) Regulations 2003, the Employment Equality (Sexual Orientation) Regulations 2003, the Employment Equality (Age) Regulations 2006, and the Equality Act (Sexual Orientation) Regulations 2007 (all as subsequently amended), plus other ancillary pieces of legislation. The Act bans unfair treatment of people because of protected characteristics (Office for Disability Issues 2010). This means that the legislation protects people with a wide range of disabilities and health conditions from unlawful discrimination. In order to avoid discrimination and to provide equal opportunities at work, employers and service providers (which includes education providers) are under a duty to make reasonable changes for disabled applicants and employees. This is known as *'reasonable adjustments'*. Reasonable adjustments to their workplaces to overcome barriers experienced by disabled people must be made. Reasonable adjustments apply to any 'provision, criterion or practice' and 'any physical feature of premises'. If any of these things place a disabled person 'at a substantial disadvantage' then the employer has to take any steps that are 'reasonable in all the circumstances' to prevent that disadvantage occurring (Equality Act 2010). The duty to make adjustments is ongoing and, subject to their effectiveness in overcoming the disadvantage, will need to be reviewed and further adjustments made. However, reasonable adjustments need to be made only if the employer is aware, or should reasonably be aware, that a worker has a disability (Equality and Human Rights Commission 2011).

The NMC (2011d) and the HCPC (2006) do not have 'blanket bans' on particular impairments or health conditions. When there is a declaration of disability or health condition, impairment of fitness to practise is considered on an individual basis as individuals may be affected differently. Rowntree (1987:60) says that to 'treat people equally is not necessarily to treat them fairly. Indeed, people being so different, equal treatment probably means injustice for most'. Rowntree's words call for the necessity for reasonable adjustment so that the same treatment is not just meted out to all. There is thus a better chance of providing equal opportunities for all students to be able to learn effectively during clinical placements. As stated above, in order to make reasonable adjustments for students, it is students' responsibility to declare the disability and the extent to which it may affect their learning, and delivery of patient care, in the clinical placement. Disclosure should be without fear of being discriminated against.

The experts in how support may best be given are the students; listen to what they have to say and develop a rapport that will be beneficial to them, the team and patient/client care. Students with particular health problems (e.g. diabetes) should be allocated the appropriate meal breaks to enable them to deal with dietary and medical needs. A student with a hearing impairment may want to sit in a certain place to make best use of hearing aids (e.g. during handovers).

Dyslexia Dyslexia is not uncommon. It can affect 5-10% of a given population. It can be inherited, and recent studies have identified a number of genes that may predispose an individual to developing dyslexia (National Institute of Neurological Disorders and Stroke, NINDS 2011). Dyslexia is perceived to be a learning disability that impairs a person's fluency or accuracy in comprehension with reading, writing or spelling (Beingdyslexic 2011). It can occur at any level of intellectual ability. Individuals with dyslexia suffer from a weakness in the processing of language-based information, which affects their ability to learn. It is now widely accepted that it can also affect a number of areas of cognitive functioning including short-term memory, mathematical calculations, personal organization and concentration span. Most dyslexic individuals have been identified as having one or more of the following deficiencies in the sub-skills that are required to acquire and use adequate literacy skills:

- A marked inefficiency in the working of the short-term memory system – this means that a dyslexic person may have problems with the amount of information that can be held and processed in the real-time, conscious memory.
- Inadequate phonological (pattern of speech sounds) processing abilities, causing problems with connecting the letter patterns with the associated sounds – this is usually due to problems with the speed in which auditory information can be processed and with accessing the memory of audio sounds to relate them to the letter pattern. This gives rise to spelling inaccuracies.
- Difficulties with automaticity – this can cause problems with sequencing, organizing and prioritizing activities.
- A range of problems connected with visual processing to do with the speed in which visual information can be processed and with accessing the memory of visual patterns.

Some individuals with dyslexia also have a specific learning difference (SpLD) as a co-morbidity. SpLD refers to a difficulty that affects a particular process. Amongst SpLD are dyspraxia and dyscalculia. *Dyspraxia* is an impairment or immaturity of the organization of movement causing individuals to appear clumsy as the brain sends the wrong signals to parts of the body in the wrong order. *Dyscalculia* is innate difficulty in learning or comprehending simple mathematics. This gives rise to difficulties in understanding numbers, learning how to manipulate numbers and learning mathematical facts.

The effects of dyslexia can largely be overcome by skilled teaching and support, and the use of compensatory strategies (Dyslexia Action 2011). There are students who will not disclose their disability for fear of unfair treatment in the workplace, ridicule or discrimination (White 2007, Illingworth 2005). Students who have dyslexia should be accorded due regard for their condition and provided with any extra support and time they may require in order to learn (Wright 2000). Due to the complexity of the nature of a learning disability, it can be difficult to determine the amount and type of support required. Not all dyslexic students are the same. Each individual may present a different combination of difficulties: support will need to be tailored to meet the individual's learning needs. The label of the disability is less important than the need to recognize the specific areas of difficulty a student is faced with. Therefore, whether the individual is diagnosed with 'dyslexia', 'dyspraxia' or 'dyscalculia' is immaterial. All of these are classed as a disability under disability legislation and individuals with any of these conditions will require understanding and support to help them to reach their potential. The Disability Act 2010 requires reasonable adjustments to be made (RCN 2010a).

The range of difficulties encountered by students is wide ranging. It will be useful for the practice educator to have a working knowledge of what these could be and some strategies to use (see Table 2.1). From the list

Table 2.1 Difficulties encountered by students

Typical problems	Strategies to help students
Literacy skills – for example, reading and writing reports. Reading and writing speeds are slower; errors in charting and writing patient/client records; late completion of care plans; deadlines missed; difficulty reading other people's handwriting; difficulty with identifying relevant information from case notes	• Make a nursing and ordinary dictionary available in the clinical area or encourage the student to carry them; a spell check dictionary is invaluable • Provide more time and a quiet environment free from distractions when doing written tasks or other activities that require concentration • Encourage students to write drafts of reports to be checked by the practice educator • Encourage students to take blank forms home and practise writing reports; check the examples • Show examples of well written reports; initially, work alongside the student to indicate what needs to be written, withdrawing direct supervision as appropriate • Assist the student in compiling a list of frequently used phrases which can be used when writing reports; devise a checklist of key areas to include in certain types of documentation
Dealing with information – difficulty with multi-tasking for example, when receiving handover report there may be inability to write down key details fast enough; handovers may be incomplete and muddled; difficulty remembering telephone conversations; difficulty with identifying relevant information from case notes	• Provide a list of common terminology used in your clinical area • Go over the key points of the patients/clients allocated to the student following the handover; assist the student to develop an action plan/work schedule • Help the student develop 'shorthand' when taking notes, for example, # for fractures, Rx for treatment • Encourage the student to write out the handover prior to giving it – this will require checking initially but once the student has demonstrated the ability to capture the salient points on paper, stop checking to allow the development of confidence; the student may wish to repeat the information back to the caller • When the student answers the telephone remind and empower the student to ask the caller to speak slowly and repeat information; encourage the student to make notes whilst talking on the telephone • Encourage the student to use a customized handover sheet developed personally or one that is already in use • Provide opportunities to discuss case notes with the student
Administering drugs – reading, spelling or pronouncing drug names; reading doctors' handwriting on prescription charts; students with dyscalculia has greater difficulty doing drug calculations	• Provide a list of commonly used drugs for your area • Encourage the student to write out the names of drugs and check the spelling; assist with the development of a personal crib sheet to help identify and learn drugs • Help with pronunciation of drug names • Encourage the student to practise saying drug names and listen to their vocalizations • Assist the student in using the formulas for doing drug calculations. Working out the drug dose methodically on paper followed by using a calculator (if its use is allowed by the Trust), or vice versa, will reinforce learning • Explain drug administration protocol and encourage the student to study this in her/his own time
Memory – difficulty remembering information or instruction, for example, passing on inaccurate/incomplete information to another team member following doctors' rounds and at handovers; giving incomplete information to patients/clients; forgetting to do things	• Provide an orientation pack with outlines of useful information and routines • Encourage the student to make notes • Support and empower the student in seeking clarification • Help the student in devising and using mnemonics
Sequencing ability – for example, when undertaking a complex activity or procedure involving many steps, the activity or procedure is carried out in the wrong sequence	• Prior to carrying out the procedure, provide written instructions of procedures for the student to study in her/his own time; create flow charts if appropriate and feasible • Explain and demonstrate the procedure at a pace that is comfortable to the student as anxiety will be increased if the student feels rushed • Provide the opportunity to practise as close as possible to the demonstration • Provide opportunities for repeated practice until the student has mastered the activity

(Continued)

Table 2.1 Difficulties encountered by students (Continued)

Typical problems	Strategies to help students
Visual orientation – confusing left and right or up and down, for example, identifying the right limb for the left limb	• Provide an orientation pack • Do a detailed orientation to the clinical area and point out salient landmarks; back up with a map or a sketch with main landmarks • Encourage the student to take the same route • Encourage the student to develop strategies for helping to remember the side of the body being treated, for example, wriggling her left limb when having to label a patient's left limb
Hand/eye co-ordination – may result in poor presentation of written work, for example, untidy and difficult to read handwritten patient/client records; difficulty in undertaking some clinical skills	• Check drafts of written reports and indicate where improvements can be made to aid tidiness and clarity • Provide opportunities to practise activities so that there is repetition • Provide alternative equipment if this constitutes reasonable adjustment
Speech – may talk in a disorganized way especially when the speech has to be spontaneous, for example, at meetings and on the telephone	• Work with the student to write down what needs to be said at handovers; rehearse handover reports
Organizational skills – poor time management and surrounding working environment can be untidy and disorganized	• Plan work to enable the student to work with small numbers of patients • Provide clear protocols for care; create flow charts if appropriate and feasible • Keep to a structured routine where possible • Encourage and assist the student to write out a work schedule – ask the student what the key activities are in the schedule; set achievable tasks for a shorter duration initially, for example, a few hours, gradually increasing to a whole morning and then a whole shift • After the shift, spend time with the student to reflect on how the student had managed her time and workload
Emotional factors – a range of emotions may be displayed such as anxiety, anger, acute embarrassment. Individuals may have a lowered self-esteem due to past difficulties with learning and failure; students may fear mispronouncing words; anxiety about negative staff attitude towards the disability	• Maintain a friendly and relaxed atmosphere; be helpful and supportive without smothering • Be approachable so that the student is not afraid to ask questions; give regular constructive feedback • Debrief regularly for example, at the end of each shift or after a complex care giving episode • Encourage other staff members to include the student as a member of the team • Introduce the student to the team

of what typical problems relate to during clinical placements (RCN 2010b, White 2007), some suggested strategies that the practice educator and students may wish to use to help make the placement experience a positive one are put forward. These have drawn upon and been adapted from publications of the RCN and the work of White (2007). These strategies are not exhaustive. Frequently, students will be aware of and have developed self-help strategies.

The reader is directed to the publication by the RCN (2010b), which provides a more comprehensive discussion of the strategies and 'tips' to help individuals with a learning disability during clinical practice.

The underpinning philosophy of support is to promote independence (RCN 2010a). Remember that you will not be there for the student after the completion of the clinical placement. The student should be encouraged and supported to participate actively and take the responsibility for learning to develop independence. However, the input from the practice educator is crucial to assist the student to learn to achieve placement learning outcomes and to enable the student to reach her/his potential (White 2007).

The following framework has been suggested by Reid & Kirk (2001) to facilitate professional development. Students can be assisted to set, monitor and evaluate their goals of learning. The following questions may be helpful:

Questions to help to become self-directing include:

- What is my goal?
- What do I want to accomplish?
- What do I need?
- What is my deadline?

Questions to assist with monitoring progress include:

- How am I doing?
- Do I need other resources?
- What else can I do?

Questions for self-evaluation include:

- Did I accomplish my goal?
- Was I efficient?
- What worked?
- What did not work?
- Why did it not work?

Moral responsibility and accountability to the student Moral responsibility and accountability are of special importance as they pervade the practice educator–student relationship. Cox (1982) makes the point that, unless students are adequately supervised and supported during clinical placements, they are getting short-changed in educational terms. What actions can practice educators take so that they do not fall short of fulfilling moral responsibilities and accountability owed to the student?

During the early days of working in a clinical area, the student is a 'guest' in that area. Special efforts should be made to make students feel welcome initially and to help them settle into the area as quickly as possible. A common anxiety of students starting new placements is to feel unwelcome and unwanted (Levett-Jones et al 2009, Phillips et al 2000). If students feel safe and that they belong, they will begin to relax and be in a better position to start learning (Maslow 1954). In the hierarchy of human needs, Maslow (1954) postulates that the basic needs must be met first in order for the higher needs to be achieved. Many students lack confidence in their ability to learn and need to be empowered to believe in their ability to succeed (Johnson & Halstead 2005).

The clinical area is anxiety-provoking for students (Johnson & Halstead 2005, Parkes 1985). The practice educator can help reduce levels of anxiety and stress for students by being aware of situations that may be stressful to students. Action can then be taken to assist students to cope with these stressors. The quality of student-practice educator interactions has the potential to have either positive or negative effects on the outcomes of the educational process by affecting student performance in the clinical setting (see, for example, Levett-Jones et al 2009, Saarikoski & Leino-Kilpi 2002, Spouse 1996,

Earnshaw 1995, Darling 1984). The practice educator has the responsibility to befriend the student so that a positive relationship can start to be fostered. Other qualities of the practice educator that a student seeks, and which directly affect learning and performance and hence the outcomes of assessment, are discussed at length by authors such as Spouse (2003) and Neary (2000). The practice educator owes it to the student to know what these are so that the student may be assisted in the most effective ways to achieve learning outcomes. This point is developed further in Chapter 8.

As we have seen in Chapter 1, the power for making assessment decisions is firmly in the hands of the practice educator as assessor. The NMC (2008a) states that the practice educator is accountable for summative assessment decisions. To be accountable one is vested with authority (see earlier discussion). The law also emphasizes the authority of the roles of the teacher and assessor (Young 1992). A student has the right to appeal only against the conduct of the assessment, but not the verdict. Within this assessment practice, several assumptions are made about the assessor (Harding & Greig 1994):

- The assessor is aware of personal limitations and can always be objective in assessment. The discussion in Chapter 5 will show that our assessments can be greatly influenced by personal biases and prejudices. This makes many assessment decisions far from the objectivity we like to espouse.
- There is a universally agreed standard of practice by which to judge a student's practice. However, standards of clinical practice vary among practitioners. Some students, therefore, may be subject to assessments that have been made based on standards of practice falling at either end of the continuum of high to low standards. In either case, the student is treated unfairly.
- Assessors possess the necessary knowledge, skills and attitudes for the supervision and assessment of learners who may be undertaking a course of training different from their own. However, many research studies have found that assessors frequently do not understand the learning needs of students they are assessing (White 2007, Duffy 2004, Fraser et al 1997, May et al 1997, Eraut et al 1995, White et al 1994, Bedford et al 1993,).
- Students receive sufficient quality teaching and supervision from their practice educators to enable them to achieve learning outcomes so that they pass their assessments. Again, findings from the above studies indicate that this is not the case. The student is generally in competition against the patient/client for the practitioner's time and the student loses out. Practice educators may also not be the best role models (Fowler 2008). The *Standards of conduct, performance and ethics* (HCPC 2008, NMC 2008b)

make it clear that the duty of care to the patient/client must always take precedence over all else.

By virtue of the authority and assumptions vested in assessors, students are owed a high level of moral responsibility and accountability. In the eyes of the law, 'educators have a duty to their students that is greater than they would have to the general public because of the teacher–student relationship' (Goudreau & Chasens 2002:43). Lello (1979:6) makes the point that 'if people are working closely together they have a continuing and permanent answerability to each other'. Who, then, is on trial, asks Rowntree (1987:9): the assessor or the student? Ponder this question posed by Rowntree in Activity 2.4.

ACTIVITY 2.4

If a student fails a placement, has the placement, and by inference the practice educator, failed in their duties towards the student, or has the student failed the placement?

Even if a student has been openly disinterested and has made no effort to learn, Rowntree cautions against placing the entire responsibility for the failure upon the student. There may be no straightforward answers to the question. It is up to the practice educator as assessor to confront the situation after considering the moral responsibility and accountability owed to the student. Issues surrounding professional moral responsibility and accountability are less tangible; it is perhaps easier for the student to obtain redress if she/he is unfairly treated as there is likely to be overt evidence of this. Moral responsibility and accountability, however, rest very much with the individual's moral code. It may not be possible for the student to obtain any form of redress if unfairness is the result of failure to exercise an appropriate level of moral responsibility and accountability towards the student.

The trust/employing authority and the higher education institution

Higher education institutions enter into contracts with their students to provide such educational experiences as are required to fulfil the aims of the programme. In the case of pre-registration health care students, where clinical experience is a requisite component of pre-registration programmes, higher education institutions in the UK require to enter into contracts with service providers such as National Health Service (HNS) Trusts and private organizations such as nursing homes to provide the clinical experiences. Such contracts are typically written and specify the management of the educational process for students during clinical practice. The specifications of the service agreement between the University of Sheffield and a National Health Service Trust (University of Sheffield 2001; reproduced with permission) is provided in detail here as an example. The agreement specifies that the Trust will provide the following:

- A high standard of teaching, learning and assessment.
- A designated supervisor who is responsible for supervising, teaching and assessing student performance.
- The supervisor is also responsible for assigning the relevant duties to the student, so that the student is given opportunities to work with a range of patients/clients.
- A liaison officer for the placement area who will liaise directly with the designated University link lecturer.
- Advising students of all local internal protocols, policies and reporting procedures relevant to the area of work.
- Ensuring that the University is notified of any accident or illness sustained by a student on placement within a timescale appropriate to the seriousness of the situation.
- Advising or instructing students to leave clinical areas if, in the Trust's view, the student is at risk or the student's health status is putting colleagues or patients at risk.
- Informing students of the specific approaches and practices for moving and handling people.
- Liability for students during the period of their placement, extending to matters of employers/occupiers liability and public liability and in respect of acts or omissions of its own employees.
- When undertaking specific procedures, the student will be provided with all protective clothing or equipment necessary for the maintenance of health and safety.
- In the event where there are reasonable grounds to suspect that a student may have committed a criminal offence or an act of serious misconduct, the Trust may immediately suspend, without prejudice, the attachment of the student and remove the student from the work area. Any such suspension must be reported to the University within 24 working hours.
- Where a student is involved in any Trust disciplinary proceedings, the University will be informed.
- There is no discrimination against any student on grounds of race, creed, gender, sexual orientation or disability and the Trust will apply its equal opportunity policy to students as it does to its own employees.
- Should service developments and changes impact on the placement educational environment in respect of both quality and capacity, the Trust will inform the University in advance of any service changes.
- The Trust will allow access to placement areas for University staff for the purposes of educational audit.

The specifications of these agreements have been provided here in detail to inform practice educators of their direct lines of responsibility and accountability to the Trust, and indirectly to the higher education institution, when supervising and assessing students. The list of specifications may appear onerous. However, if the practice educator exercises the requisite duty of care owed to students as discussed above, and follows assessment regulations laid down by the higher education institution, there will then be no necessity for concern.

Yourself, colleagues and your profession

The NMC's and HCPC's responsibilities are set out in the Nurses and Midwives Order 2001 (NMC 2001) Health Professions Order 2001, respectively. The Councils' main responsibility is to protect the interests of the public. To do this, standards for education, training and professional conduct are set for its practitioners. The NMC (2008b), the HCPC (2008) and the law make it clear that standards of clinical practice must be upheld at all times. As a practice educator then, failure to uphold standards of clinical practice may compromise not only yourself professionally and legally but also your colleagues and the profession, as your personal standard of practice is frequently reflected in your assessment decisions. Stated simplistically, a lower standard of clinical practice may result in the practice educator expecting a lower, maybe even unsafe, standard of performance of their student. You would not have fulfilled moral and professional responsibilities and accountability towards your colleagues and the profession if these compromised standards were not recognized, resulting in a failure to correct such deficits or to remove the student from training. Such unsafe students are likely to become registered practitioners on the NMC's and HCPC's professional registers. As practitioners and practice educators, we need to uphold the role of the NMC and HCPC in protecting the public by maintaining a register of people who are recommended to be practitioners who are fit to practise, and who have demonstrated fitness to practise through a qualification registered with the NMC or the HCPC. Fowler & Heater (1983:404) stated very strongly that practice educators are:

> ... *bound by a moral responsibility to the profession of nursing to give passing grades to only those students who have demonstrated clinical competence.*

In accepting the role of practice educator, the practitioner implicitly accepts the professional (NMC 2008a), and moral responsibility and accountability for maintaining standards of supervision and assessment in order that the standards of professional colleagues and the profession are protected.

ISSUES AND DILEMMA OF THE MENTOR–ASSESSOR INTERFACE

Holloway (1985) found that moral accountability to students (see discussion above) emphasizes the importance of a 'special relationship' between teacher and student. This 'special relationship' is permeated by empathy, trust and affinity. Staff–student relationships are an important influence on students' experience of belonging and the achievement of positive clinical experiences (Levett-Jones et al 2009).

The special relationship that many students expect of their practice educators is more likely to develop if students have confidence in their practice educators (Gray & Smith 2000). At the same time, students look to their practice educators for constructive feedback, which requires some judgement to be made about their performance. These challenging student expectations mean that the practice educator has to be able to maintain a professional/friend balance (Fraser et al 1997) to meet the dichotomous demands of the role of a practice educator as mentor and assessor. Good mentoring practices (discussed in Chapters 8 and 9) on the part of the practitioner as practice educator are required for the development of this 'special relationship'. At the same time, the practice educator as practitioner has professional accountabilities to fulfil. Professional accountability stresses the importance of maintaining standards of professional practice to safeguard patient/client care. The practitioner working with a student is thus required to be an assessor - to judge the student's clinical competence. This demands good supervision and assessing practices to fulfil the role of assessor. The formal role of assessor is generally not as well acknowledged as the role of mentor. Is this because practice educators are avoiding their role of assessor? In a study that examined the mentoring and assessing practices of practice educators in nursing, midwifery and medicine, Bray & Nettleton (2007) found that practice educators identified assessment as having less of a priority than the more pastoral aspects of teaching and supporting students. Likewise, practitioners failed to identify that assessment is central to being a practice educator (Chow & Suen 2001, in Bray & Nettleton 2007).

Can both moral accountability to students and professional accountability be fulfilled without causing anguish to both parties? In developing a 'special relationship' the practitioner as mentor is a 'friend' to the student (Neary 1997, Darling 1984). Enacting the role of assessor requires the practitioner to be a 'judge' (Neary 1997). Is a friend capable of being an objective judge? Students in Neary's (1997) study saw the assessor as not forming any 'special relationship' with them but as having the formal tasks of assessing skills and progress, completing assessment booklets and keeping records. They thought that mentors took responsibility for students and provided guidance, gave support, assisted the student in setting learning outcomes and subsequently acted as facilitator for learning and created learning opportunities.

Whereas it is already accepted in many practice settings that the practice educator as mentor does act as an assessor and vice versa (HCPC 2009a, NMC 2008a, Andrews & Wallis 1999, Neary 1997), should a mentor and an assessor be the same person? The student nurses interviewed in Neary's study had opinions that ranged from being happy with the same practitioner as both mentor and assessor to the other extreme of preferring the mentor and assessor to be two different people. Many of the students did not wish to be assessed summatively by their mentor, especially if the relationship was not a comfortable or relaxed one. They referred to the necessity of a good relationship for the assessment to be fair. However, when the relationship developed into friendship, some students felt that the assessor could not remain unbiased. Brown (2000) found that students' personal qualities and attributes had considerable influence on the judgements made about student performance, suggesting that judgements may be have been made on the basis of the liking for the student. Students in White et al's (1994) study also thought that the nature of the relationship between assessor and student affected the assessment process – positively in the event of a good relationship or negatively in the event of a poor relationship. However, there were students in Neary's study who expected all practice educators to remain 'professional' and to be able to assess against agreed criteria without bias or prejudice. The practitioners in Neary's study were more definite in their view about being both mentor and assessor – many found it difficult to 'wear two hats' and experienced role conflict.

Recent guidelines from the NMC (2008a) state clearly that the practice educator (termed the 'mentor' by the NMC) has the responsibility to supervise students and facilitate their learning in practice, as well assess their performance to make judgements about fitness to practise and be accountable for such decisions. The practice educator is expected to be both mentor and assessor. Prior to these guidelines, mentors were not required to assess – rather, their roles and responsibilities related directly to guiding, assisting and supporting student learning (ENB 1988, 1997).

It is my contention that if assessment processes are to assist learning (see Ch. 6) the practitioner as practice educator who is both mentor and assessor is best placed to fulfil this function of assessment. Assessment of clinical practice is a complex activity and has always been fraught with difficulties – is it ever possible to remain 'professional' and at the same time be a friend, to be able to assess against agreed criteria without bias or prejudice? What does it take to be a competent practice educator who is able to maintain the correct professional–friend balance with a student? The model of a competent midwife in Fraser et al's study (1997) comprises three main closely interlinked dimensions. These dimensions may provide some helpful parallel processes for the practice educator to draw upon in attempts to achieve the appropriate professional–friend balance.

1. **Professional–friend approach**: the midwife's ability to be autonomous and professional but 'with woman'. The competent practice educator will be responsible and accountable for mentoring and assessing practices, making formative and summative assessment decisions (see Ch. 7). The competent practice educator is pragmatic, rigorous and maintains diplomacy. In being 'with student', the practice educator advocates for students and inspires them with confidence.

2. **Individualized approach**: the midwife's ability to provide individualized care. The competent practice educator works in partnership with students and exercises non-judgemental appreciation of the differences in the personal backgrounds of students.

3. **Clinical competence**: a sound knowledge base and appropriate skills for the provision of midwifery care. The competent practice educator will have the knowledge base and skills to be both mentor and assessor to students.

In the model above it can be seen that the competent midwife is one who is aware of the importance of the professional–friend balance. Likewise, the competent practice educator needs to achieve this professional–friend balance in the roles of being both a mentor and assessor. What is important is that mentoring and assessment processes assist learning while retaining a focus on procedures (Torrance & Pryor 1998). If learning is facilitated through our assessment processes then the products of assessment – in this case the students – are more likely to be positive.

CONCLUSION

Inherent in professional practice are professional responsibilities and accountability. The nursing and midwifery professions, along with other professional groups serving our society, are increasingly held accountable for the quality of service they provide. Is society receiving the care it needs, or is it receiving the care we think it needs or deserves (Reilly 1980)? This requires an assessment of our goals, our actions, resources and outcomes of care in light of society's needs. As mentors and assessors in whatever setting we practise, we too will be held more and more accountable for our actions. We must answer to the student, to society, to our profession, to our colleagues, to our employer, to the higher education institution offering the programme, and to ourselves.

Students are the direct consumers and beneficiaries of our educational programmes. Are they getting the kind of learning that is needed or are they getting short-changed in educational terms? Before we claim that the student is indeed the beneficiary, we should try to answer the following question posed by Reilly (1980:3): 'How well do we meet our contract with the learner?'

Assessment of clinical practice is a significant responsibility and can be both challenging and time consuming. It also carries professional, contractual and moral accountability. Lello (1979) acknowledges the burden of being answerable and responsible. The strain results from the amount of responsibility shouldered rather than from the amount of work done. To achieve the purposes of clinical assessment, we need to recognize and accept the responsibilities and accountability of an assessor. Reilly (1980:3) challenges us most succinctly by posing the following questions:

We are the gatekeepers of our profession, with the power to determine who enters the profession and to define the nature of nursing [and midwifery] practice. How well are we using the power bestowed upon us?

How well do we meet the test of accountability to ourselves? Are we authentic individuals? Have we formalized for ourselves values and beliefs that guide our actions? Are we true to those values, and are we real and genuine human beings?

Reilly raised these questions to remind nursing educators in higher education institutions and practice educators involved with the evaluation of nursing and midwifery programmes that, to achieve quality in any plan for accountability, they must incorporate the concept of responsibility. Our role as assessors carries the ultimate responsibility: that of ensuring that only practitioners who are competent are allowed to register with the statutory professional body so that the public is safeguarded against unsafe and incompetent practice.

KEY POINTS FOR REFLECTION

Health care practitioners are responsible and accountable for the quality of service they provide. Within their additional role as assessors of health care students, practitioners are also responsible and accountable for the quality of the supervision and assessment of students through the exercise of educational processes. They also have a 'gatekeeping' role in the determination of who enters the profession through assessment decisions made.

In relationship to responsibility and accountability for the assessment of clinical practice, two key questions are posed:

- What are practice educators responsible and accountable for?
- Who are practice educators responsible and accountable to?

What are practice educators responsible and accountable for?

It is suggested here that the practice educator can be answerable for the following aspect of personal professional practice with its inevitable impact on learning, and the following aspects of supervision and assessment:

- Personal standards of practice – as these frequently form the basis of 'how' and 'what' are assessed.
- Standards of care delivery by learners – through supervision of learners' practice and appropriate delegation of tasks. Students are never professionally accountable and practice educators are professionally responsible for the consequences of students' actions and omissions.

- What is taught, learned and assessed – by having a full understanding of relevant aspects of the curriculumm so that learners can be assisted to achieve the programme learning outcomes.
- Standards of teaching and assessing – as learners are entitled to the best instruction available. Failure to instruct properly could be construed as a negligent act.
- Professional judgements about student performance – and accountability for the summative assessment decision; practice educators have a moral responsibility to fail incompetent students.

Who are practice educators responsible and accountable to?

Practice educators are answerable to the following individuals and organizations:

- The patient/client for both a legal and professional duty of care whose rights as a patient/client supersede at all times the student's rights to knowledge and experience.
- Students through upholding their rights as learners for the teaching, supervision and support to facilitate their learning. Assessors also have a duty of care to students.
- The Trust/employing authority and the higher education institution for upholding the conditions of the contract between these organizations to support the clinical learning of students.
- Yourself, colleagues and your profession by upholding the standards for education, training and professional conduct laid down by the statutory professional body.

REFERENCES

Allan, H.T., Smith, P., O'Driscoll, M., 2011. Experiences of supernumerary status and the hidden curriculum in nursing: a new twist in the theory–practice gap? J. Clin. Nurs. 20, 847–855.

Allen, J., Dennis, M., 2010. Leadership and accountability. Nurs. Manag. 17 (7), 28–29.

Andrews, M., Wallis, M., 1999. Mentorship in nursing: a review of the literature. J. Adv. Nurs. 29 (1), 201–207.

Armstrong, N., 2010. Clinical mentors' influence on student midwives' clinical practice. Br. J. Midwifery 16 (2), 114–123.

Ashworth, P., Morrison, P., 1991. Problems of competence-based nurse education. Nurse. Educ. Today 11, 256–260.

Baker, R., 2001. Harold Shipman's Clinical Practice 1974-1998: A Review Commissioned by the Chief Medical Officer. Stationery Office, London, Online. Available: <http://www.dh.gov.uk/assetRoot/04/06/50/46/04065046.pdf> (accessed December 2005).

Bandura, A., 1977. Social Learning Theory. Prentice Hall, Englewood Cliffs, NJ.

Baskett, M., Marsick, V., 1992. Professional Ways of Knowing. Jossey-Bass, San Francisco.

Beaumont, S., 2004. Stop incompetent nurses. Br. J. Nurs. 13 (11), 663.

Becher, T., Eraut, M., Knight, J., 1981. Policies for Educational Accountability. Heinemann Educational Books, London.

Bedford, H., Phillips, T., Robinson, J, et al., 1993. Assessment of Competencies in Nursing and Midwifery Education and Training. The English National Board for Nursing, Midwifery and Health Visiting, London.

Beingdyslexic 2011. What is dyslexia? Online. Available: at <http://www.beingdyslexic.co.uk/> (accessed August 2011).

Bergman, R., 1981. Accountability – definition and dimensions. Int. Nurs. Rev. 28 (2), 53–59.

Bray, L., Nettleton, P., 2007. Assessor or mentor? role confusion in professional education. Nurse. Educ. Today 27, 848–855.

Brown, N., 2000. What are the criteria that mentors use to make judgements on the clinical performance of student mental health nurses? An exploratory study of the formal written communication at the end of clinical nursing practice modules. J. Psychiatr. Ment. Health. Nurs. 7 (5), 407–416.

Brykczynska, G., 1995. Working with children: accountability, paediatric nursing. In: Watson, R. (Ed.), Accountability in Nursing Practice. Chapman & Hall, London, pp. 147–160.

Castledine, G., 2000. Professional misconduct case studies: nursing students' accountability. Br. J. Nurs. 9 (15), 965.

Castledine, G., 1991. Accountability in delivering care. Nurs. Stand. 5 (25), 28–31.

Champion, R., 1991. Educational accountability – what ho the 1990s! Nurse. Educ. Today 11, 407–414.

Charters, A., 2000. Encouraging student centred learning in a clinical environment. Emerg. Nurse. 7 (10), 25–29.

Clothier, C, 1994. The Allitt Inquiry: Independent Inquiry Relating to Deaths and Injuries on the Children's Ward at Grantham and Kesteven General Hospital During the Period February to April 1991. Stationery Office, London.

Cornock, M., 2011. Legal definitions of responsibility, accountability and liability. Nurs. Child. Young People 23 (3), 25–26.

Cox, C., 1982. The seeds of time. Nurse. Educ. Today 2 (6), 4–10.

DDA 1995. Disability Discrimination Act. Online. Available: <http://www.legislation.hmso.gov.uk/acts/acts1995/1995050.htm> (accessed December 2005).

Darling, L.A.W., 1984. What do nurses want in a mentor? J. Nurs. Admin., 42–44.

Davies, E., 1993. Clinical role modeling: uncovering hidden knowledge. J. Adv. Nurs. 18 (4), 627–636.

Department of Health, 1999. Making a Difference. Department of Health, London.

Department of Health, 1995. The Patient's Charter. Department of Health, London.

Dimond, B., 2011. Legal Aspects of Nursing, sixth ed. Pearson Education, Harlow, Essex.

Dimond, B., 1994. The Legal Aspects of Midwifery. Books for Midwives Press, Cheshire.

Dolan, G., 2003. Assessing student nurse clinical competency: will we ever get it right? J. Clin. Nurs. 12, 132–141.

Duffy, K., 2004. Failing Students Report. Nursing and Midwifery Council, London, Online. Available: <http://www.nmc-uk.org/nmc/main/publications/mentor_study.pdf> (accessed December 2005).

Dyslexia Action, 2011. What is dyslexia? Online. Available: <http://www.dyslexiaaction.org.uk/> accessed August 2011).

Earnshaw, G.J., 1995. Mentorship: the students' views. Nurse. Educ. Today 15, 274–279.

Emerton, A., 1992. Professionalism and the UKCC. Br. J. Nurs. 1 (1), 25–29.

ENB, 1997. Standards for Approval of Higher Education Institutions and Programmes. The English National Board for Nursing, Midwifery and Health Visiting, London.

ENB, 1988. Institutional and Course Approval/Reapproval Process: Information Required, Criteria and Guidelines. Circular 1988/39/APS. The English National Board for Nursing, Midwifery and Health Visiting, London.

Eraut, M., Alderton, J., Boylan, A., et al., 1995. An Evaluation of the Contribution of the Biological and Social Sciences to Pre-registration Nursing and Midwifery Programmes. The English National Board for Nursing, Midwifery and Health Visiting, London.

Equality Act 2010. Online. Available: <http://www.legislation.gov.uk/ukpga/2010/15/pdfs/ukpga_20100015_en.pdf> (accessed August 2011).

Equality and Human Rights Commission, 2011. The Duty to Make Reasonable Adjustments for Disabled People. Online. Available: <http://www.equalityhumanrights.

com/advice-and-guidance/new-equality-act-guidance/> (accessed August 2011).

Fowler, D., 2008. Student midwives and accountability: are mentors good role models? Br. J. Midwifery 16 (2), 100–104.

Fowler, G.A., Heater, B, 1983. Guidelines for clinical evaluation. J. Nurs. Educ. 22 (9), 402–404.

Fraser, D., Murphy, R., Worth-Butler, M., 1997. An Outcome Evaluation of the Effectiveness of Pre-registration Midwifery Programmes of Education. The English National Board for Nursing, Midwifery and Health Visiting, London.

Goclowski, J., 1985. Legal implications of academic dismissal and educational malpractice for nursing faculty. J. Nurs. Educ. 24 (3), 104–108.

Goudreau, K.A., Chasens, E.R., 2002. Negligence in nursing education. Nurse. Educ. 27 (1), 42–46.

Gopee, N., 2008. Assessing students nurses' clinical skills: the ethical competence of mentors. Int. J. Ther. Rehabil. 15 (9), 401–407.

Graveley, E.A., Stanley, M., 1993. A clinical failure: what the courts tell us. J. Nurs. Educ. 32 (3), 135–137.

Gray, M.A., Smith, L.N., 2000. The qualities of an effective mentor from the student nurses perspective: findings from a longitudinal qualitative study. J. Adv. Nurs. 32, 1542–1549.

Griffith, R., Tengnah, C., 2010. Law and Professional Issues in Nursing, Second ed. Learning Matters, Exeter.

Gunby, S.S., 2008. Legal issues in teaching nursing. In: Penn, B.K. (Ed.), Mastering the Teaching Role: A Guide for Nurse Educators. FA Davis, Philadelphia, pp. 411–421.

Hager, P., Gonczi, A., 1996. Professions and competencies. In: Edwards, R., Hanson, A., Raggatt, P. (Eds.), Boundaries of Adult Learning. Routledge, London, pp. 246–260.

Illingworth, K., 2005. The effects of dyslexia on the work of nurses and healthcare assistants. Nurs. Stand. 19 (38), 41–48.

Johnson, E.G., Halstead, J.A., 2005. The academic performance of students. In: Billings, D.M., Halstead, J.A. (Eds.), Teaching in Nursing: A Guide for Faculty. Second ed. WB Saunders, Philadelphia, pp. 41–66.

Harding, C., Greig, M., 1994. Issues of accountability in the assessment of practice. Nurse. Educ. Today 14, 118–123.

Health and Care Professions Council, 2006. A Disabled Person's Guide to Becoming a Health Professional. HCPC, London, Online. Available: <http://www.hcpc-uk.org/aboutregistration/healthanddisability/> (accessed August 2011).

Health and Care Professions Council, 2008. Standards of Conduct, Performance and Ethics. HCPC, London, Online. Available: <http://www.hcpc-uk.org/publications/standards/> (accessed August 2011).

Health and Care Professions Council, 2009a. Standards of Education and Training Guidance. HCPC, London, Online. Available: <http://www.hcpc-uk.org/publications/standards/> (accessed August 2011).

Health and Care Professions Council, 2009b. Guidance on Conduct and Ethics for Students. HCPC, London, Online. Available: <http://www.hcpc-uk.org/publications/brochures/> (accessed August 2011).

Health and Care Professions Council, 2010a. Information for Employers and Managers: The Fitness to Practise Process. HCPC, London, Online. Available: <http://www.hcpc-uk.org/complaints/> (accessed August 2011).

Health and Care Professions Council, 2010b. Fitness to practise annual report 2010. HCPC, London, Available at <http://www.hcpc-uk.org/publications/reports/index.asp?id=403> (accessed August 2011).

Health and Care Professions Council, 2011a. Standards of Proficiency. Online. Available: <http://www.hcpc-uk.org/aboutregistration/standards/standardsofproficiency/> (accessed August 2011).

Health and Care Professions Council, 2011b. Character. Online. Available: <http://www.hcpc-uk.org/aboutregistration/standards/character/> (accessed August 2011).

Health and Care Professions Council, 2011c. Fitness to Practise Annual Report 2011. HCPC, London, Online. Available: <http://www.hcpc-uk.org/publications/index.asp?startrow=11&sCategory=0&sKeyword=fitness>

to practise reports (accessed February 2012).

The Health Professions Order, 2001. Consolidated Text Incorporating Repeals and Amendments Made up to 1st April 2010. HCPC, London, Online. Available: <http://www.hcpc-uk.org/Assets/documents/10002D20HPORDER-2010CONSOLIDATION.pdf> (accessed July 2011).

Hepworth, S., 1991. The assessment of student nurses. Nurse. Educ. Today 11, 46–52.

Holloway, D., 1985. Accountability in further education: teachers' perceptions. J. Further High. Educ. 9 (2), 31–45.

Ilott, I., Murphy, R., 1999. Success and Failure in Professional Education: Assessing the Evidence. Whurr, London.

Killam, L.A., Montgomery, P., Luhanga, F.L., et al., 2010. Views on unsafe nursing students in clinical learning. Int. J. Nurs. Educ. Scholarsh. 7 (1), 1–17. Article 36.

Lello, J. (Ed.), 1979. Accountability in Education. Ward Lock Educational, London.

Levett-Jones, T., Lathlean, J., Higgins, I., et al., 2009. Staff-student relationships and their impact on nursing students' belongingness and learning. J. Adv. Nurs. 65 (2), 316–324.

Luhanga, F., Yonge, O.J., Myrick, F., 2008. Failure to assign failing grades: issues with grading the unsafe student. Inter. J. Nurs. Educ. Scholarsh. 5 (1), 1–14. Article 8.

McGaghie, W.C., 1991. Professional competence evaluation. Educ. Res. 20, 3–9.

Marks-Maran, D., 1995. Accountability in nursing education. In: Watson, R. (Ed.), Accountability in Nursing Practice Chapman & Hall, London, pp. 232–240.

Maslow, A., 1954. Motivation and Personality. Harper and Row, New York.

May, N., Veitch, L., McIntosh, J., et al., 1997. Evaluation of Nurse and Midwife Education in Scotland. The National Board for Nursing, Midwifery and Health Visiting for Scotland, Edinburgh, 1992 Programmes.

McAllister, M., Tower, M., Walker, R., 2007. Gentle interruptions:

transformative approaches to clinical teaching. J. Nurs. Educ. 46 (7), 304–312.

Neary, M., 2000. Teaching, Assessing and Evaluation for Clinical Competence. Stanley Thornes, Cheltenham.

Neary, M., 1997. Defining the role of assessors, mentors and supervisors: part II. Nurs. Stand. 11 (43), 34–38.

Nicklin, P.J., Kenworthy, N., 1995. Teaching and Assessing in Clinical Practice, second ed. Baillière Tindall, London.

National Institute of Neurological Disorders and Stroke. 2011 Dyslexia Information. Online. Available: (<http://www.ninds.nih.gov/disorders/dyslexia/dyslexia.htm> (accessed August 2011).

Nursing and Midwifery Council, 2001. The Nursing and Midwifery Order 2001 (SI 2002/253). The Stationery Office, Norwich, Online. Available: <http://www.legislation.gov.uk/uksi/2002/253/contents/made> (accessed September 2011).

Nursing and Midwifery Council, 2004. Nursing and Midwifery Council (Education, Registration and Registration Appeals) Rules 2004. Statutory Instrument 2004/1767. The Stationery Office, Norwich.

Nursing and Midwifery Council, 2005. NMC Circular 16/2005 Appendix 1: Advice and guidance for placement providers for the NMC Overseas Nurses Programme. Nursing and Midwifery Council, London, Online. Available: <http://www.nmc-uk.org> (accessed December 2005).

Nursing and Midwifery Council, 2006. Standard to Support Learning and Assessment in Practice. NMC, London.

Nursing and Midwifery Council, 2008a. Standards to Support Learning and Assessment in Practice, second ed. NMC, London, Online. Available: <http://www.nmc-uk.org/Publications/Standards> (accessed August 2011).

Nursing and Midwifery Council, 2008b. The Code: Standards of Conduct, Performance and Ethics for Nurses and Midwives. NMC, London, Online. Available: <http://www.nmc-uk.org/Publications/Standards> (accessed August 2011).

Nursing and Midwifery Council, 2008c. Delegation. NMC, London, Online.

Available: <http://www.nmc-uk.org/Nurses-and-midwives/Advice-by-topic/A/Advice/Delegation/> (accessed August 2011).

Nursing and Midwifery Council, 2009. Standards of Pre-registration Midwifery Education. NMC, London, Online. Available: <http://www.nmc-uk.org/Publications/Standards/> (accessed August 2011).

Nursing and Midwifery Council 2010a Sign-off mentor criteria. Circular 05/2010. London: NMC. Online. Available: <http://www.nmc-uk.org/Publications-/Circulars/Circulars-2010/> (accessed August 2011).

Nursing and Midwifery Council, 2010b. Guidance on Professional Conduct for Nursing and Midwifery Students, second ed. NMC, London, Online. Available: <http://www.nmc-uk.org/Publications/Guidance> (accessed August 2011).

Nursing and Midwifery Council, 2010c. Standards of Pre-registration Nursing Education. NMC, London, Online. Available: <http://www.nmc-uk.org/Publications/Standards/> (accessed August 2011).

Nursing and Midwifery Council, 2010d. Fitness to Practise: How The Process Works. NMC, London, Online. Available: <http://www.nmc-uk.org/Hearings/How-the-process-works/> (accessed August 2011).

Nursing and Midwifery Council, 2010e. Good Health and Good Character: Guidance for Approved Educational Institutions. NMC, London, Online. Available: <http://www.nmc-uk.org/Educators/Good-health-and-good-character/> (accessed August 2011).

Nursing and Midwifery Council, 2011a. Nursing and Midwifery Council: Annual Fitness to Practise Report 2010-2011. NMC, London, Online. Available: <http://www.nmc-uk.org/About-us/Statistics/Statistics-about-fitness-to-practise-hearings/> (accessed August 2011).

Nursing and Midwifery Council 2011b Online. Available: <http://www.nmc-uk.org/Students/Good-Health-and-Good-Character-for-students-nurses-and-midwives/Definitions/> (accessed August 2011).

Nursing and Midwifery Council 2011c Online. Available: <http://

www.nmc-uk.org/Get-involved/Consultations/Student-indexing/> (accessed August 2011).

Nursing and Midwifery Council 2011d NMC and the Equality Act 2010 Great Britain and disability discrimination legislation in Northern Ireland. Online. Available: <http://www.nmc-uk.org/Students/Good-Health-and-Good-Character-for-students-nurses-and-midwives/Legislative-requirements/> (accessed August 2011).

Orchard, C., 1994. The nurse educator and the nursing student: a review of the issue of clinical evaluation procedures. J. Nurs. Educ. 33 (6), 245–251.

Office for Disability Issues 2010 Equality Act 2010: Guidance. Online. Available: <http://odi.dwp.gov.uk/docs/wor/new/ea-guide.pdf> (accessed August 2011).

Ormerod, J.A., 1993. Accountability in nurse education. Br. J. Nurs. 2 (14), 730–733.

Parkes, R., 1985. Stressful episodes reported by first-year student nurses: a descriptive account. Soc. Sci. Med. 20 (9), 945–953.

Phillips, T., Schostak, J., Tyler, J., 2000. Practice and Assessment in Nursing and Midwifery: Doing it for Real. The English National Board for Nursing, Midwifery and Health Visiting, London.

Phillips, T., Bedford, H., Robinson, J., et al., 1993. Assessment of Competencies in Nursing and Midwifery Education and Training. The English National Board for Nursing, Midwifery and Health Visiting, London.

Pollard, K.C., 2008. Non-formal learning and interprofessional collaboration in health and social care: the influence of the quality of staff interaction on student learning about collaborative behaviour in practice placements. Learn. Health Soc. Care 7 (1), 12–26.

Reid, G., Kirk, J., 2001. Dyslexia in Adults: Education and Employment. John Wiley, Chichester.

Reilly, D.E., 1980. Behavioral Objectives: Evaluation in Nursing. Appleton-Century-Crofts, Norwalk.

Rowntree, D., 1987. Assessing Students: How Shall We Know Them?, second ed. Kogan Page, London.

Royal College of Nursing, 1990. Accountability in Nursing – a Discussion Document Royal College of Nursing of the United Kingdom. Scutari Press, Harrow.

Royal College of Nursing 2010a Dyslexia, dyspraxia and dyscalculia: a guide for managers and practitioners. Online. Available: <http://www.rcn. org.uk/development/publications/ publicationsA-Z#D> (accessed August 2011).

Royal College of Nursing 2010b Dyslexia, dyspraxia and dyscalculia: a toolkit for nursing staff. Online. Available: <http://www.rcn.org. uk/development/publications/ publicationsA-Z#D> (accessed August 2011).

Saarikoski, M., Leino-Kilpi, H., 2002. The learning environment and supervision by staff nurses: developing the instrument. Int J Nurs Stud 39, 259–267.

Schön, D., 1983. The Reflective Practitioner. Basic Books, New York.

Spink, L.M., 1983. Due process in academic dismissal. J. Nurs. Educ. 22 (7), 305–306.

Spouse, J., 1996. The effective mentor: a model for student-centred learning in clinical practice. Nurs. Times Res. 1 (2), 120–132.

Spouse, J., 1998. Learning through legitimate peripheral participation. Nurse Educ. Today 18 (5), 345–351.

Spouse, J., 2003. Professional Learning in Nursing. Blackwell, Oxford.

Torrance, H., Pryor, J., 1998. Investigating Formative Assessment. Open University Press, Buckingham.

UKCC, 1996. Issues Arising from Professional Conduct Complaints. United Kingdom Central Council for Nursing, Midwifery and Health Visiting, London.

University of Sheffield, 2001. Service Agreement for the Provision of Clinical Placement Services and Facilities. The University of Sheffield.

White, J., 2007. Supporting nursing students with dyslexia in clinical practice. Nurs. Stand. 21 (19), 35–42.

White, E., Riley, E., Davies, S., et al., 1994. A detailed study of the relationship between teaching, support Supervision and Role Modelling in Clinical Areas within the Context of P2000 Courses. The English National Board for Nursing, Midwifery and Health Visiting, London.

Wood, V., 1987. The nursing instructor and the teaching climate. Nurse Educ. Today 7, 228–234.

Wright, D., 2000. Educational support for nursing and midwifery students with dyslexia. Nurs. Stand. 14 (41), 35–41.

Young, A., 2009. Review: the legal duty of care for nurses and other health professionals. J. Clin. Nurs. 18, 3071–3078.

Young, A.P., 1992. Case Studies in Law and Nursing. Chapman & Hall, London.

Young, A.P., 1994. Law and Professional Conduct in Nursing, second ed. Scutari, London.

Chapter | 3 |

What do we assess?

INTRODUCTION

The health care professions have a responsibility to, and are accountable to, the public. They serve to train health care practitioners who are clinically competent and fit to practise (HCPC 2010, NMC 2001). Fraser et al (1997:51) put it very simply:

> *The public needs to be assured that those about to become midwife [or nurse] practitioners have developed the right blend of knowledge, skills and attitudes to become competent.*

However, in the nursing and midwifery professions there has been much accusation over the years that nursing and midwifery education does not produce competent nurses and midwives (Bradshaw 2000, Castledine 2000). This concern remains today (Jervis & Tilki 2011, Rutkowski 2007). It is essential that pre-registration health care students achieve the learning outcomes that will satisfy the UK Nursing and Midwifery Council (NMC) and the Health and Care Professions Council (HCPC) training requirements (HCPC 2011a, NMC 2010, 2009). It is necessary to measure and assess the standards of proficiency so that the practitioner who qualifies is clinically competent and fit to practise.

The issue of being clinically competent is not just restricted to newly qualified practitioners. Nurses and midwives and registrants on the HCPC register are required to maintain their professional knowledge and competence (HCPC 2008, NMC 2008). However, the NMC (2011a) reported that approximately 37% of cases referred when the registrant's fitness to practise is in doubt related to a lack of competence of the practitioner and not to professional misconduct. Over a decade ago, the United Kingdom Central Council (UKCC 1999) reported similar findings: there was lack of competence in a significant number of cases. In the case of registrants on the HCPC register (HCPC 2011), 19% of allegations concerned issues of lack of competence.

It is therefore important to consider carefully what it means to be clinically competent.

In this chapter, the use of competency statements and a competency-based model of assessment are suggested as means to be clear about what we want to assess (Hager & Gonczi 1996). The key features of the National Vocational Qualification (NVQ) system are described to illustrate how a tight structure and format for assessment can be constraining, but has the potential advantages of validity and reliability of assessment. The nature of competencies, what it means to be clinically competent and their assessment in professional practice are explored. The competency-based model of assessment is critically evaluated as an assessment tool for assessing professional practice.

PRE-REGISTRATION HEALTH CARE EDUCATION REQUIREMENTS IN THE UK

The nursing and midwifery professions in the UK regulated by the Nursing and Midwifery Council, and professions in the UK regulated by the Health and Care Professions Council, came into being through Acts of Parliament. The Nursing and Midwifery Order 2001 and the Health and Care Professions Order 2001 require these statutory bodies to establish standards of education and training necessary to achieve the standards of proficiency in order to be admitted to the professional registers. The standards of proficiency are set at a 'threshold' level, as this is the minimum level for safe and effective practice in order to protect the public.

Before a higher education institution (HEI) can provide and run a pre-registration health care course of the professions regulated by the NMC and the HCPC, the course must be validated by the relevant statutory body and the HEI. The process of conjoint validation frequently brings competing sets of demands in relation to course assessment strategies (Bedford et al 1993). The NMC and HCPC are concerned that assessment strategies are sensitive to the demands of professional practice. On the other hand, HEIs' concerns focus on academic credibility and the extent to which assessment strategies are sensitive to intellectual competence. In the case of nursing and midwifery, in the document *Fitness for Practice*, the UKCC (1999) set out a radical agenda in order to refocus nursing and midwifery education to meet the needs of the rapidly changing health service by ensuring that nurses and midwives are fit to practise. The Commission recommended that pre-registration nursing and midwifery education should utilize:

outcomes-based competency principles to ensure that students develop not only higher order intellectual

skills and abilities but also the practice knowledge and skills essential to the art and science of nursing and midwifery (p.4).

This agenda is endorsed by the NMC. By refocusing pre-registration education on outcomes-based competency principles, the NMC believes that the needs of the three key stakeholders of pre-registration education – namely the NMC, the prospective employers and the HEIs – are more likely to be met. These needs underpin the NMC's and HCPC's requirements for pre-registration programmes (HCPC 2011, NMC 2010a, 2009). The needs of each of the stakeholders are set out below:

- **Fitness to practise**. The NMC and HCPC are primarily concerned about fitness to practise – should the student be issued with a 'licence' to practise?
- **Fitness for purpose**. Prospective employers are primarily concerned about fitness for purpose – is the newly qualified practitioner able to function competently in clinical practice?
- **Fitness for award**. Higher education institutions are primarily concerned about fitness for award – has the student attained the appropriate level, breadth and depth of learning to be awarded a diploma or degree?

Gilbert Jessup, who is viewed as the most prominent English advocate of competency-based testing, argued that 'the measure of success for any education and training system should be what people learn from it, and how effectively. Just common sense you might think…' (Jessup 1991:3). Jessup suggests that professional training frequently fails to make explicit statements as to what professionals should know, understand and be able to do. Practitioners need to know, with confidence, the 'right blend of knowledge, skills and attitudes to become competent' (Fraser et al 1997:51) and the standard at which they are safe and effective. This knowledge will enable practice educators to conduct assessments and make assessment decisions with the assurance that students who qualify are fit for both practice and purpose.

The use of an outcomes-based competency approach allows the different stakeholders to agree a set of competencies and outcomes for pre-registration programmes to cover the knowledge, understanding, skills, abilities and values expected of newly qualified practitioners (UKCC 1999). Using these competencies and outcomes, referred to as *Standards* by the NMC (NMC 2010a, 2009), there is a requirement for pre-registration nursing and midwifery programmes are designed to prepare the student to be a practitioner who can apply knowledge, understanding and skills to perform to the standards required in employment, and to provide care safely and competently, thereby assuming the responsibilities and accountability necessary for public protection. Jessup's measure of success may thus be fulfilled!

Whilst the HCPC does not state explicitly that an outcomes-based competency principle is used in its pre-registration courses, like the NMC it requires *Standards* to be achieved in all the pre-registration courses of the professions it regulates. An examination of these standards indicates that all the elements of outcomes-based competency principles (to be discussed below) are implicit in the *Standards* (HCPC 2011).

THE NATURE OF COMPETENCE

Two major concepts now require exploring: the nature of competence and the outcomes-based competency approach. I start this discussion by posing the question: *What does it mean to be professionally competent?* The NMC (2008) stipulates that competence is the individual practitioner's responsibility. On completion of a nursing updating course in order to return to practise after a career break, Bradshaw (2000:319) came to this conclusion:

> ... *I had no objective measures or standards by which to judge what I knew, what I should know, and most importantly, what I did not know ... [it] left me unsure about my competence in the practicalities of caring for patients ... gradually I realized that I had no idea whether I was competent in the new*

> *techniques and technology which I was expected to use [original emphases]*

What, indeed, does it take to be a professionally competent nurse or midwife, or paramedic, or occupational therapist? You may wish to discuss the questions in Activity 3.1 with your colleagues.

ACTIVITY 3.1

What does professional competence mean and entail?
What does it mean to be professionally competent?
What does it take to be a professionally competent nurse or midwife or paramedic or occupational therapist?

You may have discovered that the concept of professional competence resists straightforward answers or categorization. Debates that I held with groups of nurses and midwives about the meaning of professional competence gave me much room for thought. The main aspects elicited are shown in Figure 3.1. These aspects point to the multifaceted and complex nature of competence, and what it means to be a professionally competent health care practitioner. Research in the nursing and midwifery professions by Watson et al (2002), Fraser et al (1997) and Bedford et al (1993) concluded that there is no commonly shared definition of a competent nurse or

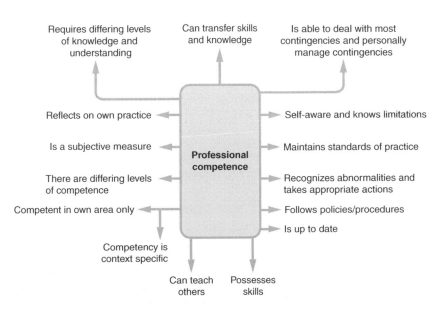

Figure 3.1 Aspects of professional competence.

a competent midwife. Bedford et al (1993:40) think that there are:

many different aspects of this wide-ranging and complex concept … there is more to competence than simply what can be easily observed and measured.

Wolf (1995), who is viewed as one expert in the field of competency-based assessment, wrote that 'competence' and 'competencies' are vexed terms – acres of print continue to be expended over their definitions. Rather than take the reader on a tedious trawl of these definitions, I have selected those that I see are pertinent to the discussion of competence in the health care professions.

Jessup (1991:26) defines both occupational and job competence. Note that his concept of occupational competence is broader:

A person who is described as competent in an occupation or profession is considered to have a repertoire of skills, knowledge and understanding that he or she can apply in a range of contexts and organizations. To say that a person is competent in a 'job', on the other hand, may mean that their competence is limited to a particular role in a particular company.

Jessup's definition of competence is stated simply as 'the ability to perform to recognized standards' (1991:40). He goes on to say that 'these standards are those used to maintain or improve "quality" in the relevant occupation or profession'. Here, Jessup reiterates the expectation of the Manpower Services Commission (1985, in Wolf 1995:31) of someone who is competent – 'by competent we mean performing at the standards expected of an employee doing the same job'.

Eraut's (1998:135) definition of competence as 'the ability to perform the tasks and roles required to the expected standard' reflects the definition of competence that underpins the thinking of those professions in Australia that have established competency standards. Gonczi et al's (1993:5) definition is as follows:

A competent professional has the attributes necessary for job performance to the appropriate standards.

The definition of competence by Gonczi et al (1993) possesses three key components:

- attributes
- performance
- standards.

Attributes

Professionals are competent as a result of possession of a set of relevant attributes such as knowledge, understanding, skills, personal traits, attitudes and values. These attributes, which jointly underlie and determine competence, are referred to as *competencies*. A *competency* is therefore a combination of attributes underlying some aspect of successful professional performance.

Performance

In competency-based assessments, competence is focused on *performance* of a role or sets of tasks (Gonczi et al 1993). Performance is directly observable, whereas competence is not: rather, it is inferred from performance, which is why competence is defined as a combination of attributes that underlie successful performance. There are numerous professional roles, such as nurses, midwives, doctors, pharmacists, physiotherapist, teachers and so on. Roles consist of a multitude of tasks, which can be further divided into sub-tasks. The approach taken by the NVQ movement in the UK focuses on the performance of discrete tasks and sub-tasks: each NVQ covers a particular area of work at a specific level of achievement (Wolf 1995). The professions in Australia have taken what Gonczi et al (1993) describe as the 'integrated approach' – analysis into tasks ceases at the level of relatively complex and demanding professional activities. Competency standards consider the complex combinations of attributes that are required for effective professional activities.

Gonczi et al (1993) stress that both the attributes of the practitioners and their performance of key professional tasks are essential to their definition of competence; this means that attributes of individuals do not in themselves constitute competence. Nor is competence the mere performance of a series of tasks. Rather, the notion of competence integrates attributes with performance; that is, the competent practitioner is not only able to perform, but is also capable (Worth-Butler et al 1994). Competence assessment that incorporates both performance and capability underpin the notion of 'fitness to practise'.

The NMC (2008) and the HCPC (2008) require health care practitioners to integrate attributes with performance in their definition of 'fitness to practise'. Their notion of 'fitness to practise' means having the skills, knowledge, good health and good character to practise safely and effectively (HCPC 2010, NMC 2010b). The NMC adds that this practice is to be without supervision.

Standards

The judgement of the performance of a role and its associated tasks is either competent or incompetent – competence therefore requires that the performance be judged against pre-specified 'standards'. Standards specify the skills, knowledge and understanding that underpin performance in the workplace (Wolf 1995). The 'standards' embody and define competence in the relevant

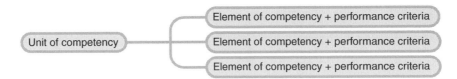

Figure 3.2 A competency standard.

occupational context. A 'competency standard' consists of a unit of competence (representing a wide work function), which is subdivided into smaller elements of competence (tasks within the wider function) with their associated performance criteria (the standards by which the competence in the task will be judged) (Hager & Gonczi 1996). This is the framework in both England and Australia. This framework is illustrated in Figure 3.2.

An example of a unit of competency and its associated elements of competency is shown in Appendix 2.

THE OUTCOMES-BASED COMPETENCY APPROACH TO PROFESSIONAL EDUCATION AND ASSESSMENT

An outline of the background of competency-based assessment

Modern competency-based assessment (in association with competency-based education) first became important in the early 1970s in the context of American teacher education and certification (Wolf 1995). In response to mounting public attacks on the quality of teacher education, the federal government became involved in education reform – competency-based teacher education was seen as a major panacea for the improvement of American education. In the late 1980s in Australia, there was considerable pressure from the national government on industry and the professions to adopt a competency-based approach to education, staff development and performance appraisal (Sutton & Arbon 1994). Consequently, most of the professions have developed competency-based standards (statements) and competency-based assessment strategies (Hager & Gonczi 1996). In the UK in the 1980s, following a Scottish lead, the government launched a huge programme of 'standards development' – this produced 'standards of competence' in a big range of occupational sectors, each with its associated NVQ award, or in Scotland the Scottish Vocational Qualification (SVQ). Although NVQs were approved by a national body, the Qualifications and Curriculum Authority (QCA), the actual processes of supervision and assessment were carried out by 'awarding bodies' such as the City and Guilds of London Institute. The new qualifications framework for England, Wales and Northern Ireland, the Qualifications and Credit Framework (QCF), has developed new qualifications to replace the Health and Health and Social Care suite of NVQs (Skills for Health 2012). Whilst the qualifications in the QCF units are competence based, QCF units differ from NVQ units in that they contain learning outcomes instead of knowledge and performance criteria statements. The reader is directed to the work of Wolf (1995), who gives a critique of competency-based assessment and the NVQ system.

Competency-based assessment is a form of assessment that emphasizes the outcomes of achievement. These outcomes are specified to the point where they are clear and 'transparent', so that assessors, assessees and 'third parties' can all make reasonably objective judgements with respect to their achievement or non-achievement. Certification is made on the basis of demonstrated achievement of these outcomes (Wolf 1995).

Using competency-based assessment in professional health care education

Can a case be made for using the competency-based approach in the health care professions? Thirty years ago, Patricia Benner (1982:303, 309) had this to say about using this approach in nursing education:

> *The quest for competency statements and competency-based exams in nursing has led to what seems to be a premature faith in the current state of the art and capability of competency-based performance examinations in nursing. Carried along by a technological, measurement-oriented age, we have been convinced that many of our problems in nursing education and practice will be solved when we have mastered the current measurement technology available – when we can simply and unequivocally describe the competencies involved in the practice of nursing and measure them. Some of us have gone so far as to say that any area of practice that cannot be so defined, described, and measured does not legitimately belong in the arena of professional practice.*
>
> *Unfortunately, this faith in the feasibility of competency examinations does not come to grips with the difficulties and issues inherent in the methodology … to overestimate the power of competency-based testing will cause an undesirable reductionism in nursing.*

Notwithstanding Benner's warning about competency-based education in nursing, one recommendation made in the reports *Making a Difference* (Department of Health 1999) and *Fitness for Practice* (UKCC 1999) was to refocus pre-registration nursing and midwifery education on an outcomes-based competency approach. This recommendation is endorsed by the HCPC (HCPC 2011) and the NMC (NMC 2010a, 2009). Is this recommendation justified? What are the implications of using competency-based assessment of clinical practice? An examination of two particular ways of using competency-based assessment may provide some answers: these are the NVQ system in the UK and the 'integrated' approach used by the professions in Australia.

Competency-based assessment for NVQs

The NVQ framework represents a very particular application of competency-based assessment (Wolf 1995). This section will provide an outline of the basic structure of NVQs and discuss the principles underlying competency-based assessment for NVQs. The process of assessment within the competency-based framework is discussed in Chapter 6. Inferences will then be drawn about the appropriateness of the NVQ system for the assessment of professional practice, such as in the nursing and midwifery professions.

An NVQ comprises several units and their associated elements to be achieved at one of the five pre-specified levels (DfES 2005). A unit consists of a group of 'elements of competence' and their associated performance criteria and knowledge specification. Each unit reflects a discrete activity or sub-area of competence – each is worthy of separate accreditation, much like an academic module in fact (NCVQ 1991). An element of competence is a description of something that a person who works in a given occupational area should be able to do; it encompasses some action, behaviour or outcome. Competency-based assessment for NVQs is made concrete through highly specified performance criteria and knowledge specification. The element of competence is assessed and validated against these performance criteria and knowledge specification. Appendix 2 provides an example of a unit, its associated elements and one element of competence with its performance criteria.

Assessment requires that the individual demonstrates successfully that he/she has met every one of the performance criteria and knowledge specification, as these are the statements by which an assessor judges whether the evidence provided by the individual is sufficient to demonstrate competent performance (Wolf 1995). The NVQ approach requires assessment to be centred on whether performance meets the pre-specified standards. Performance is judged to be either competent or not yet competent only – the individual has either consistently demonstrated workplace performance that meets the specified 'standards' or has not yet been able to do so. Grading is rejected – the individual either has or has not reached the required level of the NVQ.

Up until 2005, each element of competence with its associated performance criteria had an associated 'range'. These ranges officially 'elaborate the statement of competence by making explicit the contexts to which the element [of competence] and performance criteria apply. Also, they put limits on the specification to ensure a consistent interpretation' (NCVQ 1991:14). Contextualizing the performance criteria identifies the different contexts in which the individual is expected to achieve competent performance. This means that competence must also be assessed 'across the range' and performance evidence is 'normally required for every performance criteria [sic] across as much of the range as possible' (City and Guilds 1992). Following the review of the National Occupational Standards in Health and Social Care and the launch of the new Health and Social Care N/SVQs in February 2005 (Skills for Health 2005), the 'range' has been replaced by the 'scope'. The statements in the scope do not appear to be as specific as the range statements. The scope is intended to give guidance on possible areas to be covered in the unit. It specifies a list of options linked with items in the performance criteria. Evidence is required for any option related to the candidate's work area. The specification of the scope for the unit HSC35 can be found in Appendix 2.

In its early years, NVQs were criticized for producing people who might be able to demonstrate performance but would have no understanding of what they were doing (Norris 1991). To fend off mounting attacks on NVQs as undemanding, and to ensure that individuals have an understanding of what they are doing (Wolf 1995), NCVQ added a separate 'knowledge/understanding' list to every element of competence. Candidates are required to demonstrate that they understand all the items listed under knowledge evidence and supporting evidence. From 2005, knowledge and understanding are specified at unit level. Appendix 2 contains the 'knowledge and understanding' statements required for unit HSC35.

NVQs are offered at five levels to cover progression from routine and predictable work activities to the complex and unpredictable (Directgov 2012, DfES 2005). Box 3.1 details the summary of each level.

It can be seen that the NVQ system applies competency-based assessment in a very tightly defined format. It embraces the performance philosophy of competency-based systems to the very core (Wolf 1995). Thus, its notion of competence is 'the ability to perform the activities within an occupation' (Wolf 1995:31). While competency-based systems vary in their interpretation of what outcomes may be (see, for example, Gonczi et al 1993), the learning outcomes in NVQs relate directly to performance – what counts as an outcome is thus very highly constrained. An

Box 3.1 **Summary of the five NVQ levels**

Box 3.1 **Summary of the five NVQ levels**

- **Level 1** Competence that involves the application of knowledge in the performance of a range of varied work activities, most of which may be routine and predictable.
- **Level 2** Competence that involves the application of knowledge in a significant range of varied work activities, performed in a variety of contexts. Some of these activities are complex or non-routine and there is some individual responsibility or autonomy. Collaboration with others, perhaps through membership of a work group or team, may often be a requirement.
- **Level 3** Competence that involves the application of knowledge in a broad range of varied work activities performed in a wide variety of contexts, most of which are complex and non-routine. There is considerable responsibility and autonomy and control or guidance of others is often required.
- **Level 4** Competence that involves the application of knowledge in a broad range of complex, technical or professional work activities performed in a variety of contexts and with a substantial degree of personal responsibility and autonomy. Responsibility for the work of others and the allocation of resources is often present.
- **Level 5** Competence that involves the application of a range of fundamental principles across a wide and often unpredictable variety of contexts. Very substantial personal autonomy and often significant responsibility for the work of others and for the allocation of substantial resources feature strongly, as do personal accountabilities for analysis, diagnosis, design, planning, execution and evaluation.

element of competence must encompass some action, behaviour or outcome that is contextually related to that occupational sector through its range statement. The elements of competence referred to in Unit HSC35 are legitimate as being outcome-based because they involve an *active verb* and an *object* and relate directly to performance. Each element of competence is specified in such a way that there can be no doubt about what constitutes satisfactory performance. For example, competence in Element HSC35a requires the person to be able to 'develop supportive relationships that promote choice and independence'.

Arguments for and against the NVQ system for assessing professional practice

As stated earlier, the NVQ framework represents a very particular application of competency-based assessment that can be summarized as follows:

- the elements of competence define the performance requirements
- the performance criteria describe competent performance
- the scope specifies the list of options for which assessment evidence is required
- statements of knowledge and supporting evidence define the underpinning knowledge and understanding required
- levels specify the nature of work activities for competent performance, ranging from the routine and predictable to the complex and unpredictable.

A contentious issue about what is to be assessed concerns the optimum level of specificity. Storey et al (1995:382) say that 'if there is too little specificity, the result may be a lack of clarity, poor communication and diminished credibility'. This is the criticism directed at earlier pre-registration nursing and midwifery competencies and outcomes. On the other hand, too much specificity can lead to assessment criteria that take too long to read and are cumbersome to use by busy practitioners. This criticism has been directed at the NVQ system. However, you may agree that the NVQ approach has the attraction of precision and clarity as to *what* is to be assessed to achieve competence. Advocates of this approach also emphasize its potential contribution to effective training and learning. Storey et al (1995) and Fletcher (1991), for example, argue that specific criteria for assessing competence are provided, thereby giving the much-desired guidance for assessees and assessors. Individuals know exactly what they have to achieve and assessors can provide specific guidance and feedback. Educational provisions and employment needs can be brought together.

The appropriateness of the NVQ approach for assessing professionals such as in nursing and midwifery has been criticized (Le Var 1996, Norris 1991). What could be the trouble with an approach where the assessment of competence is grounded in performance in the workplace? The NVQ model is seen by Norris (1991:334) to be 'highly reductive, providing atomised lists of tasks and functions'. He elaborates further:

> the sum of the parts rarely if ever represents the totality of good practice … in their tidiness and precision, far from preserving the essential features of expertise, they distort and understate the very things they are trying to represent.

Competence is conceived of in terms of the discrete behaviours associated with the ability to complete individual tasks. This approach is unconcerned with the connections between tasks and ignores the possibility that the coming together of tasks could lead to their transformation (Hager & Gonczi 1996). Le Var (1996) feared that the care activities in nursing and midwifery would become fragmented if students were trained within this approach. If holistic care is to be valued and provided, care activities need to be designed and integrated around the needs of the client at that particular time. Unless professionals are involved in the planning and evaluation of total care, they cannot engage in the processes of critical analysis and synthesis that lead to the development of theories and principles of practice. If this 'atomized' approach of the NVQ system is used by professionals, qualifications could be in danger of being reduced to a list of technical skills (Storey et al 1995). Hager & Gonczi (1996) and Le Var (1996) echo this concern when they point out that this approach ignores the complexity of performance in the real world and the role of professional judgement. Furthermore, the practice and assessment of 'components of care' do not engender the development of problem-solving skills. Watson et al (2002) also argue that being competent requires something greater than the demonstration of correct procedure, as the competent practitioner needs to be able to intertwine the unpredictable and elusive aspects of human care with the flexible application of technical and psychological skills.

So far, a number of general concerns have been raised about the use of a competency-based approach to nursing and midwifery education. The degree to which competencies can be used to describe professional practice is questionable (Watson et al 2002, Sutton & Arbon 1994, Benner 1982). The practice of health care professionals is undeniably complex and competency-based statements can provide only a limited view of this practice – they cannot be used to reflect the complexities of practice with accuracy. They must, by their very nature, provide a reductive analysis of practice (Sutton & Arbon 1994), which excludes learning derived from a whole performance (Benner 1982). Although competency statements purport to describe the attributes, including knowledge and skills necessary for effective and/or superior performance, the testing of intangible attributes such as attitudes is still subjective (Ashworth & Morrison 1991, Benner 1982). Benner pointed out the difficulties of testing some attributes and abilities such as empathy and the ability to relate to others, as learning the behaviour does not guarantee the possession of the accompanying attitude and/or values.

If we return to the definition of a competent professional offered by Gonczi et al (1993) above, you will notice that the competent professional should also possess the appropriate underlying personal attitudes and traits. The assessment of these aspects of competence is not given due consideration in the NVQ system. The Training Agency (1988) states that competence should take into account the 'qualities of personal effectiveness that are required in the workplace to deal with co-workers, managers and customers'. Underlying attributes and qualities may include interpersonal and social skills, attitudes, perceptiveness, receptivity, creativity and maturity as well as knowledge, understanding and critical thinking capacity (Ashworth & Morrison 1991). These underlying attributes of the practitioner are crucial to effective performance (Hager & Gonczi 1996) and are fundamental to excellence in clinical practice (Novak 1988).

If the NVQ system for assessing professional practice is used, the reader is left to ponder the answers to the following questions:

- The NMC and HCPC are concerned about 'fitness to practise': Will the student who is assessed using this system be 'fit for practice' and be allowed to register?
- Employers are concerned about 'fitness for purpose': Will the newly-qualified nurse or midwife or dietitian or orthoptist and so on, be able to function competently in clinical practice? Can the new practitioner fulfil the NMC's and HCPC's expectation of competence – that is, possess the 'skills and abilities required for lawful, safe and effective professional practice without direct supervision'? Due to the speed of change in the context and content of health care, fitness for purpose is an evolving entity: it is not fixed, and depends on the 'commitment of employers and employees to constant updating' (UKCC 1999:34). Having trained and been assessed using the NVQ system during clinical practice, how likely is the new practitioner in making this commitment?

The case for an integrated competency-based approach for assessing health care practice

The UKCC Education Commission recommended refocusing pre-registration education on 'outcomes-based competency principles to ensure that students develop not only higher order intellectual skills and abilities but also the practice knowledge and skills essential to the art and science of nursing and midwifery' (UKCC 1999:4). These recommendations are endorsed by the NMC (2010a, 2009).

In refocusing pre-registration education on outcomes-based competency principles, the NMC believes that the needs of the three key stakeholders of pre-registration education – the NMC, the prospective employers and the HEIs – are more likely to be met. This belief reinforces Hager & Gonczi's (1996) views that a competency-based approach to education and training potentially provides a framework for bringing together professional policies for training and employment requirements. Competencies provide consumers and professionals with some common understanding of standards expected of professionals, and may thereby enable both parties to relate to each other more successfully.

The nursing profession of Australia (Sutton & Arbon 1994) views competency development as one means by which the profession can monitor and maintain its own professional standards and thus enhance its accountability to the public. Hager & Gonczi (1996), however, recommended that any assessment strategy that utilizes the outcomes-based competency model should be 'holistically orientated' – a holistic/integrated competency-based model is more valid and reliable than current ways of assessing professionals. It enables us to come closer than we have in the past to assessing what we want to assess (i.e. the capacity of the professional to integrate knowledge, values, attitudes, skills and other attributes in the real world of practice). It is therefore important that any holistic/integrated model of assessment utilizing the outcomes-based competency approach to the assessment of professional practice takes into account the following:

- effective performance of work activities in a range of contexts
- the exercising of cognitive skills such as integration of theory with practice, critical analysis, problem solving and synthesis
- the ability to provide holistic care
- the underlying attitudes and traits of the learner
- that practice is up to date.

A holistic/integrated competency-based approach considers the complex combinations of attributes (knowledge, understanding, skills, personal traits, attitudes and values) that are used to understand and function within the particular situations in which professionals find themselves. The abilities of practitioners are considered in relationship to the tasks that need to be performed in particular situations. The notion of competence is relational – it is conceived of as the complex structuring of attributes needed for intelligent performance in specific situations. It incorporates the idea of professional judgement. Many authors (e.g. Eraut 1998, Jessup 1991, McGaghie 1991, Black & Wolf 1990) also consider that, other than practical skills and knowledge, professional judgement is an important underpinning of competence. Jessup (1991:127) describes it thus:

> *An analysis of the knowledge which people actually draw upon, and need to draw upon, to perform competently, may not appear in what is taught as the body of knowledge underpinning a profession or occupation, or if it is covered, may not be accorded the priority it deserves. Competent professionals tend to acquire a set of guiding principles, of which they are often partially conscious, derived largely from their experience. These may build upon 'academic' theories and knowledge or be only loosely related. While this is recognized in areas such as management, it also appears to be true in well-established professions such as medicine.*

The holistic/integrated approach is to conceive of competent care as the capacity of the practitioner to employ a complex interaction of attributes in a range of contexts. Thus, a knowledge base and possession of a repertoire of practical skills will need to mesh with, among other things, ethical values and interpersonal skills. Practitioners may then be able to 'perform the task with desirable outcomes under the varied circumstances of the real world' (Benner 1982:304). Adapting the definition of competence used by Queensland Nursing Council 2009,

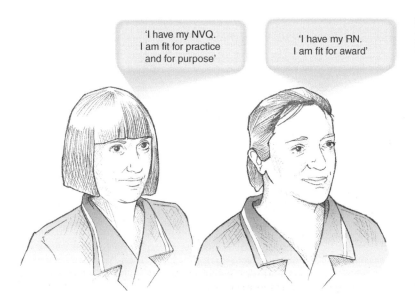

Figure 3.3 The NVQ represents a very particular application of competency-based assessment.

the NMC (2010a) states that competence is a requirement for entry to the NMC register. It is a holistic concept that may be defined as 'the combination of skills, knowledge and attitudes, values and technical abilities that underpin safe and effective nursing practice and interventions'. It can be seen that there is thus a common expectation of a practitioner who is supposed to be competent.

The real world of health care is dynamic, complex and unpredictable. Health care professionals face challenging and unique situations within practice and need flexible ways of responding to, and learning from, these situations. It follows then that competence is also developmental in orientation – never a total accomplishment, always looking forward to better performance, improved decision-making and greater quantity of outcome (Bedford et al 1993). The holistic/integrated competency-based approach allows the incorporation of ethics and values as elements in competent performance, the need for reflective practice, the importance of context and the fact that there is more than one way of conceptualizing competence. In the nursing context, the holistic/integrated approach views that competence is (Percival et al 1994:139):

The ability of a person to fulfil the nursing role effectively and/or expertly. It is an inner, highly differentiated characteristic of a person which is applicable to the very demanding and very specific context of nursing. It is an ability that effectively encompasses the entire demands of the nursing role; and therefore nursing competence itself possesses a complexity that increases with experience, and as responsibilities become more intricate.

The qualities expected by practising nurses and midwives of the competent professional nurse or midwife (see Figure 3.1) have many similarities to the holistic/

integrated way of conceptualizing competence. Another inference that can be drawn from the information in Figure 3.1 is what Gonczi et al (1993:13) said of clinical competence – that is: 'clinical competence is a complex phenomenon, which almost always requires the practitioner to use a combination of attributes simultaneously and, in addition, that the practitioners need to adapt their practices to different contexts'. It seems that if a competency-based model for assessing health care practice is used then adopting the concepts of competence inherent in the holistic/integrated approach is the way forward. In her critique of the use of the competency-based model for the nursing profession, Le Var (1996) came to the conclusion that the holistic/integrated approach is in keeping with, and will also help fulfil, the current assessment philosophy and practice in professional nursing.

The components of the holistic/integrated competency-based model can be summarized as:

- a complex combination of attributes – knowledge, attitudes, personal traits, values, skills and understanding
- exercising cognitive skills – e.g. using professional judgement in specific situations
- effective performance on different occasions in different contexts
- developmental in orientation to emphasize the need for reflective practice.

Utilizing these components, an integrated competency-based model for assessing nursing and midwifery practice can be constructed, as shown in Figure 3.4.

It is suggested here that, if assessment is unified by using the holistic/integrated competency-based model, health care practitioners are more likely to develop the requisite technical competence and scientific rationality, as well as fulfil the paradoxical expectation of meeting the holistic care needs of patients and clients (Department of

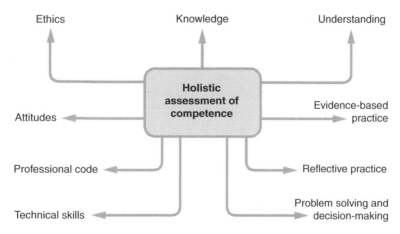

Figure 3.4 The components of a holistic/integrated competency-based model of assessment.

Health 1999). Practitioners will thus achieve 'fitness to practise' and not just be 'fit for practice' as, according to Moore (2005), there is a fundamental difference between the two terminologies. Moore suggests that the term 'fitness for practice' appears to be used to refer to the professional who has sufficient knowledge and skills to be able to practise safely, and the term 'fitness to practise' is more frequently associated with health and conduct. Therefore, it seems reasonable to assume that someone who is not fit for practice is not fit to practise. On the other hand, someone who is not fit to practise may still be fit for practice (Moore 2005). More recently, both the NMC and HCPC have defined fitness to practise as having the skills, knowledge, good health and good character to practise safely and effectively (HCPC 2010, NMC 2010b).

For the purposes of the discussion on assessment methodology (see Ch. 4) the components of professional competence are grouped into the category of *reflective practice* and the three domains of learning classified by Bloom et al (1956):

- *cognitive domain*: knowledge, understanding, problem solving, decision-making, professional code
- *affective domain*: attitude, ethics, professional code
- *psychomotor domain*: technical skills.

Using the holistic/integrated approach for competency-based assessment of clinical practice

The holistic/integrated approach to competency-based assessment used by the professions in Australia seeks to identify attributes as well as key functions and activities, and to combine these in an integrated set of competency statements (Gonczi et al 1993). This has meant that analysis into tasks has ceased at the level of relatively complex and demanding professional activities – typically, a profession does not develop more than 30-40 competencies.

Competencies should be designed to reflect the holistic nature of a profession and should represent the practice repertoire of the newly qualified practitioner (Hager & Gonczi 1996).

The UKCC (1999), endorsed by the NMC (2009, 2010a), provided the following guiding principles that should be reflected in pre-registration nursing and midwifery programmes:

- nursing and midwifery are practice-based professions that recognize the primacy of patient and client well-being and respect for individuals
- the *Code: Standards of conduct, performance and ethics for nurses and midwives* (NMC 2008) applies to all practice interventions
- the importance of lifelong learning and continuing professional development are recognized
- skills and knowledge are transferable
- practice is based on the best available evidence.

Additionally, the Department of Health (1999) called for an increase in practical skills within training programmes. Thus, a strategy similar to that used by the nursing profession in Australia has been used by the NMC in developing the standards for both the pre-registration nursing and midwifery programmes (NMC 2010a, 2009). Adapting the definition of competence used by Queensland Nursing Council 2009, the NMC states that competence is a requirement for entry to the NMC register. It is a holistic concept that may be defined as 'the combination of skills, knowledge and attitudes, values and technical abilities that underpin safe and effective nursing practice and interventions'. The NMC has defined a competency framework for pre-registration nursing education. Within this framework, there are *sets of competency* requirements for each field (branch) of nursing. Each *set of competency* comprises generic and specific *standards for competence* plus related generic and specific *competencies* for that field of nursing. Each set of competency is laid out under the four domains of professional values, communicate and interpersonal skills, nursing practice and decision-making and leadership, management and team working. Essential skills clusters (see below) support the development and achievement of learning outcomes in each set of competency. Whilst the competency framework for the pre-registration midwifery programme does not specify the standard for competence, it specifies competencies, which are laid out under the four domains of effective midwifery practice, professional and ethical practice, developing the individual midwife and others and achieving quality care through evaluation and research. Essential skills clusters support the development and achievement of learning outcomes in the competencies.

The need for an integrated competency-based approach for the assessment of clinical practice has been highlighted. This has now been adopted by the NMC as described above. Within an integrated assessment framework, assessment approaches can assess a range of elements and performance criteria, rather than collect evidence for each element and performance criterion (Gonczi et al 1993). For example, in the case of a student midwife on a community placement, home visits of women and their babies can be used to assess elements such as the practical skills of examination of the woman and/or baby, conducting interviews, monitoring progress and compiling case records and reports. The performance on these visits can also be used to measure a number of attributes at the same time, such as communication and interpersonal skills, underpinning knowledge, understanding, problem solving and so on.

In Chapter 4, there is a consideration of assessment methods that are available and how these may be used to generate the assessment evidence required to infer, and confer, competence. In Chapter 6, there is a discussion of how the components of the holistic/integrated competency-based model of the assessment of clinical practice can be incorporated and used within a learning contract.

A 'clinical skills checklist' for pre-registration nursing and midwifery education

While the holistic/integrated competency-based approach to the assessment of clinical practice will concomitantly assess practical skills, it may not identify the nature and repertoire of the skills which the student has become competent in. Moreover, the acquisition of skills is not straightforward during clinical practice. Farley & Hendry (1997) suggested that the presence of a patient will detract from the focus on the technical aspect of the procedure as the student has to interact with the client/patient. Having to concentrate on two separate and different aspects of care may affect the student's ability to do both well. In 1999, the UKCC expressed concern and unease about the lack of essential practical nursing skills of newly qualified nurses (UKCC 1999). Although concerns about the practical skills of newly qualified midwives were not as marked as those for nursing, they remain significant because of the requirement of midwives to practise autonomously on registration. Both the UKCC (1999) and the Department of Health (1999), then, called for an increase in the level of practical skills during pre-registration training. Similar concerns were still expressed by the NMC (2005). This concern has resulted in the introduction of *essential skills clusters* (ESCs) in pre-registration nursing and midwifery programmes in 2007. The ESCs give specific guidance on the skills development required at specified progression points in the programme and for entry to the register. The ESCs for nursing are:

- care, compassion and communication
- organizational aspects of care
- infection prevention and control
- nutrition and fluid management
- medicines management.

  Those for midwifery are:

- communication
- initial consultation between the woman and the midwife
- normal labour and birth
- initiation and continuance of breast feeding
- medical products management.

The use of a 'clinical skills checklist' will help both the student and the practice educator keep track of clinical experiences and care giving situations that the student needs to engage in to acquire the skills within the ESCs. It is emphasized that the checklist should not fragment the clinical experience and assessment of the student – rather, it should be used as a guide to planning clinical experiences so that the student has the opportunity to engage in those clinical activities to enable the development of the skills required for the achievement of the statutory

standards of pre-registration programmes. The checklist should be seen as a formative tool used towards the achievement of these statutory standards as the 'assessment of competence cannot be reduced solely to an assessment of a student's ability to carry out certain tasks' (UKCC 1999:38).

Following an extensive review of the literature and consultation with assessors, mentors, students and newly qualified staff nurses, Hilton (2004) developed several checklists of clinical skills to help students' and practice educators' direct learning in relation to the development of these essential skills. These checklists will also assist in the keeping of a record of achievement and progress. The clinical skills are framed around the 12 'Activities of Living' model of Aggleton and Chalmers (Hilton 2004) and are to be achieved at five levels:

- *Level 1* – have observed the procedure in the practice setting
- *Level 2* – have participated in the skill under direct supervision
- *Level 3* – have performed the skill on a number of occasions and required minimal supervision
- *Level 4* – can perform the skill safely and competently giving the rationale for their actions
- *Level 5* – have taught the skill to others.

Hilton (2004) makes the important point that the lists of skills are not exhaustive and students and practice educators are encouraged to include skills that are unique to a particular clinical setting. The checklists of clinical skills developed by Hilton (2004) around the 12 activities of living can be found in Appendix 3.

Levels of performance

Phillips et al (2000) and Gerrish et al (1997) raise many issues surrounding the assessment of levels of clinical practice. Some of these are framed in the following questions:

- Is there any purpose in attributing levels to practice in nursing and midwifery education?
- If we accept the viability of the use of levels criteria to differentiate practice, what constitutes evidence of movement from one level of practice to another?
- Does learning in the practice setting progress in a linear fashion, as implied by assessment tools which apply Steinaker & Bell's (1979) taxonomy of experiential learning?
- If practice is assessed only in relation to a competent/incompetent distinction, as in the NVQ system, what are the criteria that constitute competent versus incompetent performance?

Pre-registration nursing and midwifery curricula generally prescribe the expected level of competent performance at pre-specified points of the programme (Phillips et al 2000, Gerrish et al 1997). Within a consideration of *what to assess* in clinical practice of a pre-registration programme is the necessity to determine whether a student is achieving competent practice as the training progresses. Bradshaw (1998) is concerned that we are able to state that the nurse or midwife has reached certain minimum standards of competence in the practical knowledge and skills needed to care for patients. It is necessary to decide whether the student is learning, and therefore achieving, the competencies within the student's expected capability: this is generally determined by the stage of training the student is at. This assessment necessarily involves the use of criteria to decide how a competent/incompetent distinction can be made, and whether the student has made the requisite progress at the level specified at a particular stage of the course. These aspects of assessment are seen as part and parcel of the monitoring of progress of students and are discussed in detail in Chapter 7.

Professional conduct, values and ethics

In the health care professions, competence to perform complex and technical problems only is now increasingly challenged by the public and the professions themselves. There is an expectation that the personal attributes of practitioners are also developed as these are necessary for effective professional practice (NMC 2010a, 2009, HCPC 2009, Toohey 2002), as it is universally argued that whatever knowledge and skills students possess on qualification are no good without the right values and attitudes (Roberts 2009). The issue of impairment of fitness to practise in pre-registration health care students is complex. Fitness to practise means having the skills, knowledge, good health and good character to practise safely and effectively (NMC 2010c, HCPC 2009). Fitness to practise is questioned when there are allegations of misconduct, lack of competence and ill health. This means that a student's professional conduct, values and ethics can be questioned. There is little published research on allegations of undesirable professional conduct, values and ethics in pre-registration health care students where future professional suitability is in doubt. From the nursing literature in the UK, Braithwaite et al (1994) and Hutt (1988) reported disciplinary proceedings for students discontinuing their course. Also of interest is 'personality disorders' as a reason for discontinuation of the course (Lindop 1987).

More recent studies on undesirable professional conduct, values and ethics come from the United States in the field of medicine. One study reported that over a 10-year period from 1990 to 2000, 95% of disciplinary actions taken by the Medical Board of California were for deficiencies in professionalism (Papadakis et al 2004). Compared with a control group, the disciplined doctors were twice as likely to have had 'concerns/problem/extreme' excerpts recorded in their medical school

profiles. In a later study, three types of unprofessional behaviour whilst a medical student had a significant association with being disciplined as practising doctors (Teherani et al 2005). The unprofessional behaviours reported were poor reliability and responsibility, lack of self-improvement and adaptability and poor initiative and motivation. Another study in the United States also found that disciplinary action by a medical board was strongly associated with prior unprofessional behaviour in medical schools (Papadakis et al 2005). Severe irresponsibility and severe diminished capacity for self-improvement were most strongly linked to disciplinary action.

The argument for formalizing the development and assessment of personal attributes is that these translate into certain kinds of desirable professional values and ethics, which then ensure that the student achieves fitness to practise (Miller 2010, Hilton & Slotnick 2005, Toohey 2002). We need practitioners who are willing to look carefully and analytically at their own practice and mistakes; we want professionals who are prepared to acknowledge their limitation and call in a second opinion; we want practitioners who can work within a team so that care is coordinated with the patient/client in mind. In the main, opportunities for students to learn about such aspects of professional practice are informal and opportunistic (e.g. by learning from role models in the workplace). Although the learning from positive role models may be significant, it may not be sufficient. It would also be naïve to think that all role models are positive ones.

In their studies, Fraser et al (1997) and Hart et al (2001) identified some key personal attributes that professional midwives should possess. There are many similarities between these and those identified by Hilton & Slotnick (2005) in the medical profession; these authors have grouped these personal attributes into the two broad categories of 'personal (intrinsic) attributes' and 'cooperative attributes'. Each category encompasses three domains, as shown below.

Personal (intrinsic) attributes

- *Ethical practice* – the foundation on which agreement exists between patient/client expectations and what professionals expect to provide.
- *Reflection/self-awareness* – necessary in order to deal with complex clinical problems.
- *Responsibility/accountability for actions (commitment to excellence, lifelong learning, critical reasoning)* – must be well developed to fulfil the high expectations placed on professionals.

Cooperative attributes

- *Respect for patients* – demands an understanding of patient/client needs and an appreciation of how professionals' behaviours can be interpreted.

- *Working with others (teamwork)* – has become an essential requirement in recent times.
- *Social responsibility* – through the 'social contract' with society, professionals must be aware and sensitive to the range of views on health issues.

How can these personal attributes be best assessed? This is an area of assessment that continues to challenge assessors of professional health care students. Toohey (2002:533) suggests that the purpose of such assessment is not to certify competence but to 'harness and direct the powerful effects of assessment onto an important aspect of practice and to provide opportunities for students to reflect, self-evaluate and receive feedback'. Toohey's formative assessment of personal attributes utilized various educational and assessment strategies. Readers are directed to the discussion of assessment methods in Chapter 4 for suggestions on how to approach the assessment of personal attributes.

As well as considering the approach to this aspect of assessment, it is also important to set criteria to guide students and assessors towards the development and assessment of personal attributes. Using the empirical evidence from the work of Fraser et al (1997) and Hart et al (2001) and the behaviours identified by practice educators as 'essential' behaviours that a student midwife should demonstrate, a tool termed the 'professional behaviours inventory' is proposed to facilitate the development and assessment of pre-specified behaviours expected of a professional exhibiting the accepted conduct of a midwife. These professional behaviours reflect the professional conduct expected of health care students as laid down by the NMC (2011b) and the HCPC (2008). The professional behaviours consist of highly specified descriptors that are observable and can be readily used by the student, practice educator and other members of the team working with the student. The professional behaviours inventory may be used as one component of the assessment of practice of pre-registration health care students. As such, it may serve as both a formative and a summative tool. This assessment tool is shown in Appendix 4.

CONCLUSION

To achieve the aim of preparing health care practitioners who are 'fit to practise' it is necessary to be clear about *what* we want to assess in the clinical setting. The NMC and HCPC specify statutory standards for pre-registration education. These are to be achieved through the principles of a competency-based model of assessment. Two particular applications of this model have been described in this chapter. First is the NVQ system, which is seen to focus almost exclusively on the performance of discrete tasks and is therefore reductionist in nature. This application of the competency-based model is therefore not entirely appropriate for assessing professional health care education such as nursing and midwifery. Secondly, the other application of the competency-based model utilizes the holistic/integrated approach as used by the professions in Australia (Gonczi et al 1993), and now endorsed by the NMC. This approach conceives of competent health care as the capacity of the practitioner to employ a complex interaction of attributes needed for intelligent performance in a range of contexts. Thus, a knowledge base and the possession of a repertoire of practical skills will need to mesh with, amongst other things, ethical values and interpersonal skills. Clinically, the assessment can be integrated by using those methods that assess a number of elements and all their performance criteria simultaneously, so that evidence towards the achievement of one or several competencies can be generated. The holistic/integrated competency-based approach is recommended for the assessment of students in the health care professions.

All existing methods of clinical assessment are potentially appropriate for use in the holistic/integrated competency-based approach. This is because it is not the methods that are competency-based, but the way they are used, the emphasis given to each method and the way in which the results are interpreted that are important. The following chapter examines the range of methods available and how these can be used in competency-based assessment.

KEY POINTS FOR REFLECTION

A competency-based approach to education and training potentially provides a framework for bringing together professional policies for training and employment requirements so that practitioners are both 'fit to practise' and 'fit for purpose'.

A competent professional has the attributes necessary for job performance to the appropriate standards. This encompasses the three key components of attributes, performance and standards:

- **Attributes**: professionals are competent as a result of possession of a set of relevant attributes such as

knowledge, understanding, skills, personal traits, attitudes and values. These attributes, which jointly underlie and determine competence, are referred to as *competencies. A competency* is therefore a combination of attributes underlying some aspect of successful professional performance.

- **Performance**: is directly observable, whereas competence is inferred from performance. The notion of competence integrates attributes with successful performance.

- **Standards**: specify the skills, knowledge and understanding that underpin performance in the workplace. The judgement of the performance of a role and its associated tasks is either competent or incompetent – competence therefore requires that the performance is judged against pre-specified 'standards'.

The National Vocational Qualification (NVQ) framework represents a very particular application of competency-based assessment. It applies competency-based assessment in a very tightly defined format and embraces the performance philosophy of competency-based systems to the very core. The NVQ model is criticized as being highly reductive, providing atomized lists of tasks and functions. Competence is conceived of in terms of the discrete behaviours associated with the ability to complete individual tasks. There is a danger that this will fragment the learning of care activities by health care professionals.

The holistic/integrated competency-based model is more valid and reliable than current ways of assessing professionals. It enables us to come closer than we have in the past to assessing what we want to assess (i.e. the capacity of the professional to integrate knowledge, values, attitudes, skills and other attributes in the real world of practice). This model requires the components shown in Figure 3.4 to be considered.

The specification of component skills that contribute to being competent would enable students to develop the essential practical skills required of the competent practitioner. These skills could be in the form of a 'clinical skills checklist', which in turn can be grouped into 'essential skills clusters' (e.g. communication, management of a group of patients/clients). These essential skills should be assessed at pre-specified standards commensurate with the stage of the education programme.

The assessment of personal attributes is a challenge. The specification of criteria will guide students and practice educators towards the development and assessment of personal attributes that are essential for effective professional practice.

REFERENCES

Ashworth, P., Morrison, P., 1991. Problems of competence-based nurse education. Nurse. Educ. Today. 11, 256–260.

Bedford, H., Phillips, T., Robinson, J., et al., 1993. Assessing Competencies in Nursing and Midwifery Education: Final Report. The English National Board for Nursing, Midwifery and Health Visiting, London.

Benner, P., 1982. Issues in competency-based testing. Nurs. Outlook. 30, 303–309.

Black, H., Wolf, A., 1990. Knowledge and Competence: Current Issues in Training and Education. Employment Department, Sheffield.

Bloom, B.S., Engelhort, M.D., Furst, E.J., et al., 1956. Taxonomy of Educational Objectives, Handbook 1: Cognitive Domains. Longman, London.

Bradshaw, A., 1998. Defining competency in nursing (part II): An analytical review. J. Clin. Nurs. 7, 103–111.

Bradshaw, A., 2000. Editorial. J. Clin. Nurs. 9, 319–320.

Braithwaite, D.N., Elzubeir, M., Stark, S., 1994. Project 2000 student wastage: a case study. Nurse. Educ. Today. 14, 15–21.

Castledine, G., 2000. New nurse competencies: are they adequate? Br. J. Nurs. 9 (5), 314–315.

City and Guilds, 1992. 3033: Care – NVQ Level 2. City and Guilds of London Institute, London.

Department of Health, 1999. Making a Difference. Department of Health, London.

Department of Health, 2004. The NHS Knowledge and Skills Framework (NHS KSF) and the Development Review Process. DH, London, Online. Available: <http://www.dh.gov.uk/assetRoot/04/09/08/61/04090861.pdf> (accessed December 2005).

DfES, 2005. NVQ: Department for Education and Skills Online. Available: <http://www.dfes.gov.uk/nvq/what.shtml> (accessed May 2005).

Directgov, 2012. Online. Available: <http://www.direct.gov.uk/en/EducationAndLearning/QualificationsExplained/DG_10039029> (accessed March 2012).

Eraut, M., 1998. Concepts of competence. J. Interprof. Care. 12 (2), 127–139.

Farley, A., Hendry, C., 1997. Teaching practical skills: A guide for preceptors. Nurs. Stand. 11 (29), 46–48.

Fletcher, S., 1991. NVQs Standards and Competence. A Practical Guide for Employers, Managers and Trainers. Kogan Page, London.

Fraser, D., Murphy, R., Worth-Butler, M., 1997. An Outcome Evaluation of the Effectiveness of Pre-registration Midwifery Programmes of Education. The English National Board for Nursing, Midwifery and Health Visiting, London.

Gerrish, K., McManus, M., Ashworth, P., 1997. Levels of Achievement: A Review of the Assessment of Practice. The English National Board for Nursing, Midwifery and Health Visiting, London.

Gonczi, A., Hager, P., Athanasou, J., 1993. The Development of Competency-Based Assessment Strategies for the Professions. National Office of Overseas Skills Recognition, Research Paper No. 8. Australian Government Publishing Service, Canberra.

Hager, P., Gonczi, A., 1996. Professions and competencies. In: Edwards, R., Hanson, A., Raggatt, P. (Eds.), Boundaries of Adult Learning Routledge, London, pp. 246–260.

Hart, A., Lockley, R., Henwood, F., et al., 2001. Evaluation of the Effectiveness of Midwifery Education in Preparing Midwives to Meet the Needs of Women from Disadvantaged Groups. The English National Board for Nursing, Midwifery and Health Visiting, London.

Health and Care Professions Council, 2008. Standards of conduct, performance and ethics. HCPC, London, Online. Available: <http://www.hcpc-uk.org/publications/standards/ (accessed August 2011).

Health and Care Professions Council, 2009 Guidance on conduct and ethics for students. HCPC, London. Available at http://www.hcpc-uk.org/publications/brochures/ (accessed August 2011).

Health and Care Professions Council, 2010a. Fitness to Practise Annual Report 2010. HCPC, London, Online. Available: <http://www.hcpc-uk.org/publications/reports/index.asp?id = 403> (accessed August 2011).

Health and Care Professions Council, 2010b. Information for Employers and Managers: The Fitness to Practise Process. HCPC, London, Online. Available: <http://www.hcpc-uk.org/complaints/> (accessed August 2011).

Health and Care Professions Council 2011. Standards of Proficiency. Online. Available: <http://www.hcpc-uk.org/aboutregistration/standards/standardsofproficiency/> (accessed August 2011).

The Health and Care Professions Order, 2001. Consolidated text incorporating repeals and amendments made up to 1st April 2010. HCPC, London, Online. Available: <http://www.hcpc-uk.org/assets/documents/10002D20HPORDER-2010CONSOLIDATION.pdf> (accessed July 2011).

Hilton, P.A., 2004. Record of achievement. In: Hilton, P.A. (Ed.), Fundamental Nursing Skills Whurr, London, pp. 306–313.

Hilton, S.R., Slotnick, H.B., 2005. Proto-professionalism: how professionalisation occurs across the continuum of medical education. Med. Educ. 39, 58–65.

Hutt, R., 1988. Lasting the course, Part IV: findings and conclusions. Senior Nurse. 10 (3), 4–8.

Jervis, A., Tilki, M., 2011. Why are nurse mentors failing to fail student nurses who do not meet clinical performance standards? Br. J. Nurs. 20 (9), 582–587.

Jessup, G., 1991. Outcomes: NVQs and the Emerging Model of Education and Training. The Falmer Press, London.

Le Var, R., 1996. NVQs in nursing, midwifery and health visiting: a question of assessment and learning? Nurse. Educ. Today. 16, 85–93.

Lindop, E., 1987. Factors associated with student and pupil nurse wastage. J. Adv. Nurs. 12, 751–756.

McGaghie, W.C., 1991. Professional competence evaluation. Educ. Res. 20 (1), 3.

Manpower Services Commission, 1985. Guidance Notes for Two-Year Youth Training Schemes. Manpower Services Commission, Sheffield.

Miller, C., 2010. Literature review: improving and enhancing performance in the affective domain of nursing students. Contemp. Nurse. 35 (1), 2–17.

Moore, D., 2005. Assuring fitness for practice: a policy review. Nursing and Midwifery Council Task and Finish Group, London.

NCVQ, 1991. Guide to National Vocational Qualifications. National Council for Vocational Qualifications, London.

Norris, N., 1991. The trouble with competence. Camb. J. Educ. 21 (3), 331–341.

Novak, S., 1988. An effective clinical evaluation tool. J. Nurs. Educ. 27 (2), 83–84.

Nursing and Midwifery Council, 2001. The Nursing and Midwifery Order 2001 (SI 2002/253). The Stationery Office, Norwich, Online. Available: <http://www.legislation.gov.uk/uksi/2002/253/contents/made> (accessed September 2011).

Nursing and Midwifery Council, 2005. Consultation on Proposals Arising from a Review of Fitness for Practice at the Point of Registration. NMC, London, Online. Available: <http://www.nmc-uk.org> (accessed December 2005).

Nursing and Midwifery Council, 2007. Essential Skills Clusters for Pre-registration Nursing Programmes. NMC, London, Online. Available: <http://www.nmc-uk.org/Documents/Circulars/2007circulars/NMCcircular07_2007.pdf> (accessed September 2011).

Nursing and Midwifery Council, 2008. The Code: Standards of Conduct, Performance and Ethics for Nurses and Midwives. NMC, London, Online. Available: <http://www.nmc-uk.org/Publications/Standards> (Accessed August 2011).

Nursing and Midwifery Council, 2009. Standards of Pre-registration Midwifery Education. NMC, London, Online. Available: <http://www.nmc-uk.org/Publications/Standards/> (accessed August 2011).

Nursing and Midwifery Council, 2010a. Standards of Pre-registration Nursing Education. NMC, London, Online. Available: <http://www.nmc-uk.org/Publications/Standards/> (accessed August 2011).

Nursing and Midwifery Council, 2010b. Fitness to Practise: How the Process Works. NMC, London, Online. Available: <http://www.nmc-uk.org/Hearings/How-the-process-works/> (accessed August 2011).

Nursing and Midwifery Council, 2010c. Guidance on professional conduct for nursing and midwifery students, 2nd edn. NMC, London. Available at www.nmc-uk.org/Publications/Guidance (accessed August 2011).

Nursing and Midwifery Council, 2011a. Nursing and Midwifery Council: Annual Fitness to Practise Report 2010-2011. NMC, London, Online. Available: <http://www.nmc-uk.org/About-us/Statistics/Statistics-about-fitness-to-practise-hearings/> (accessed August 2011).

Nursing and Midwifery Council, 2011b. Guidance on Professional Conduct for Nursing and Midwifery Students. NMC, London, Online. Available: <http://www.nmc-uk.org/Publications/Guidance/> (accessed September 2011).

Papadakis, M.A., Hodgson, C.S., Teherani, A., et al., 2004. Unprofessional behaviour in medical school is associated with subsequent disciplinary action by a state medical board. Acad. Med. 79, 244–249.

Papadakis, M.A., Teherani, A., Banach, M.A., et al., 2005. Disciplinary action by medical boards and prior behaciour in medical school. N. Engl. J. Med. 353, 2673–2682.

Percival, E., Anderson, M., Lawson, D., 1994. Assessing beginning level competencies: The first step in continuing education. J. Contin. Educ. Nurs. 25 (3), 139–142.

Phillips, T., Schostak, J., Tyler, J., 2000. Practice and Assessment in Nursing and Midwifery: Doing it for Real. The English National Board for Nursing, Midwifery and Health Visiting, London.

Roberts, D., 2009. Editorial: newly qualified nurses – competence or confidence? Nurse. Educ. Today. 29, 467–468.

Rutkowski, K., 2007. Failure to fail: assessing nursing students' competence during practice placements. Nurs. Stand. 22 (13), 35–40.

Skills for Health, 2005. National Occupational Standards and National Workforce Competences. Online. Available: <http://www.skillsforhealth.org.uk/frameworks.php> (accessed December 2005).

Skills for Health 2012. Helping you get the most out of your education and training. Online. Available: <http://www.skillsforhealth.org.uk/getting-the-right-qualifications/> (accessed March 2012).

Steinaker, N., Bell, M., 1979. The Experiential Taxonomy: A New Approach to Teaching and Learning. Academic Press, New York.

Storey, L., O'Kell, S., Day, M., 1995. Utilising National Occupational Standards as a Complement to Nursing Curricula. Department of Health, London.

Sutton, F.A., Arbon, P.A., 1994. Australian nursing – moving forward? Competencies and the nursing profession. Nurse. Educ. Today. 14, 388–393.

Teherani, A., Hodgson, C.S., Banach, M., et al., 2005. Domains of unprofessional behaviour during medical school associated with future disciplinary action by a state medical board. Acad. Med. 80 (suppl.), 17–20.

Toohey, S., 2002. Assessment of students, personal development as part of preparation for professional work – is it desirable and is it feasible? Assess. Eval. High. Educ. 27 (6), 529–538.

Training Agency, 1988. Development of Assessable Standards for National Certification. Guidance Note 1: A Code of Practice and a Development Model. Training Agency, Sheffield.

UKCC, 1999. Fitness for Practice. United Kingdom Central Council for Nursing, Midwifery and Health Visiting, London.

Watson, R., Stimpson, A., Topping, A., et al., 2002. Clinical competence assessment in nursing: a systematic review of the literature. J. Adv. Nurs. 27 (5), 519–524.

Wolf, A., 1995. Competence-Based Assessment. Open University Press, Buckingham.

Worth-Butler, M., Murphy, R., Framer, D., 1994. Towards an integrated model of competence in midwifery. Midwifery 10, 225–231.

Chapter | 4 |

How do we assess?

INTRODUCTION

It is discussed in Chapter 3 that competence is a construct that is not directly observable, but rather, is inferred from performance. Assessing performance will therefore be important to infer clinical competence. Equally important will be the requirement to gather sufficient evidence to justify the inference and, in particular, that a safe inference has been made (Gonczi et al 1993). Clinical competence is a complex entity and it almost always requires the practitioner to use a combination of attributes simultaneously and adapt practices to different contexts. Thus, the assessment of clinical competence is not straightforward and no one method can hope to assess overall competence. Moreover, some competencies are less easily assessed through performance than others. Hager & Gonczi (1996) state that it is not enough merely to observe performance in the complex world of professional work – a breadth of evidence is required to enable practice educators to make a sound inference that pre-registration health care students can perform competently in the variety of clinical situations in which they can find themselves.

What is therefore needed is a 'range of forms of evidence' (Bedford et al 1993) to provide this breadth so that practice educators can make valid and reliable inferences. Following their extensive review of the literature on assessment of competence to practise, Redfern et al (2002) drew the conclusion that a multi-method approach enhances validity and ensures comprehensive assessment of the complex range of skills required of pre-registration nursing students. Consequently, it is necessary to use planned combinations of a variety of methods of assessment to obtain this 'breadth of evidence' to evaluate overall clinical competence, so that assessors of clinical practice know with confidence that the student has the necessary knowledge, skills and attributes to ensure public safety and protection. In the standard to support learning and assessment in practice, the Nursing and Midwifery Council (NMC 2008) requires practice educators to consider how evidence from various sources might contribute towards making a judgement on performance and competence. Bedford et al (1993) suggest that the strategy of triangulation is utilized to obtain this breadth of evidence.

There is one key similarity between the processes of clinical assessment and research: simplistically, both seek to obtain data or evidence to add to the knowledge base about the subject and/or prove or disprove the case under investigation. In clinical assessment we seek data by which we obtain clearer perspectives of our learners, and evidence to confirm the achievement of competence for safe practice. When conducting clinical assessment there is much to be learnt from the rigour with which research studies are generally conducted in order to achieve validity and reliability of results. One rigorous research strategy is the use of triangulation.

In this chapter the importance of using the strategy of triangulation to achieve validity and reliability of assessment is explored. In research, the technique of triangulation is used to obtain more valid and reliable research data. The principles guiding the use of this technique will be extrapolated for use in assessment so that assessments can also be conducted with the same degrees of validity and reliability as in research. The uses, merits and limitations of a range of methods that can be used in the competency-based approach for the assessment of clinical practice are also explored and debated. To reflect the principle of integration through the use of the holistic/ integrated competency-based model of assessment (see Figure 3.4), integrated assessment approaches that use a combination of methods are put forward so that a number of competencies and their performance and knowledge outcomes can be assessed simultaneously.

TRIANGULATION

The theoretical perspectives of the term 'triangulation' are drawn from the literature on research, as literature that relates this term to the conduct of assessment is perfunctory and indirect (see, for example, Bedford et al 1993). Triangulation is a term borrowed by the social sciences from surveying and navigation. It refers to the principle of geometry that the third point of a triangle can be plotted using the two known points as the vertices (Fielding & Fielding 1986, in Redfern 1994). This concept of triangulation was first applied to research methodology by Campbell & Fiske (1959, in Redfern 1994) in psychological research as a metaphor to describe the use of several methods to measure a single construct in order to confirm a hypothesis. Triangulation in this context then does not mean three. Later researchers such as Denzin (1989) argue that triangulation is more than the use of several methods – it is the combination of '*methodologies*' used to investigate the same phenomenon. These 'methodologies' are referred to as '*types of triangulation*': four of them are described by Denzin (1989). From the work of Denzin, three types of triangulation are selected for exploration here, as these are seen to be relevant and applicable for the conduct of integrated assessments: they are therefore discussed and extrapolated to our discussion on assessment in this chapter. The types of triangulation are:

- method triangulation
- data triangulation
- investigator triangulation.

Method triangulation

There are two kinds of method triangulation: *within-methods* and *between-methods*.

Within-methods triangulation is the application of different types of the same method to measure a phenomenon. An example is that of using different scales to measure pain, such as a visual analogue scale, a Likert-type scale and a semantic differential scale. All these scales are different in the way they assess the amount and/or the quality of pain, but they are all examples of the same kind of method (i.e. *scales*). As a test of validity, the issue is whether they come up with the same answer when applied to the same patients at the same time.

When a student is assessed whilst caring for patients experiencing pain, the student can be observed by the assessor during clinical practice when caring for these patients. Arrangements can also be made for the student to be observed by a second assessor, thus generating evidence of performance using the 'testimony of others'. Both assessors are using the same assessment method (i.e. *observation*). As a test of validity, the issue is whether they come up with the same or similar answers of what the student is able to perform.

Between-methods triangulation uses different methods to measure the same phenomenon. The important point about using between-methods triangulation is that it is much more than the mere combination of several methods. Rather, the methods should be selected as a combined strategy so that the strengths of each are maximized and their limitations are minimized. Linking the data in a coherent and systematic way is essential. In the case of the student assessment above, an example of using between-methods triangulation is to ask questions about care you have observed the student giving. Questioning will establish, for example, whether there is a sound understanding of the needs of the patients who are experiencing the pain, which in turn should influence the care given. It may also reveal the attitudes of the student on this aspect of care or his/her attitudes towards the patients. The strengths and weaknesses of observation in determining performance evidence are complemented by the strengths and weaknesses of questioning in determining knowledge and understanding. As a test of validity, the answers of the student will augment the assessor's observation of performance.

Data triangulation

Data triangulation refers to the use of multiple data sources, with each source focused upon the phenomenon of interest (Denzin 1989). These data sources can differ by person, time or place. For example, data can be collected from different people or during different times or at different locations. The aim is that the data sources provide unique and diverse views about the same topic to contribute to validity and reliability: this enables the researcher to discover the dimensions of a phenomenon that are similar and dissimilar. As shown below, it is appropriate to make use of the three data sources as described by Denzin (1989) for the purposes of clinical assessment:

- *Person* – assessment evidence is collected from other assessors and/or student self-evaluation.
- *Time* – assessment evidence is collected on different clinical shifts over a period of time.
- *Place* – assessment evidence is collected from the different instances of practice provided within the range of context in the learning contract (see Ch. 6).

If we return to the example of assessing the student caring for patients who are experiencing pain, we can see how evidence from the three data sources can provide the assessor with diverse views about the student when caring for patients experiencing pain. Evidence provided by the testimony of the second assessor and student self-assessment will contribute to the validity and reliability of assessments of the student. If all sources agree that the student has achieved the performance and knowledge outcomes and is able to care for this category of patients, the assessment is likely to have validity. Conversely, if there is disagreement, the assessment could lack validity and/or reliability. The use of continuous assessment of practice will help to ensure that evidence collected on different clinical shifts reflects a wide range of conditions. Caring for different patients, working at different times of the day and working with different environmental stresses such as noise and busyness of the ward are factors that may influence how the student practises. The evidence collected from a range of occasions when the student cared for patients experiencing pain will provide information about the quantity and quality of learning. It will also serve to identify the strengths and weaknesses of the student in this aspect of care. For instance, does the student provide better care for the younger than the older patient? How well does the student cope when caring for these patients? Is the student able to assess the patient's need for pain relief with accuracy? Is the student able to plan care for these patients so that they are as comfortable as possible?

Investigator triangulation

Investigator triangulation occurs when the different knowledge and expertise held by members of the research team are used in the analysis of raw data. When several investigators are involved in a study, this type of triangulation helps reduce the potential bias that occurs when only a single investigator is involved. In clinical assessment, investigator triangulation takes place when the range of evidence contributed by different assessors is used in the analysis of student competence. This will help reduce the potential bias of a single assessor. In their research report on the assessment of competence, Bedford et al (1993) recommend that:

> *Assessment documentation should be broadened to include evidence contributed by more than one accredited witness ….*

These 'witnesses' could be the assessor, other clinical colleagues, the clinical link lecturer and the service user. Each person is likely to 'know' the student in slightly different ways and be able to contribute to identification of the range of learning that has taken place, what the strengths and weaknesses of the student are and so on. Investigator triangulation may be particularly valuable when attempting to evaluate the student's attitudes. Several people's views are likely to have been collected after independent assessment of the student, thus reducing biases and adding to the reliability of the assessment (Phillips et al 2000). Whilst there is a requirement for service user and carer involvement in all aspects of the social work degree (Department of Health 2002), the involvement is not well tested as a valid source of witness testimony (Rhodes 2012, Elliott et al 2005, Edwards 2003). The use of evidence from the service user will be considered later in the chapter.

So far, then, triangulation is about:

- the use of different assessment methods or ways of collecting assessment evidence
- ensuring that different assessment methods complement each other.

The main aim of using triangulation in clinical assessment is to obtain as complete a picture as possible of the student's achievement of competence, so that the assessment is valid and reliable. It is therefore important to remember that triangulation is more than just obtaining three (or more) sources or types of evidence: the evidence also needs to be linked so that an integrated and comprehensive assessment of the student is made.

Advantages and limitations of triangulation

Practically triangulation may be quite straightforward to arrange when plans are made for the supervision and assessment of students. Using triangulation to the extent that an integrated and comprehensive assessment of the student is made can prove to be challenging, which may be construed to be a limitation by some. However, the use of triangulation carries many advantages. Advantages and limitations are now considered.

You may wish to try Activity 4.1.

ACTIVITY 4.1

From the discussion so far on triangulation, what advantages and limitations can you elicit? Make a list of them. Compare your responses with the feedback in the text.

Advantages

1. *It allows confirmation of assessment evidence and increases confidence in the assessment decision made.* By combining the types of triangulation – that is, method, data and investigator triangulation – a fuller and more complete picture of the student's achievement or non-achievement is obtained. Different aspects of the student's competence can be identified so that there is a richer and deeper understanding of the student's learning, be it performance or knowledge and understanding or the development of some attitude or a set of values, which confirms our assessment of the student. This therefore increases our confidence when we are making the assessment decision. Consider this scenario: you have a student who is not achieving several competencies. You have come to this decision over several weeks of observing the student in practice and asking her questions about her practice. You wonder whether your decision is influenced by the fact that you do not like the student's green and red hair! Another assessor provides assessment evidence that confirms your decision. You probably breathe a sigh of relief and say: 'I'm not biased after all'. The testimony provided by another assessor increases your confidence in your assessment decision. *Does this enhance the validity, or reliability, or both, of your assessment?* (See discussion in Ch. 5.)

2. *It guards against a blinkered perspective.* The use of triangulation can potentially help to overcome the bias of 'single-method, single-observer' assessments (Redfern 1994). However, Redfern warns that the use of several methods and assessors may not compensate for assessor bias. It can be difficult to overcome strong likes and dislikes.

3. *It is more likely to portray a 'whole picture' of the student.* Rowntree's (1987) book has this question as the title: *Assessing Students: How Shall We Know Them?* Attempting to 'know' students so that we are fair in our assessments of them requires us to understand a complex and multidimensional being. Furthermore, competencies are generally complex, which requires the student to learn and develop several attributes concurrently (see Ch. 3 for a discussion of the holistic/integrated competency-based model). A range of assessment evidence will provide a richer and deeper understanding of the student's strengths and weaknesses and what has and has not been achieved, so that a fuller picture of the student's achievement is obtained. We will then be in a better position to provide the guidance and support that the student requires in order to learn and achieve some more.

4. *It allows divergent evidence to enrich explanation.* When triangulation is used we are more likely to obtain or be given unexpected and divergent assessment evidence about the student. This should be regarded as a bonus (Redfern 1994), as such evidence may explain some aspect of the student or the student's performance that has been eluding us. For example, a colleague who was working with your student may report to you that your student was observed to have been in tears when caring for a patient with terminal cancer. The student subsequently revealed that a close friend had recently died of cancer. For several weeks you have been attempting to involve the student in this aspect of care, but had been unsuccessful as the student was always reluctant. You were getting concerned that the student is not learning about care of patients with terminal cancer. The evidence from your colleague has served as a source of divergent evidence.

Limitations

1. *It is expensive on resources.* When using triangulation, arrangements need to be made for the student to learn and practise over a range of contexts over time. Several assessment methods, including other assessors, need to be used: more resources, such as time and extra assessors, are required. In today's climate of health care, where such resources are in scarce supply, the need for student supervision and assessment competes with the need to deliver care. It would be tempting, and certainly easier, to ignore the use of triangulation when assessing students! As was practised by the General Nursing Council for England and Wales in the 1970s, the use of 'one-off' assessment when student nurses were assessed on four 'one-off' occasions, for a stated period of time on each occasion, for four aspects of learning, was much more economical on resources: *Have you experienced this form of assessment? And how valid and reliable were the assessments?*

2. *It cannot compensate for assessor bias.* If we cannot overcome our biases, or if we are not aware of them, the use of triangulation will not help us achieve the validity and reliability we desire in our assessment.

3. *It may compound sources of error:* This point relates to Point 2 above. If we hold some biases and the other assessor also holds some biases that are different from ours, our assessment evidence will not be as objective as we perceive. In fact, the student could

be more disadvantaged than if we had not used the evidence from the other assessor.

4. *Methods selected may be inappropriate.* As discussed earlier, the assessment methods selected should complement each other so that a 'rich' range of evidence is provided to allow the development of professional competence to be assessed fully (Fotheringham 2010). This means we have to assess the development of knowledge, attitudes, skills and attributes. The selection of methods should allow the assessment of those areas of learning, performance and development equally, and not focus on the assessment of one or two domains of learning. For example, if we use observation to assess the student's performance, the testimony of another assessor was also based on observation of practice and simulation as our assessment methods, we have assessed very well the student's abilities to perform, but may not have assessed attributes such as understanding and attitudes well, if at all.

5. *Triangulation is no use with the 'wrong' research question.* This limitation is equally relevant to assessment. If we are not clear about *what* we want to assess, then triangulation is not going to enhance the validity and reliability of the assessment. It is therefore important to define, and describe clearly, the competency statement, the knowledge and performance outcomes we wish students to achieve.

You may wish to try Activity 4.2.

ACTIVITY 4.2

Debate the following with your colleagues:
  The limitations of the different types of triangulation are real and daunting. What can be done to reduce these limitations?

Despite the challenges and difficulties associated with the use of triangulation, the advantages of using this strategy indicate that it can give better opportunities to achieve validity and reliability of assessment. What this means when using the holistic/integrated competency-based approach to assessment is that both the *attributes* of the learner and the *performance* of key professional tasks are assessed. The discussion of competence in Chapter 3 stated that the attributes of individuals do not in themselves constitute competence. Nor is competence the mere performance of a series of tasks. Rather, the notion of competence integrates attributes with performance. Another point about competence to be reiterated is that competence is a construct that is not directly observable, but is inferred from successful performance. Therefore, combinations of assessment methods need

to be considered and used so that a range of evidence is provided to enable a safe judgement of competence to be made (Gonczi et al 1993).

ASSESSMENT METHODS

This section starts with Activity 4.3.

ACTIVITY 4.3

What methods do you frequently use to assess students you work with? Can you give reasons for your selection?

In my experience, the following methods are the most commonly used by assessors:

- working with the students and observing their practice
- asking questions leading to reflective discussions on contextualized practice
- obtaining the opinion (testimony) of other assessors
- checking care records made by the students.

Gonczi et al (1993) say that all existing methods of assessment used by a profession are potentially appropriate for use in the competency-based approach to assessment. They go on to explain that it is not the methods themselves that are competency-based but the *way* they are used, the *emphasis* given to the methods and *how results* are interpreted that are important in competency-based assessment. The uses, merits and limitations of a range of methods that can be used for the assessment of the different components of professional competence are now explored.

Observation of practice

Observation simply means watching and noting what you see (Stoker 1994). Stoker (1994:iv) says that 'observation is an essential tool in assessment – it is one of the most effective ways of finding out whether learning has taken place'. It is an NMC (NMC 2008) requirement that confirmation of clinical competence is made through direct observation of a student's delivery of care in the practice setting.

There is a better chance of making more accurate assessments if observation is part of a continuous process of working with the learner. Learners can be assessed on a number of occasions in their everyday working environment while they are performing in their 'natural' surroundings to give us a picture of their ability to perform a variety of real tasks so that direct evidence of competence can be collected. As the learner is watched in action, direct evidence of behaviours and behavioural patterns is obtained.

Far more reliable judgements about professional competence are therefore possible than with assessments conducted in limited time periods on limited ranges of context. Assessments are also more likely to have predictive validity.

There are two ways we can observe the learner's performance: by participant and non-participant observation. Working directly with the learner is known as *participant observation*. In research, during participant observation, researchers join the group, often keeping their identities a secret to try to minimize any changes in behaviour that participants may be inclined to make as a result of being observed (Swanwick 1994). In clinical assessment, however, the identity of the assessor cannot be made a secret! Therefore, the effects of being observed – the *observer effect* – may affect the learner's performance. The observer effect is discussed in Chapter 5. Another important point to bear in mind when observing practice is that of *observer bias* and how this may affect assessment; this is also discussed in Chapter 5.

Try Activity 4.4.

ACTIVITY 4.4

If you were being directly observed, how might your performance be affected?

The fact that someone is looking at us may make us nervous. Our actions may not be as smooth as usual, or we may have lapses of memory. I can recall an instance when I was observed during teaching practice – I dropped all my papers and acetates during the middle of the teaching session and I felt that I stuttered for the whole hour! *Have you had similar experiences?* On the other hand, we may exercise more attention to the task than we normally would. Again, I can recall many instances of teaching practice when I knew in advance that I would be observed and assessed. I have never since prepared my lectures, audiovisual aids, handouts and so on as meticulously, and lost so many nights of sleep!

In the above instances, we are obviously not giving a true picture of the way we practise. Is the validity, or reliability, or both, affected?

Observing the learner 'from a distance' is known as *non-participant observation*. In research, the researcher does not interact with the participants unless approached. If this happens, interaction is kept to a minimum (Swanwick 1994). During clinical assessment, we may observe the learner caring for a patient while we are performing another activity such as dispensing medications, talking to someone else and so on. What strategies have you used for observing a learner 'from a distance'?

Using the standards and performance criteria in a checklist

Fletcher (1991:66) stated that in competence-based assessment 'it is individual performance which is judged – and judged against explicit standards which reflect … the expected outcomes of that individual's competent performance …'. When assessing for the

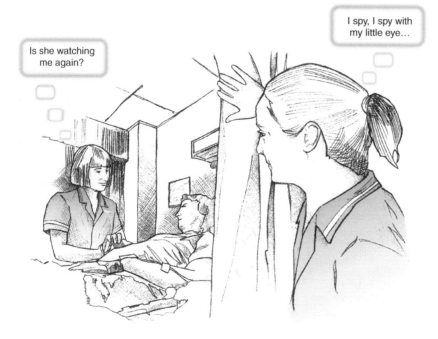

Is she watching me again?

I spy, I spy with my little eye…

Figure 4.1 Nerve wracking – or an opportunity to outshine?

development and achievement of a professional competency, the assessor looks for pre-specified behaviours such as the ways a skill is performed, or the ways the learner interacts with a patient, or how care is being given. These criteria are used to determine whether learning has taken place. When using observation to assess performance, noting these criteria in the form of a mental or written checklist (Stoker 1994) will guide the assessor's observation. Dawson (1992) says that:

The use of observation schedules in assessment is quite acceptable, and accurate, when the observer is seeking to identify pre-specified behaviours concerned with a given operation.

Ewan & White (1996) recommend the use of written checklists, as they have a high inter-observer agreement. They also have the advantages of ensuring *validity*, *discriminatory power* and *feasibility* (Stoker 1994), concepts that are discussed in Chapter 5. As checklists are generally detailed, they provide a useful profile of performance that can be discussed with the learner and other assessors.

When using written checklists, the following points may be useful to remember (Ewan & White 1996):

- longer checklists tend to be more reliable than shorter ones
- as checklists require the observer to judge whether certain behaviours have taken place, they are most effective where components of performance are specified in detail
- it is possible to include behaviours that may underpin aspects of attitudes and interpersonal relationships
- have three options for recording (i.e. *observed, not observed, not applicable*)
- important errors should also be noted
- if any essential component of the performance is omitted, the learner is assessed as *not yet competent* and is re-assessed.

In particular instances it becomes necessary to assess the process of performance (Gonczi et al 1993). When observing these instances of practice, the ways of performing a task can also be included in a checklist, such as:

- accuracy or lack of error
- speed of performance
- choice of the correct techniques
- the proper sequence of techniques
- adherence to regulatory and policy requirements.

Although the use of checklists has advantages, Ewan & White (1996) warn that if the criteria in the checklist emphasize the performance of a specific skill then beginning students may become fixated on specifics rather than learning the perspectives of care as a whole. Conversely, Benner (1984) thinks it necessary to break a psychomotor skill down into sequenced elements that the student can grasp in order to become technically competent as a beginning practitioner in the real world of clinical practice. One key facilitation skill of the practice educator is to be able to coach the student through the necessary paces to learn the psychomotor skill and, at the same time, learn about how to care for the patient.

Allow enough time for observation

Assessments, in general, sample only a fraction of what a learner is expected to know. This is inevitable as it is not feasible or desirable to attempt to assess every aspect of learning; for example, it would be impractical to attempt to assess a pharmacist's knowledge of every drug that could be encountered in everyday practice. Likewise, when assessing the competent clinical practice of students, inference of competence is inevitably based on a sampling of performance. Fish & Twinn (1997:114) made this important point about observing practice: 'all seeing is selective, and all reporting of what is seen is interpretive; there is no such thing as purely objective factual observation'. It is important to remember that competence is a construct that is not directly observable, but is inferred from successful performance. There must therefore be enough evidence so that we are confident that it is safe to make the inference that the learner is competent. The assessor must therefore allow enough time to observe the learner on a number of occasions so that it is possible for sufficient evidence of learning to be demonstrated. It is an NMC requirement (NMC 2008) that most assessment of competence should be undertaken through direct observation in practice. It is also a requirement that, whilst giving direct care in the practice setting, at least 40% of a student's time must be spent being supervised by the named practice educator. This working arrangement will give the practice educator more time to work with the student so that learning and progression can be monitored with accuracy.

How does the assessor know when there is enough evidence? Making an assessment decision based on concrete evidence is one of the key principles of competency-based assessment. This important aspect of competency-based assessment is discussed in Chapter 7.

So far, there has been a consideration of how to use observation as an assessment method, its usefulness or otherwise in ascertaining a true picture of the learner's ability in 'natural' surroundings and some of the difficulties associated with its use. To summarize, effective observation (Stoker 1994) requires you to:

- use a checklist
- allow enough time for observation
- be aware of observer bias
- be aware of observer effect.

Which components of competence can be assessed with any accuracy using observation? When a learner's performance is observed, only overt behaviours and behavioural patterns exhibited by the learner when care is performed can be seen. Although behavioural patterns may indicate the underlying attitude (Andrusyszyn 1989), inwardly held beliefs, values or feelings cannot be seen (Dawson 1992), nor can knowledge and understanding of the care or task be determined. As an observer, one can only say that the observable performance is mainly a reflection of the possession of skills. Observation is therefore useful only for the assessment of the skills developed that are contributing to effective performance at the time. Gonczi et al (1993), however, claim that observation allows assessment of attitudes and interpersonal skills.

Try Activity 4.5 on the use of observation as an assessment method.

ACTIVITY 4.5

Make a list of the uses/merits of observation and another of the limits of observation.

Advantages of observation of practice

- *Can provide a high level of integrated assessments.* As the learner is observed performing care and tasks, it is possible to use evidence of performance to assess several competencies and several components of competence simultaneously.
- *Allows assessment of attitudes and interpersonal skills.* Attitudes can be inferred from behaviours and behavioural patterns. Interpersonal skills can be directly observed.
- *Offers realistic evidence of competence.* Competence-based assessment uses explicit standards of occupational performance as its foundation. The logical way to assess whether someone is meeting those standards is to watch them working in that occupation (Fletcher 1991).
- *Allows evaluation of problem solving.* As the learner is observed managing a situation, it is possible to assess how well the learner has managed the situation. From this, it can be inferred that the learner has been able to solve the problem.
- *Mistakes in performance can be corrected.* Direct observation and supervision of practice will enable the practice educator to identify and correct any mistakes at the time or immediately afterwards.

Disadvantages of observation of practice

- *Circumstances of observation may be too specific.* Evidence obtained about the ability to perform in care situations that occur rarely generally cannot be used with any degree of validity towards the assessment of many competencies.

- *Requires lengthy and costly assessments for reliability.* The learner needs to be observed on more than one occasion to ensure reliability. This means that the period of assessment is longer rather than shorter and is therefore costly in terms of time and effort required.
- *Gives indirect evidence of knowledge/understanding only.* If a learner is able to perform the care or task, it can only be inferred that knowledge/understanding underpins that performance.
- *Does not assess ability to learn through practice.* Even if a learner is able to perform a task, or care for a patient, it cannot be assumed that the learner can transfer this performance to another situation and perform to the same standards another time.
- *Subject to observer bias and observer effect.* Polit et al (2010) state that one of the most pervasive problems with observation is the vulnerability of observational data to distortions and biases – human perceptual judgemental errors can pose a serious threat to the validity and accuracy of observational information.

In summary, direct observation of clinical practice is used primarily to obtain evidence of ability to perform when we assess the learning of practical skills and behaviours and behavioural patterns, which may indicate the underlying attitudes and value systems held by the learner.

An ability to perform is only one component of competence. Evidence of achievement of the other components of competence needs to be obtained using other assessment methods. Questioning frequently complements observation in that we are obtaining the 'indirect evidence' of competence, which is 'hidden' and not open to observation (Stoker 1994).

'Examination of products'

There are occasions when evidence of ability to perform may be inferred from an examination of the product of the learner's work – items that the learner produced or has worked on (e.g. a made bed and the surrounds, the bandaged stump of a below-knee amputation and so on). The level of achievement is judged by assessing the quality of the piece of work.

Questioning

It is discussed in Chapter 1 that one of the purposes of assessment is to maximize learning. Gipps (1994:15) made the point that 'assessment alone will not develop higher-order skills in the absence of clearly delineated teaching strategies that foster the development of higher-order thinking in pupils'. Asking questions is an integral part of teaching and learning, and places students in the role of active learners (De Young 1990). It is one teaching/learning strategy to help students develop higher level cognitive skills. Questioning can also serve as positive reinforcement for students when we indicate that answers are correct and/or insightful. This gives feedback to the student that material has been understood and higher level thought processes were used (Activity 4.6).

ACTIVITY 4.6

For what purposes have you used questioning?

In clinical assessment, questioning can be used for the following purposes:

- To assess baseline knowledge (e.g. knowledge of the stages of the grieving process).
- To assess ability to form links between previously isolated information (e.g. if a student midwife is learning how to support women in labour, questions could be asked about the support strategies used for the individual woman and how well these worked for that woman; further questioning could then lead the student to explore those common strategies that work, or do not work, for a number of women the student has looked after).
- To assess application of theory to practice (e.g. using the policy on infection control you had previously discussed with the learner, ask your learner to discuss the actions he/she would take when preparing for the admission of the next patient who requires barrier nursing).
- To assess understanding of care given (e.g. the rationale for using certain communication skills when comforting the dying patient; if the learner understands the *why* behind the use of these ways of communicating, it indicates that theory underpins practice).
- To assess problem solving skills (e.g. by posing: ... What's the real issue here? What other information do you need before you can solve this problem? How else could you ... ? Give reasons for .... What would happen if you tried ... ? What other options do you have?).
- To assess decision-making skills (e.g. by posing: ... What action would you take if ... ? Give reasons .... What do you intend doing about it?).
- It is possible to obtain an indication of underlying attitudes, values and beliefs (e.g. by posing: ... What do you think of euthanasia? ... detaining psychiatric patients under the Mental Health Act? Do you agree with Jenny's opinions? Why?).
- It is possible to assess verbal communication skills by the ability of the student in verbalizing responses.

From the above discussion of the uses of questioning, it can be seen that learning in the cognitive domain and affective domain (Bloom et al 1956) – and thus several attributes of competence – can be assessed using

this assessment method. When we assess learning in the cognitive domain, it is important to assess not only the knowledge base but also higher level thinking, so that the range of cognitive skills is assessed. The kinds of questions asked will stimulate different kinds and levels of thinking and the learner will then become aware of the kind and level of thinking expected (Perrott 1982). Formulating questions to assess higher level thinking can be tricky. An understanding of how questions can be classified may assist in the framing of those questions that are necessary to elicit the level of thinking required of the learner.

The most popular classification system is based on Bloom's taxonomy of educational objectives (Bloom et al 1956). Although the taxonomy was developed to classify educational objectives, questions can be related to each level of the taxonomy. Table 4.1, adapted from De Young (1990), lists the cognitive activity at each level, as well as some sample questions.

With the assistance of the information in Table 4.1, try Activity 4.7.

ACTIVITY 4.7

Examine one learning outcome that a learner has to achieve. Formulate one question at each level of Bloom's taxonomy so that you can assist your learner to develop the range of higher level cognitive skills.

The aim is to structure questions so that they define a linking path, as these are more valuable in assessing the quality of learning and helping the learner to develop higher-level thinking (Minton 1997). Do not be too concerned if you have had difficulties formulating the questions. Many trained teachers manage only to ask questions predominantly at the lower cognitive levels (De Young 1990). In view of the high-level thinking required of health professionals, however, it is beneficial to assess students at the application through to evaluation levels (see Table 4.1). Stoker (1994) says that using questions effectively is an essential skill in assessment. This skill should, and can, be developed. The reader is referred to the chapter on questioning in De Young (1990) for a further discussion of how to frame and ask questions.

It is important to remember that, when questioning is used in clinical assessment, the main aim is to gain evidence about how much learning has taken place (i.e. how much of the competency the student has achieved). Questions asked should therefore be related to the competency and be based on the context of the practice event. The following checklist on the use of questioning may be helpful. It builds upon the work of Stoker (1994):

- Are the questions relevant to the learner? Do they relate to things the learner needs to know and should know rather than focusing on unusual aspects of the subject?

Table 4.1 Question classification according to Bloom's taxonomy

Category	Cognitive activity required	Sample question words	Examples of questions
1. Knowledge	Recall	What	What is the definition of glaucoma?
	Questions, regardless of complexity, can be answered by simple recall of previously learnt material	Identify Define When Describe List Which Who	At what age do infants begin to crawl?
2. Comprehension	Understanding	Compare	What does the nursing process have in common with the scientific method?
	Questions can be answered by merely restating and reorganizing material in a rather literal manner to show that there is understanding of the essential meaning	Contrast Differentiate Explain Extrapolate	Why does intravenous tubing have to be free of air?
3. Application	Solving	Apply	Given these arterial blood gas results, what nursing interventions are needed?
	Questions involve problem solving in new situations with minimal identification or prompting of the appropriate rules, principles or concepts	Consider How would Checkout	How would you obtain a blood pressure reading on a person with third-degree burns of all extremities?
4. Analysis	Exploration of reasoning	Support your	What is the major premise behind Kubler-Ross's theory of death and dying?
	Questions require the student to break an idea into its component parts for logical analysis, facts, opinions, logical conclusions, etc.	What assumptions What reasons	What data would you need to support this nursing diagnosis?
5. Synthesis	Creating	Think of a way	Given all of the data in this case study, what nursing diagnoses can be developed?
	Questions require students to combine ideas into a statement, plan, product, etc., that is new for them	Create Propose Plan Suggest	Think of a way that we could research the relationship between those variables.
6. Evaluation	Judging	Judge	Of the two possible nursing interventions in this situation, which would be more appropriate?
	Questions require students to make a judgement about something using some criteria or standard by making their judgement, principles, or concepts	Which would Consider Defend What is the most appropriate	

(Adapted with permission from Craig & Page 1981.)

- Are the questions appropriate for the stage of the course of the student?
- Is the wording clear? Does it indicate what sort of answer you require?
- Have you provided some sort of feedback at the time? Be especially aware of how you deal with incorrect or incomplete answers. Try not to let your reaction have the effect of demotivating the learner.
- Be careful not to make learners feel that you are trying to catch them out.

The limitations of using questioning for assessing clinical practice are:

- Questions cannot assess attitudes, values and beliefs with accuracy, as what the learner says may not be a reflection of inwardly held beliefs.
- The learner may feel threatened. This may affect the responses, and an inaccurate picture is formed of the student's ability.
- Inappropriately framed questions may not elicit the correct responses.
- Questioning can be time consuming.
- It may not have predictive validity. Correct responses to questions may not reflect the ability to perform.

As the use of questioning in the clinical setting is frequently related directly to the care-giving experiences of the learner, questioning sessions may lead to a discussion of these instances of practice. It is generally believed that *reflection on practice* – where the thinking done in one situation is made explicit and built on to be used in another – should be developed through discussion that takes place away from the arena of care activity (Bedford et al 1993). The use of discussions in clinical assessment is now examined.

Discussion around care and care activities

De Young (1990) says that topics that are most suitable for discussion are controversial issues, clinical or professional problems, and emotionally laden topics such as death and dying. After deciding on which clinical event you wish to explore further with the student through discussion, you need to provide some structure for the discussion. De Young (1990:87) made this important point about the use of discussion: 'Good discussions do not just happen spontaneously; they require careful planning'. She suggests making the following arrangements before you start:

- Be clear about what you want the student to learn – set some objectives.
- Plan the physical environment – use a room where you will not be interrupted; ensure that the seating is adequate.

During the discussion, take on the role of the facilitator (Rogers 1983). As you work with students during discussions, you can assess their development of those attributes desirable of a competent practitioner. Depending on the topic and the skills of the facilitator (De Young 2009, 1990, Ewan & White 1996, Oliver & Endersby 1994), students may have the following learning opportunities:

- To consider and explore the principles, concepts and theories used in that particular practice situation and transfer such learning to new and different situations.
- To clarify information and concepts.
- To develop critical thinking skills, leading to the development of problem-solving and decision-making skills. Bedford et al (1993) emphasize the importance of post-event discussion in fostering the development of high-quality decision-making and problem-solving skills.
- To develop and evaluate their beliefs, values and attitudes, leading to attitude change. The use of discussion to bring about attitude change is well documented (De Young 1990). As students are facilitated to give and take during the discussions, they learn whether the stance they take on a particular issue is clear, logical and defensible.

Bedford et al (1993:139) advocate that discussions should be critical and take place *before*, *during* and *after* an activity 'through which the activity is reviewed and analysed'. They say that these critical discussions move the assessment activity from being mere surveys of 'activities "done" and skills "covered" to a collaborative, analytical discussion about practice' and divorce criticism from personal attack. Bedford et al (1993:136) emphasized that it is 'assessment discussion' rather than simple discussion that complements observational data in the assessment of competent practice:

> *Through discussion about a particular event, students can demonstrate the knowledge, understanding and values that have informed their actions in the clinical area on a given occasion, enabling assessors to test their own observation-based judgements about the quality of those actions. The great advantage of assessment dialogue, as opposed to simple discussion, is that it facilitates learning as part of the assessment process.*

Assessment discussions can help students to develop 'situational understanding' that will help them live with, and negotiate a way through, the competing and contradictory values they encounter as they perform care (Phillips et al 2000). Among others, Elliott (1991) and Schön (1987) postulated that professional practice is learned and developed through 'doing' and 'reflection on doing'. During the course of assessment discussions then, students are allowed to voice their understanding, views and opinions, disagreements and doubts, their *range of cognitive skills* and *attitudes, values and beliefs* can be assessed.

Assessment discussions around practice can thus be held:

- *Before* an activity – when the student is being prepared for taking part in the care. The student's knowledge, understanding and perhaps attitude, values and beliefs can be assessed when questions are asked during discussions
- *During* an activity – as the student performs, discussions can be held to check understanding. Care has to be taken that there is minimal interruption to the student's attention and concentration on the performance.
- *After* an activity – when care is reviewed and analysed. During the analysis, the range of cognitive skills, such as knowledge, understanding, problem solving and attitudes, values and beliefs developed or altered as a result of the experience can be discussed. Post-activity discussion should be held as soon as possible after the experience, while events are still fresh in the mind, to allow more accurate recall of details and for any feedback to have more impact.

Learning diary

Assessment discussions can also be conducted using the student's learning diary entries as the basis. In proposing that reflective understanding should be developed around written evidence of practice, Bedford et al (1993) call for assessment documentation to require:

> *… written accounts of analytical reflection on the relationship between particular clinical events and general nursing and midwifery principles.*

They believe that documentation – in this instance the student's learning diary – that requires discussion between the practice educator and student is more likely to promote assessment discussion on practice. Learning diaries can offer insight into how students make sense of and feel about their practice. It is possible that students may choose to write only that which they want to be read (Phillips et al 2000). Nevertheless, it provides an evidence base and focus for dialogue (Phillips et al 2000) and gives a starting point from which to begin an assessment discussion with the student. As a source of evidence of practice, learning diaries can be considered by more than one assessor. The creation of a databank of sharable evidence was advocated by Bedford et al (1993). The views of another assessor would enrich the assessment evidence base on the student and is one way of achieving investigator triangulation.

Facilitating and assessing learning through reflective assessment discussions using the student's diary is not straightforward (Stuart 1997). Flexibility and abilities to deal with the unexpected are required. When 'working' with a student's diary entry, the following framework may assist in carrying out the reflective assessment discussion with intent:

1. Consider the level of detail in the student's account of the incident.
   - Is there any description/discussion of the incident in relationship to personal involvement?
   - Have the actions taken by the student been discussed in terms of the negotiation undertaken within the situation (Phillips et al 2000)?
   - Is there any description/discussion of the incident in relationship to the involvement of others?
   - What suggestions would you make so that the quality of the account could be enhanced?
2. Consider the ways in which the student has explored personal behaviours, feelings and thoughts and those of others involved.
   - Is there a constructive exploration of behaviours and actions, thoughts and feelings?
   - How perceptive is the student?
   - Was there an objective appreciation of how and why self and others behaved, felt and thought as they did?
   - Was there any indication of how these affected the incident?
   - What suggestions would you make to help the student explore these further?
3. Consider the ways in which the student has used or referred to relevant theory and literature.
   - Is relevant underpinning knowledge identified?
   - Is there any indication of application of theory to practice?
   - Has the student critically analysed theory and current literature and their relationship to practice?
   - What broad theoretical areas may be included in order to explore the incident further?
   - What broad professional issues may be brought into this incident?
4. Consider the amount of learning the student has extracted through the incident.
   - Has the student identified any implications for future practice?
   - Does the student specify how own practice can develop?
   - Does the student integrate any 'new' learning with previous knowledge to reach different/new perspectives about care?
   - Have any assumptions about current practice been critically appraised?
   - Has the student suggested alternative ways for practice?
   - What influenced the choices made about the way care was done (Phillips et al 2000)?
   - What constraints affected any decisions made (Phillips et al 2000)?
   - What suggestions would you make to help the student develop the above issues further?

Try Activity 4.8. Do not rush it.

ACTIVITY 4.8

Obtain a learning diary entry of a student. Using the above framework, work through the diary entry with a colleague.

Diaries are considered to be an effective way of encouraging active reflection on experience, particularly where a review takes place with the assessor at some point in the future (Boud et al 1985). As the basis for reflective assessment discussion, it will allow the student opportunities to justify personal actions by giving the rationale for choices in different circumstances. The student is likely to feel valued, as the incident under discussion has been personally identified as important. To an extent, the student is taking control of personal learning by identifying what is important. By an inclusion of the requirement to record not only behaviours and actions but also feelings and thoughts, the student may indicate attitudes, values and beliefs held about particular situations. Although diaries can be used to assess attitudes, values and beliefs, Dawson (1992) says that any such assessment should be formative, as attitude is dynamic and changes over time.

What aspects of learning can be assessed through the reflective assessment discussion of a student's diary? Assessing learning through this process is complex (Boud et al 1985). In using the framework suggested above to facilitate the reflective discussion, the following aspects of learning may be assessed:

- the perceptiveness of the student in the situation
- the self-awareness of the student
- communication and interactive skills
- unobserved practical skills
- underpinning knowledge
- ability to apply theory to practice
- higher level cognitive skills such as problem solving and decision-making
- attitudes, values and beliefs.

Every assessment method has disadvantages and limitations! There are several limitations of using the student's learning diary for assessment:

- it does not assess ability to perform in the practical setting
- it can be time consuming
- it may not have predictive validity
- it may not have reliability, as each incident is different
- it may not elicit the appropriate responses if the assessor is unskilled in facilitating reflective assessment discussions.

Testimony of others

Harlen (1994:3) observed that 'all forms of assessment are subject to human judgement and thus require some form of moderation'. In the section on triangulation, the use of investigator triangulation was suggested as a means of reducing the potential biases of a single assessor. The potential diversity of views from more than one assessor would also enrich and strengthen the assessment database on the learner. This section will consider the use of testimony of others as an assessment method.

Testimony from other practitioners

As the student's key practice educator, you need to take into account the several perspectives about the achievement of the student and, during that process, draw out both commonalities and points of disagreement (Bedford et al 1993). In practice, explicit arrangements are made for the student to work with other professional colleagues who may assess the student by observing the student's practice. Evidence from observation can be complemented with evidence from other assessment methods. When students spend time working with members of the multidisciplinary team, these members of the team may also be called upon to provide assessment evidence. Making arrangements for the student to work with, and be assessed by, others has the advantage of making the assessment more feasible, as the student will have more opportunities to practise. As the key assessor, you are responsible for coordinating learning and assessment activities so that they are purposeful – the student will then have a fair chance of achieving learning outcomes and competencies. The arrangements you make with other practitioners should include:

- briefing them about the learning experiences that the student needs
- the learning outcomes and competencies to be achieved
- the level of performance expected of the student.

Ewan & White (1996) and Bedford et al (1993) caution that we have different standards of practice, which may lead to inconsistent expectations, and judgements of our student. These issues may be compounded if practice educators lack confidence in their professional expertise and feel threatened by students with a more theoretical orientation (Jervis & Tilki 2011). The reliability of assessments will be reduced and validity may be compromised.

Duffy (2004) found that one of the reasons that assessors were not failing students was that they had inadequate knowledge of the assessment process of students they were assessing. Later studies, for example, by Jervis & Tilki (2011) and Luhanga et al (2008) found that assessors lacked confidence in making decisions to refer students. In these instances where unsafe students are passed, the reliability and validity of assessment are clearly compromised.

Try Activity 4.9.

ACTIVITY 4.9

Make some suggestions to reduce inconsistencies among practice educators and thus increase the validity and reliability of your assessment.

Some suggestions you and your team of assessors may wish to consider are:

- regular practice educator meetings to confer on criteria for high standards of practice
- regular practice educator meetings to confer on the expected levels of performance in comparison with an ideal standard; having a common standard among practice educators will help to rate a student's performance at the level expected of students for that stage of the training, which has the advantage of ensuring that assessments have discriminatory power (see Ch. 5 for a discussion of this)
- using a checklist for observation
- discussing the criteria in the checklist with the other practice educators to avoid multiple interpretations
- appropriate training and regular updating of practice educators
- openly discussing personal biases with each other so as to deal with them objectively
- soliciting the assistance of the link lecturer from the higher education institution.

Assessment evidence from others – termed 'witness testimonies' – should be collated by the key assessor. This could be in the form of verbal discussions or in a written format. Written witness testimonies are a requirement of the National Vocational Qualification (NVQ) system (DfES 2005). The assessment process in the new Health N/SVQs and Health and Social Care N/SVQs launched in February 2005 (Skills for Health 2005) encourages the use of expert witnesses to provide evidence in the form of witness testimonies that contributes to the assessment of the competence of the candidate. Expert witnesses who have current expertise and occupational competence are to be used if there are no occupationally competent assessors for those occupationally specific units.

Testimonies should:

- be specific to the clinical activity
- give a brief description of the background and circumstances of practice
- identify the aspects of competence demonstrated
- state the standard achieved by the student – that is, how well the student has performed.

Box 4.1 is an example of a witness testimony.

Box 4.1 **Witness testimony on student nurse Mary**

During an afternoon shift, Mary was assisting in the care of clients on the short-term area of the unit. When sitting with a client called Joseph during tea time, Mary observed him having an epileptic seizure. I was away from the area at the time, so Mary immediately called for help. On entering the dining room, I observed that Mary had moved Joseph's food and drink away from him and was supporting his upper body and head while offering reassurance. It was obvious to me that Joseph was experiencing a series of seizures as he appeared to regain consciousness for a short time and then enter into another seizure. Both of us continued to support him until he had fully recovered.

During the discussion that followed this incident, I praised Mary for acting quickly by calling for help and ensuring a safe environment by removing the food and drink, which may have harmed Joseph. Although Mary could not name the specific type of seizure, she was able to describe the client's behaviour, which allowed me to assess the type of seizure. More important, Mary had remembered the importance of maintaining the safety of the client by supporting his upper body and head to ensure a clear airway. Mary also reported that she had made a note of the time and duration of the seizure and was able to explain the reasons for recording such information in the client's care file.

Mary acted in a competent and professional manner during this incident and followed the correct procedure when administering first aid.

Testimony from users

Another group of people who could potentially provide testimonies about student performance are the users. Users are patients, clients and carers who are current or recent recipients of a service (Jones et al 2009). There is an increasing impetus to involve users in all aspects of health and social care education (Department of Health 2002, 2009, NMC 2010). The pre-registration degree in social work requires service user and carer involvement in all aspects of the course (Department of Health 2002). In 2005 the NMC explored ways of involving lay people in the assessment of practice by, for example, directly soliciting feedback from patients/clients and carers on care given by students, or indirectly by contributing to examination boards and moderating panels as members. More recently, in its *Standards for Pre-registration Nursing Education*, the NMC stated that *programme providers must make it clear how service users and carers contribute to the assessment process* (NMC 2010).

As recipients of care given by students, users are a legitimate source of assessment data. Who can say with more accuracy whether the nurse was kind or gentle, or explained and reassured before giving the injection? Neary (2001:9) found that patients and clients do assess students informally as illustrated by this statement from a patient: 'Nurse [name] took me for a bath today. I feel safe with her, the way she encouraged me into the bath, … I was frightened I'd fall … Nurse [name] never left my side, gave me confidence, she did, good lass that she is'. A study by Redfern and Norman (1999a,b) found that the congruence between patients' and nurses' perceptions of quality care was high and significant. There is also evidence from the field of medicine where the high scores given by patients on the performance of medical students correlated well with the scores given by the doctors (Braend et al. 2010). This suggests that user assessment of student performance is likely to be valid and reliable. User comments and complaints (following the appropriate investigations) could, feed into the assessment of individual students.

However, formalizing and gaining access to this source of assessment evidence can be fraught with difficulties around organizational barriers, professional and academic politics (Repper & Breeze 2007). Moriaty et al (2010) report that the most frequent type of involvement was informal feedback with some service users completing a 'compliments form' and feedback forms where their involvement was formalized. From their work on developing a user testimony tool to assess the clinical practice of pre-registration nursing students, Chapman et al (2011) identified that communication, comfort and treating individuals with respect are areas of care that could be assessed by users. These areas fit well with the competency domains of professional values, communication and interpersonal skills and nursing practice and decision-making (NMC 2010). It is suggested here that some of the items in the *Professional Behaviours Inventory* contained in Appendix 1 may be adapted for use within a user testimony tool.

Testimony from the student's peers

Another group of possible assessors comprises the student's peers. Peer reviews are becoming an increasingly important feature of professional practice (Lankshear & Nicklin 2000). Peer assessment during training provides opportunities for students to learn to rate the work of other students, helping students to develop collaborative skills; it builds on the skills of giving feedback and develops professional responsibility (Papinczak et al 2007, Gomez et al 1998), thereby preparing aspiring professionals for evaluating the work of others. Stengelhofen (1993) says that peer feedback is important in laying down the concept that it is part of professional work to be observed and evaluated by one's own colleagues. A criticism of student peer assessment is that students are not experts – so this is a case of the 'blind leading

the blind' (Jarvis & Gibson 1997). If students are to be expected to perform peer assessment, training should be provided.

The student's peers have a useful contribution to make in the overall assessment process of both theory and practice. Peers frequently work for sustained periods in close proximity; they therefore have the opportunity to make assessments that may be inaccessible to others. Burke (1969, in Rowntree 1987) found that students are realistic when assigning grades to their peers. However, Gomez et al (1998) report that peers may be biased in providing only favourable information because of not wanting to cause trouble for someone, or having unrealistic expectations of their peer. A later study by Papinczak et al (2007) found that scores from student peer assessment were significantly higher than those from tutor assessments.

It is suggested here that peer assessment is used to contribute to the formative assessment process whereby students may be assisted by peers to develop more accurate impressions of themselves and their abilities.

Simulation

In some situations it may not be possible to assess learners' performance in the real situation as exemplified in Box 4.1. Reasons may be a shortfall of learning opportunities(e.g. dealing with emergency situations), or it may not be desirable to assess learners' performance with real patients or in real situations because of risks or discomfort to patients or the learner. In midwifery education, student midwives could qualify without having had experience in dealing with obstetric emergencies (Westwood-Timms 1995). In these instances, the same simulation exercises used for teaching can be used to assess learning (De Young 1990). This section discusses the use of simulation to provide another source of assessment evidence.

A simulation is the reproduction of the essential features of a social or physical reality that corresponds to a real-life situation that a student or client might encounter. During a simulation learners can be put into a situation where they can experience some aspect of the real situation by becoming involved in activities that are closely related to it. Advances in technology during the last decade have generated opportunities to create realistic simulations during which pre-registration health care students can develop and demonstrate clinical skills without endangering real patients. Gibbs (1988) maintains that simulation is an invaluable substitute for experience. When using simulations, the aim is to create a scenario that resembles the real-life situation as closely as possible so that the learner's responses and behaviours can be assessed with some degree of validity and reliability (De Young 1990). Such learning is more likely to be transferred to the real setting.

All simulated activities cannot take account of the complexities of the 'real' clinical environment. The amount of learning that can be transferred to the real-life setting is debatable (Fero et al 2010, Shepherd et al 2010, Wotton et al 2010, Quinn 2000). Shepherd et al also state that learning within different domains requires different forms of simulated teaching.

Rethans et al (1991, cited in While 1994) claim that assessments of students during simulated activities have predictive validity for performance in actual practice. Research on the use of simulations as an assessment activity has shown that achieving reliability is generally not a problem (De Young 1990). What is questionable is the validity of this testing procedure. At the very least, students will have had the opportunity to experience, and perhaps internalize, the actions and reactions required of a given situation.

Simulated activities can give more control over what happens in the assessment as consistent and comparable experiences can occur for all students. For example, if the same scenario to assess the achievement of several students is used, the conditions of performance and the criteria for assessment will remain the same. The assessment is more likely to be reliable. The validity of the assessment can be increased by close representations of simulations to actual practice situations (Forker & McDonald 1996).

Simulations can take the following formats:

- enacting a simulated clinical situation
- analysing a simulated clinical problem
- using educational models
- using computer-based simulation
- objective structured clinical examinations.

Enacting a simulated clinical situation

This format can be used for many social and emergency situations. It closely resembles the use of role play, except that the learner will 'play' the part of the health professional and someone else will 'play' the part of the patient or relatives or some other role. In simulating the clinical situation, we should remember that we are assessing the learner's development into the health professional – this, therefore, requires the learner to play that role. Quinn (2000) states that one of the hallmarks of simulating the clinical situation is that the learner is not expected to act out any kind of script but, rather, is expected to behave and react in a way that is thought and felt to be appropriate. It therefore involves learners to be themselves and to deal with situations using their repertoire of normal everyday professional behaviour and clinical skills.

Hoban & Casbergue (1978, cited in DeTornyay & Thompson 1987) put forward four principles to consider when using simulations:

- The responses and behaviours – knowledge, attitude, skills – that are expected at the end of training should be specified, as well as the minimal acceptable level of performance the learner is required to demonstrate.

- The simulation should represent reality with enough fidelity to ensure face validity of the test of the learner's performance.
- The simulation being used to assess performance should be standardized for all learners to achieve validity and reliability of assessment.
- Decisions regarding the purpose of the assessment should be made before a simulation is used.

An activity is now used to illustrate how a simulated exercise of a clinical situation can be carried out (Activity 4.10).

ACTIVITY 4.10

You are planning to involve your learner in a simulated exercise to give her practice in explaining aftercare and home visits to a patient following discharge from the ward. How should you plan for and conduct the simulation?

There are several key steps to follow:

1. Thoroughly prepare the scenario, including setting learning outcomes for enacting the simulated clinical situation. In Activity 4.10, you will need to collect information about the patient and any problems the patient may encounter at home, the illness of the patient, the home and surrounding environment, any social support and so on. Creating a simulation as near as possible to the real-life situation that the learner will encounter enhances retention so that the established behaviours can be transferred more easily to the real setting (Quinn 2000).
2. Brief the learner, and the person who is playing the part of the patient. The learner and the 'patient' need to be prepared, particularly if they have not been involved in a simulated exercise before. This involves thorough briefing about the roles they will be playing, the intended learning outcomes to be achieved and agreeing any ground rules. Briefing ensures that the learner is more likely to benefit from the activity.
3. Allow sufficient time to carry out the activity. The learner is expected to behave and react in any way she/he feels is appropriate, as the simulation is not scripted. As discussed above, a simulation involves the learner in 'being herself/himself' and dealing with the situation using her/his natural reactions and behaviours. The success of the exercise therefore depends to a large extent on the selection of the simulated 'patient' (Ewan & White 1996). A 'patient' who is a good role player will put the student through her/his paces!
4. Debriefing and processing the learner's responses and behaviours to give feedback is an important final step.

Debriefing should be immediate and is the key to successful simulation (Wotton et al 2010). It should facilitate reconstruction of real-time representations of students' interactions and build on existing knowledge to form mental representations of clinical problems. The following points may be used to guide the debriefing:

- allow the student to self-evaluate
- identify the concepts learned
- relate learning to the outcomes of the exercise
- discuss any problems encountered
- discuss application to clinical practice
- give feedback (e.g. discuss if the student needs to do it differently).

What aspects of learning can be assessed using enactment of a simulated clinical situation?

What can be assessed will depend on the simulated activity. In the example above, it is possible to assess the following aspects of learning:

- knowledge of how the illness has affected the patient
- knowledge of resources and social and support services for the patient
- knowledge of the arrangements to be made prior to discharge of a patient
- communication and interpersonal skills
- decision-making and problem-solving skills
- attitude about discharge planning.

If a scenario requires the performance of physical activities such as enacting the drill for an emergency situation, as in a cardiac arrest, responses and reactions during an emergency can be assessed. In these simulated clinical situations, the use of the 'thinking aloud' technique is helpful in developing knowledge and clinical reasoning processes (Corcoran-Perry & Narayan 2000). The 'thinking aloud' technique requires the learner to think aloud while making decisions: this makes the reasoning process of the learner explicit and transparent. In their study, Corcoran-Perry and Narayan tape-recorded the thinking aloud verbalizations for later transcription. Analysis of the transcripts revealed the cues attended to, the inferences generated and the actions proposed.

Analysing a simulated clinical problem

This format can be used for many social and emergency situations. A written simulated clinical problem, as close to life as possible, is presented to the learner, who analyses the problem and discusses how the problem would be managed. De Young (1990) recommends that written simulated clinical problems have these features:

- Use real cases as far as possible – these are better because of the wealth of information from which to draw; fabricated cases too often become just summaries of what supposedly happened. The more

complex simulations should be based on real cases with all the variables that were involved. Phillips et al (2000:161) recommend that 'assessees should be enabled to work with accounts of practice that tell it like it is and thereby map real practice problems with richly described contextual details'. The assessment is more likely to be valid by focusing on the reality of practice rather than idealized versions.

- The cases that you choose should not be esoteric or unique – the purpose of simulations is to teach and assess learners to solve typical problems and confront commonplace information that they can transfer to their clinical practice.
- The case should be appropriate for the learner's level of knowledge and experience. Cases that are too easy are boring and are also not likely to stimulate thinking. Those that are too difficult may defeat the objectives – the emphasis in simulations is on the learning process; the learning of content should be a by-product (Ewan & White 1996, De Young 1990).

De Young suggests that simulations can be taken home for the learner to work on for subsequent presentation, or they can be used for 'on-the-spot' assessment. Westwood-Timms (1995) reports the use of written simulations in midwifery education to assess student midwives' ability to manage obstetric emergencies. These were used for 'on-the-spot' assessment; these assessments were reported to have reliability. The validity of these assessments was not reported. Box 4.2 gives an example of a clinical problem used by Westwood-Timms.

What aspects of learning can be assessed using analysis of a simulated clinical problem? To analyse a simulated clinical problem successfully, the student requires prior knowledge and, perhaps, practical experience of similar situations. During the analysis, and the subsequent solving of the problem, the student has to exercise higher level cognitive skills. Westwood-Timms (1995) devised assessment criteria to assess the full range of cognitive skills, including the higher cognitive skills of

---

Box 4.2 **Undiagnosed twin births**

It is fairly busy on the labour ward in a consultant obstetric unit. There are three midwives on duty, including you and two student midwives. One of the student midwives is with you for the shift.

You admit a 30-year-old multigravida at 36 weeks of pregnancy in advanced labour. She is accompanied by her husband. A female baby is delivered soon after admission. The baby appears smaller than you would expect for the gestation. On palpation of the mother's abdomen, a second fetus is detected. Fortunately, the oxytocic drug has not been administered.

How would you manage this situation?

analysis, evaluation and synthesis. In the scenario given in Box 4.2, it is possible to assess the following aspects of learning:

1. Underpinning knowledge, ability to assess the situation and planning the care
   - analysis of the facts presented
   - formulation of an action plan
   - rationale for the choices and strategies in the action plan.
2. Problem-solving and decision-making skills
   - ability to predict potential problems and/or complications
   - ability to select relevant cues and to discriminate in order to reach an appropriate decision
   - ability to prioritize actions and the rationale for the decisions
   - ability to delegate care.

It is possible to assess attitudes and values held by the student. Practical skills cannot be assessed. Gipps (1994) warns us that intentions to measure higher-order thinking can be subverted by repeated practice on the task. Intended higher-order tasks such as analysis of a simulated problem can be turned into rote tasks. If many opportunities are provided to practise a task so that the criteria for its assessment are learned – such as how to resuscitate a person – that task is then learned through rote learning.

Try Activity 4.11 with your colleagues.

ACTIVITY 4.11

Compile a list of problems that you and your colleagues have dealt with that can be used for simulated problem solving and management. Include the details of each problem. This will form a set of teaching/learning resources that can be kept in a file and be added to.

Using educational models

Educational models may be used to assess skills such as cardiopulmonary resuscitation, suctioning, catheterization, dressing change, administration of injections and so on. In midwifery education, models may be used to assess a learner's ability to perform complex skills and manoeuvres such as performing a breech birth or managing a shoulder dystocia. Fletcher (1995, in Medley & Horne 2005) used the term 'fidelity' to describe the degree of accuracy between the simulation and the real experience. Static or low-fidelity models are used for the practice and testing of specific skills, whereas high-fidelity models challenge students to make clinical decisions based on data obtained from assessments

and interventions made on the model. Features of high-fidelity models such as palpable pulses, visible respirations, measurable blood pressure and pulse oximetry are programmed by computer. High-fidelity simulators imitate most physiological responses, and some simulated patients can initiate conversation and respond verbally.

Aspects of learning that can be assessed are:

- ability to perform the care and practical skill correctly and in the right sequence
- other aspects of performing the procedure correctly, such as maintaining cleanliness or asepsis, using the right equipment, preparation of the environment, disposal of used equipment and so on
- attitudes towards the performance of the skill (e.g. the importance attached to the observation of maintaining asepsis)
- if the 'thinking aloud' technique is used (see above), the 'thinking' of the learner can be assessed while the procedure or skill is being performed
- if observation is supplemented by the use of questioning, it is possible to assess knowledge and understanding of performing that skill.

What are the advantages and disadvantages of learning to perform a skill using a model?

- patient safety is not compromised
- patient rights are protected
- learner anxiety is reduced, as practice is in a protected environment
- 'unlimited' and protected opportunities for practice until 'perfection' is achieved!
- errors can be corrected and discussed immediately
- likely to have reliability, as consistent and comparable experiences can occur for all students
- may not have predictive validity, as the complexities of the real world are absent
- communication skills and interpersonal skills cannot be assessed.

Using computer-based simulation

Computers are used increasingly to provide sophisticated simulations of clinical events, both for training and for assessment purposes. As mentioned above, computers program high-fidelity models to simulate realistic clinical situations and challenge students to make clinical decisions based on data obtained from assessments and interventions made on these models. Students' understanding of the systems and concepts upon which the simulations are based can be assessed in a conventional way such as using a written test.

There are, however, a variety of ways of designing assessment directly around the use of computer simulations. Using computer graphics, realistic patient care situations similar to those likely to be encountered in clinical practice are presented that closely represent actual reality. Learners are assessed managing that simulated situation by their responses to a series of cues and changes in variables of the patient condition. Responses are recorded and a print-out is then handed in for assessment. Patient management problems can also be used to assess problem-solving skills. In medical training, such problems typically begin with a patient's presenting complaint (Cantillon et al 2004). Learners then select appropriate items of history, examination and investigation before making a diagnosis and outlining a management plan. As the ability to solve problems is generally context specific, a larger number of patient management problems are usually necessary to ensure reliability of the test.

An example of a high-fidelity computer simulation is MACPUFF, which was developed by Manchester University Medical School for learning about and assessing the management of patients with respiratory problems (Brown et al 1996). The simulated patient can be set up with a chosen set of respiratory variables in a particular atmospheric environment. The patient is then 'run' for several minutes to see what happens to various vital indicators of physiological functioning. Biochemical measures are calculated, listed every 3 seconds and plotted on graphs. The complex chemical interactions involved in maintaining a stable and healthy respiratory state can thus be observed. Students' understanding of these interactions, which inform the management of the patient, can be assessed by setting up the patient using different variables. The student is then required to manipulate conditions such as the amount of oxygen required to stabilize the patient's condition. The assessment of the student could include the requirement to stabilize the patient's condition within certain parameters and within a certain time limit. Such a goal cannot be achieved by trial and error, but only through an understanding of the biochemistry of respiration. The variable patient conditions during the simulations help to ensure the validity and reliability of assessments.

Aspects of learning that can be assessed using computer-based simulations are discussed in 'Analysing a simulated clinical problem' above. It needs to be acknowledged that, to implement computer-based simulation, students and assessors must be conversant with the use of both the software and hardware, and adequate computing facilities should be available.

Objective structured clinical examinations (OSCEs)

In their literature review on the use of OSCEs, Redfern et al (2002) reported that, following its introduction by Harden et al in Scotland in 1975, the OSCE is now widely used in medicine in Canada, the USA, the Netherlands and elsewhere. An OSCE is not an assessment method in the same way as observation or question and answer. It is basically an organization framework comprising multiple testing points called 'stations' around which students rotate. Students perform at these stations and are assessed on specific tasks. The OSCE is best suited to the testing of clinical, technical and practical skills and can do so across a broad range, often with a high degree of fidelity (Newble 2004). OSCEs have been used predominantly by teaching staff in university laboratory settings to assess competence in performing psychomotor skills, ability to analyse and interpret data, take a patient's history, identify and solve problems, make clinical decisions and the use of interpersonal and communication skills (see, for example, Meechan et al 2011, Rentschler et al 2007, Govaerts et al 2001, Phillips et al 2000, Ladyshewsky 1999, Fahy & Lumby 1988). The assessment evidence of competence from this source can supplement other sources of evidence.

As students have to be tested at each station in turn, it means that several students can be tested simultaneously during each OSCE – in practice, the number of stations set up will determine the number of students going round during the OSCE. The conventional use of an OSCE is to rotate students through a series of 5-10-minute stations where standardized simulated professional tasks are performed under the observation of one or two assessors, who score the performance against a checklist on a marking sheet. Questions may be asked during the performance to supplement evidence obtained through observation.

There are alternative ways of conducting an OSCE. For example, stations may be much longer and examiners may not be present if the simulated patient on whom the task is performed undertakes the marking. Another variant is the inclusion of stations where multiple-choice questions or other forms of written responses are required (Newble 2004). Nicol & Freeth (1998) report the use of an OSCE that utilized one station only. The station was a simulated hospital or community setting where the student 'cared for' one simulated patient only for 30 minutes while working alongside the assessor. Communication skills, prevention of cross infection and recording of vital signs were assessed in all students as they were considered to be core skills. Other skills assessed depended on the needs of the patient and were drawn from a pre-determined schedule of skills that students at that stage of training were expected to be able to carry out at the appropriate level of performance. Performance was evaluated by the student, 'patient' and the assessor. Standardized questions prompted students to evaluate their own performance and opportunities given to correct poor or incorrect performance. The student self-evaluation fed into the summative rating of the performance that was done in consultation with the simulated patient.

A sample of performance was audio- and video-taped for validation and evaluation by an external examiner. It was concluded that this OSCE has high fidelity, avoids lengthy, task-oriented checklists and face, content and construct validity and inter-rater reliability are acceptable. Nicol & Freeth claim that the inter-rater reliability was enhanced by the requirement to use a 'prompt list' of expected behaviours when assessing students for that station and assessment of 10% of students by independent moderators who were experienced assessors.

One key limitation of assessment evidence from OSCEs is that the performance of students under laboratory conditions may not reflect their performance in real clinical settings. Furthermore, ability to perform the specific task or solve the specific problem at one station is a very poor predictor of ability to perform another, even similar, task or problem (Newble 2004). This means that wide sampling across problems is required to obtain an adequate level of reliability and content validity. Other limitations are that students find it stressful (Phillips et al 2000); it focuses more on the assessment of basic and technical skills rather than complex cognitive skills (Sharp et al 1995 in Redfern et al 2002); it compartmentalizes the clinical assessment of patients and students may therefore not learn to assess patients holistically (Harden et al 1975) and it may be too expensive for regular formative assessment (Blake et al 1995).

Evidence of the reliability and validity of assessment evidence from OSCEs is conflicting. Nicol & Freeth (1998), Govaerts et al (2001) and Ladyshewsky (1999) report high reliability and validity of this test procedure, whereas Phillips et al (2000) report that as a form of assessment it is seriously flawed, having neither inter- nor intra-assessor reliability. While acknowledging the value of intense psychometric research since the introduction of OSCEs, Walsh et al (2009) and Hodges (2003) also question the validity and reliability of OSCEs. Hodges stated that an OSCE is a 'social drama' with 'scripts and parts for actors to play' and 'students modify their performance in order to convey the impressions they believe their audience desires' (Hodges 2003:1134, 1136). The following measures have been reported to increase the validity and reliability of the use of OSCEs:

Reliability is increased when:

- Assessors are carefully trained (Nicol & Freeth 2002, Redfern et al 2002).
- Assessors are experienced (Nicol & Freeth 2002).
- There is more than one assessor (Weinrott & Jones 1984).
- Scoring is standardized (Nicol & Freeth 2002, Harden & Gleeson 1979. This could be in the form of checklists. Newble (2004) however, warns that the phenomenon of 'trivialization' could occur when using checklists: this is when detailed checklists do produce reliable scores but which do not truly reflect the examinee's performance of the task; only criteria that are easy to define are included at the expense of equally or more important criteria and appropriate weightings of the criteria are not made. He suggests that, within the framework of structured tasks, the use of global ratings by informed or trained assessors may be as reliable or even more reliable.

- A large number of stations are used to enable wide sampling across problems and learning tasks (Newble 2004).
- A separate written test is added to the requirement to perform at the stations (Redfern et al 2002, Verhoeven et al 2000).
- There is periodic review of assessment procedures to confirm that testing remains unbiased (Humphris & Kaney 2001).

Newble (2004) suggests that validity is increased when:

- Problems that learners need to be competent in dealing with are generated by expert groups or by more formal studies based on observation and analysis of what that group of learners will have to undertake.
- Tasks within the problems or conditions in which the student is expected to be competent are defined. For example, if the problem was 'dyspnoea', tasks might include taking a history from a patient with dyspnoea, performing and interpreting a pulmonary function test, demonstrating competence in assisting a patient into the optimal position for minimal respiratory effort, demonstrating competence in the administration of oxygen using the range of equipment available and educating a patient about the use of medication for the relief of dyspnoea and, if appropriate, health promotion measures to prevent the deterioration of the respiratory illness.
- A 'blueprint' is constructed. This is a way of including the sample of items to be included in the test. The simplest form is a two-dimensional matrix with one axis representing the generic competencies such as history taking, communication skills, management skills and care planning skills. The other axis represents the problems or conditions on which the competencies will be demonstrated.
- There is wide sampling across the competencies.

Readers are referred to the text by Abbatt & McMahon (1993) for the logistics of staging an OSCE. The papers by Walsh et al (2009), Hodges (2003) and Redfern et al (2002) provide literature reviews of research on OSCEs.

The next three methods of assessment to be considered will focus on the use of written evidence of competence. These methods are:

- care records made by the learner
- case study presentation by the learner
- project or assignment compiled by the learner.

Care records made by the learner

This section starts by considering a scenario: try Activity 4.12.

ACTIVITY 4.12

You wish to assess your learner's ability to record an accurate history, assess, plan and document the care needs of a client admitted to the unit. How can the learner be assessed?

The learner has to demonstrate the ability to obtain the history in the first instance, and subsequently to record the history, assessment of the client and plan of care in writing. The most appropriate way to assess this is to observe the student taking the history and then to examine the written records made by the learner. The activity of interviewing a client to obtain a history followed by the formulation and documentation of a care plan is one way of integrating assessment so that several competencies can be assessed concurrently.

What can we find out about the learner?

The observation will tell us how the student attempted to establish rapport and develop a relationship with the patient, how and what type of communication skills were used, the accuracy of the questioning and so on. The care plan and records made by the learner will tell us whether:

- all the relevant information has been obtained
- the student is able to analyse and synthesize the information in a meaningful way, resulting in an accurate assessment of care needs
- the student is able to plan care using the above information
- the student has achieved the standards of record keeping required; in the case of nurses and midwives these standards are laid down by the Nursing and Midwifery Council (NMC 2007).

Subsequently, as the learner cares for the client and is able to maintain a continual review of care needs, this should be reflected in the changes made to the care plan. In this instance, we will be able to assess the learner's ability to:

- evaluate the effectiveness of care given
- solve any problems
- involve the patient/client in planning care
- make decisions about client needs
- manage change
- work as a member of the multi-professional team as most patient/client needs require input from a range of professionals.

Most of these are higher-level cognitive skills that the beginning student may not have acquired. It would therefore be inappropriate to assign such a task to a junior student. There are other areas of learning that can be assessed through a student obtaining a client history with the subsequent development of a care plan:

- underpinning knowledge of the condition or illness
- knowledge of the history to be taken and effective communication skills in order to obtain an accurate and comprehensive history; an understanding of the information obtained and the ability to analyse the information in order to synthesize information meaningfully
- problem-solving and decision-making skills in order to evaluate and make changes to care as required
- effective written communication skills in order to maintain standards of record keeping
- the standards of the records may tell us about how important the student views record keeping.

Examination of care records, however, may not tell us about the student's attitudes towards the task. Rowntree (1987) gives the example of the ability of a medical student in eliciting information from the case histories compiled, but the fact that he antagonized each and every one of the patients by his arrogant and insensitive manner was concealed.

Case study presentation by the learner

Case studies provide students with the opportunity to carry out an in-depth study of one particular patient/client in their care over a period of time. In the written format this method of assessing learning is more frequently used for the assessment of theory. However, the evidence of learning provided by a case study can be used as one source of evidence for the assessment of competence in the clinical setting. This evidence can be examined in the written format or be presented verbally by the student. Some elements guiding the compilation of a case study are:

- an orientation to the patient/client
- the socioeconomic background of the patient/client and the influence of this on the development of the condition/illness
- draw on and integrate theory from a range of subjects to explain the nature and cause of the condition/illness
- the problems/difficulties encountered by the patient/client and the care required
- the rationale for the care, management and treatment
- contributions made by other members of the multidisciplinary team and their importance
- identify services available
- evaluate the effectiveness of care.

What aspects of competence can be assessed using a case study?

These include:

- knowledge base surrounding the case study
- an understanding of that knowledge
- application of theory to practice
- ability to assess, plan, implement appropriate care and evaluate care
- possibly assessment of attitudes and interpersonal skills.

Practical skills cannot be assessed. A difficulty when assessing the case study is that it may reflect idealized standards of care rather than actual care given (Lankshear & Nicklin 2000). This will then reduce the validity and reliability of that assessment.

Project or assignment compiled by the learner

It is possible to arrange for the learner to carry out a small-scale project or assignment. On completion of the work it is usual to provide a written record for assessment. Rowntree (1987) suggests that, if students are allowed to set their own objectives and how to achieve them, we can assess not only the product but also, more importantly, the process of learning. Like the case study, a project or assignment is more frequently used for the assessment of theory. The evidence of learning, however, can be used as one source of evidence for the assessment of competence in the clinical setting to give us a more holistic measurement of competence. Through examination of a project or assignment, it is possible to assess the following (Quinn 2000, Rowntree 1987):

- knowledge and understanding of the subject under investigation
- application of theory to practice
- creativity
- independence and resourcefulness
- how the situation was managed (e.g. coming up with solutions to problems will be indicative of problem-solving and decision-making skills).

The above qualities and attributes are some of the hallmarks of a competent practitioner and are therefore important for the student to develop. Practical skills and attitudes cannot be assessed with accuracy.

SELECTING AND COMBINING METHODS OF ASSESSMENT

Gonczi et al (1993) say that, in competency-based assessment, the methods selected should be most direct and relevant to the nature of the competency being assessed. Some methods of assessment are simply inappropriate for the assessment of certain aspects of competence. For example, interpersonal communication skills cannot be assessed using written assessment methods; manual dexterity and psychomotor skills cannot be assessed through verbal assessment methods. Attitudes, the most difficult aspect of competence of all to assess, may elude assessment altogether if special care is not exercised. The careful selection of method is thus required so that the assessment method matches the type of attribute being assessed. An examination of the uses, advantages and limitations of the assessment methods discussed in this chapter will help you consider which combination of methods will be most suitable to assess the particular attributes of competence.

When selecting methods for use in the holistic/integrated competency-based assessment system, Gonczi et al (1993:20) provide two guiding principles:

1. The assessment should be as integrated and holistic as possible (i.e. combinations of attributes should be assessed simultaneously). For example, when a student is observed admitting a patient, attributes such as knowledge of the admission procedure, communication and interpersonal skills, record keeping skills and so on can be assessed simultaneously.
2. The assessment should be as direct as possible (i.e. as close as possible to the real-work situations in which these combinations of attributes are employed).

The key question arising is this: How well will the methods assess the capacity to function appropriately across the uncertain situations of professional practice? Redfern et al (2002) found that the use of a multi-method approach enhances validity and ensures comprehensive assessment of the complex repertoire of skills required of students in nursing. Whilst this may be the case, inevitably, not all the professional attributes needed to function in the dynamic world of practice can be assessed holistically and directly. Therefore, combinations of methods need to be considered which will provide the range of evidence on which a judgement of competence can be made. The principles underpinning the use of the strategy of triangulation should also be taken into account when selecting and combining methods.

Other factors to be considered when selecting methods are:

- The time available to assessors – busy practitioners are generally hard-pushed for time to be assessors to learners who end up competing for the practitioner's time (Beskine 2009, Phillips et al 2000, Bedford et al 1993).
- The confidential nature of some aspects of work limits the capacity to undertake assessment in the

real situation, e.g. when learning counselling skills in the mental health setting, it may not be desirable to learn the skills and be assessed when working directly with these clients. Simulated activities may be required.

- The methods are not biased against particular groups of learners. Rowntree (1987:60) made the point that 'to treat people equally is not necessarily to treat them fairly. Indeed, people being so different, equal treatment probably means injustice for most'.
- The methods should be acceptable to the learners (e.g. not all learners feel comfortable taking part in enacting simulated clinical situations).

The following combinations of methods are suggested for assessing the components of competence discussed in Chapter 3.

1. To assess the components of competence in the cognitive domain use:
   a. questioning
   b. assessment discussion
   c. analysis of simulated clinical problems
   d. computer-based simulation
   e. OSCE
   f. care records
   g. testimony of others
   h. project or assignment
   i. case study.
2. To assess technical skills and performance use:
   a. direct observation of practice
   b. examination of work products
   c. testimony of others
   d. simulation of clinical situations
   e. OSCE.
3. To assess reflective practice use:
   a. questioning
   b. assessment discussion
   c. testimony of others
   d. care records
   e. case study
   f. project or assignment.
4. To assess attitudes and ethics of care use:
   a. questioning
   b. assessment discussion
   c. observation
   d. testimony of others
   e. simulation of clinical situations.

Assessment of attitudes and ethics of care abound with difficulties (Dawson 1992, Andrusyszyn 1989), and frequently pose a 'gap' in assessment strategies (Fraser 2000). Toohey (2002) warns that what we do not assess sends a particular message to students, as they tend to view that only what is assessed deserves their time, attention and effort. It is difficult to assess and measure attitudes, beliefs and values directly. We can, however, observe behaviours and behavioural patterns that may be reflective of their personal attributes (Toohey 2002), and the underlying attitudes and values held by the students (Andrusyszyn 1989). As discussed in Chapter 3, the use of criteria in the format of pre-specified behaviours expected of a professional exhibiting the appropriate conduct may assist.

CONCLUSION

In a system of competency-based assessment, any of the assessment methods described in this chapter can be used. From the discussion on the uses and limitations of the range of assessment methods, it can be seen that no one method will enable the assessment of all the components of competence. It is of course neither desirable nor economical to use all the assessment methods. It is, however, important to select and combine methods so that their strengths and weaknesses complement each other and methods are relevant to the nature of the competency being assessed. In choosing the methods to be used there will always be a need to balance the competing demands of resources and availability of learning opportunities and the necessity to obtain the range of evidence required to make a judgement of competence.

In general, a move in the direction of competency-based assessment requires the greater use of more direct methods of assessment that more closely match the kinds of day-to-day tasks undertaken by professionals. This emphasizes the importance of the use of methods that directly assess performance and the other attributes of competence and requires clinical assessors to make professional judgements in interpreting what the minimum acceptable levels of competence are in respect to professional standards. Assessment methods that are 'subjectively scored', such as observation and simulation of practice, need to be managed to ensure reasonable reliability to accompany greater validity. A high level of professional expertise is required to assess the work of others (Luhanga et al 2008, Phillips et al 2000, Gerrish et al 1997, Bedford et al 1993). Being an expert in a profession is essential, but is not enough. It is important to have some level of expertise in the assessment process. The next chapter addresses issues relating to the management of the assessment process, in particular the competency-based assessment system, so that assessments can be made with validity and reliability.

KEY POINTS FOR REFLECTION

Competence is a construct that is not directly observable, but is inferred from successful performance. Therefore, combinations of assessment methods need to be considered and used so that a range of evidence of capable performance is provided to enable a safe judgement of competence to be made.

- The strategy of triangulation in clinical assessment is to combine the use of several methods of assessment to obtain as complete a picture as possible of the student's achievement of competence. Methods selected should complement each other so that a 'rich' range of evidence is obtained.

- Triangulation allows confirmation of assessment evidence and increases confidence in the assessment decision made; guards against a blinkered perspective; is more likely to portray a 'whole picture' of the student and allows divergent evidence to enrich explanation.

- However, it is expensive on resources; it cannot compensate for assessor bias; it may compound sources of error, it is of limited use if assessment outcomes are unclear and assessment methods selected are inappropriate.

- In competency-based assessment, it is not the methods themselves that are competency based; rather it is the *way* they are used, the *emphasis* given to the methods and *how results* are interpreted that are important.

- Assessment methods selected should be most direct and relevant to the nature of the competency being assessed. Combinations of methods need to be able to obtain and provide the range of evidence on which a judgement of competence can be made.

- When selecting and combining methods, ask how well the methods will assess the capacity to function appropriately across the uncertain situations of professional practice.

OBSERVATION

- This is an essential tool in assessment – it is one of the most effective ways of finding out whether learning has taken place as direct evidence of competence can be collected.

- Working directly with the learner is known as *participant observation*, but beware of observer effect and observer bias.

- Observing the learner 'from a distance' is known as *non-participant observation*.

- Using checklists contributes to validity and reliability of the observation.

- Allowing enough time makes the use of observation more effective.

QUESTIONING

- Asking questions is an integral part of teaching, learning and assessment, and places students in the role of active learners, assisting them to develop higher level cognitive skills.

- Structure questions so that they define a linking path, as these are more valuable in assessing the quality of learning and helping the learner to develop higher level thinking.

- Questioning is used to assess learning in the cognitive and affective domains, thus assessing several attributes of competence.

DISCUSSION

- The discussion of a particular care event can assess the knowledge, understanding and values that have informed their actions in the clinical area on a given occasion, enabling assessors to test their own observation-based judgements about the quality of those actions.

- During these assessment discussions students should be facilitated to voice their understanding, views and opinions, disagreements and doubts.

- Assessment discussions can also be conducted using the student's learning diary entries as the basis.

TESTIMONY OF OTHERS

- All forms of assessment are subject to human judgement and thus require some form of moderation.

- The student's key assessor needs to take into account the perspectives from other assessors about the achievement of the student and, during that process, draw out both commonalities and points of disagreement. These 'witness testimonies' are then collated.

- Testimonies should be specific to the clinical activity, give a brief description of the background and circumstances of practice, identify the aspects of competence demonstrated and state the standard achieved by the student: that is, how well the student has performed.

- It is possible to use testimonies from patients/clients and their carers, and the student's peers.

SIMULATION

- A simulation is the reproduction of the essential features of a social or physical reality that corresponds to a real-life situation that a student might encounter. During a simulation, learners can be put into a situation where they can experience some aspect of the real situation by becoming involved in activities that are closely related to it.

- Simulated activities cannot take account of the complexities of the 'real' clinical environment. The validity of this testing procedure is questionable as the amount of learning that can be transferred to the real-life setting is debatable.

- Simulations can take the following formats:
  - enacting a simulated clinical situation
  - analysing a simulated clinical problem
  - using educational models
  - using computer-based simulation
  - objective structured clinical examinations.

CARE RECORDS MADE BY THE LEARNER

Formulating, documenting and making changes to a care plan is one way of integrating assessment so that several competencies can be assessed concurrently.

CASE STUDY PRESENTATION BY THE LEARNER

Case studies provide students with the opportunity to carry out an in-depth study of one particular patient/client in their care over a period of time. It is possible to assess attitudes, interpersonal skills, knowledge, understanding, the ability to assess, plan, implement and evaluate care surrounding the case study.

REFERENCES

Abbatt, F., McMahon, R., 1993. Teaching Health-care Workers: A Practical Guide, second ed. Macmillan Education Limited, London.

Andrusyszyn, M.A., 1989. Clinical evaluation of the affective domain. Nurse. Educ. Today. 9, 75–81.

Bedford, H., Phillips, T., Robinson, J., et al., 1993. Assessment of Competencies in Nursing and Midwifery Education and Training. The English National Board for Nursing, Midwifery and Health Visiting, London.

Benner, P., 1984. From Novice to Expert: Excellence and Power in Clinical Practice. Addison-Wesley, Menlo Park, CA.

Blake, J.M., Norman, G.R., Kinsey, E., et al., 1995. Report card from McMaster: Student evaluation of a problem-based medical school. Lancet 345 (8 April), 899–902.

Bloom, B.S., Engelhart, M.D., Furst, E.J., et al., 1956. Taxonomy of Educational Objectives Handbook I: Cognitive Domain. Longman, London.

Boud, D., Keogh, R., Walker, D., 1985. What is reflection in learning?. In: Boud, D., Keogh, R., Walker, D. (Eds.), Reflection: Turning Experience into Learning. Kogan Page, London, pp. 7–17.

Braend, A.M., Gran Frandsen, S., Frich, J.C., et al., 2010. Medical students' clinical performance in general practice – triangulating assessments from patients, teachers and students. Med. Teach. 32, 333–339.

Brown, S., Race, P., Smith, B., 1996. 500 Tips on Assessment. Kogan Page, London.

Burke, R.J., 1969. Some preliminary data on the use of self-evaluation and peer-ratings in assigning university course grades. J. Educ. Res. 62 (10), 444–448.

Beskine, D., 2009. Mentoring students: establishing effective working relationships. Nurs. Stand. 23 (30), 35–40.

Campbell, D.T., Fiske, D.W., 1959. Convergent and discriminant validity by the multi-trait, multi-method matrix. Psychol. Bull. 56, 81–105.

Cantillon, P., Irish, B., Sales, D., 2004. Using computers for assessment in medicine. Br. Med. J. 320, 606–609.

Chapman, L., James, J., McMahon, K., 2011. Involving patients in assessment of students. Nurs. Times. August 30, **107**, 34.

Corcoran-Perry, S., Narayan, S., 2000. Teaching clinical reasoning in nursing education. In: Higgs, J., Jones, M. (Eds.), Clinical Reasoning in the Health Professions. Butterworth-Heinemann, Oxford, pp. 249–254.

Craig, J.L., Page, G., 1981. The questioning skills of nursing instructors. J. Nurs. Educ. 20, 20.

Dawson, K.P., 1992. Attitude and assessment in nurse education. J. Adv. Nurs. 17, 473–479.

Department of Health, 2002. Requirements for social work training. Department of Health, London.

Department of Health, 2009. Education Commissioning for Quality. Department of Health, London.

Denzin, N., 1989. The Research Act, third ed. McGraw Hill, New York.

DeTornvay, R., Thompson, M.A., 1987. Strategies for Teaching Nursing, third ed. John Wiley & Sons, New York.

De Young, S., 2009. Teaching Strategies for Nurse Educators, second ed. Prentice Hall, Harlow.

De Young, S., 1990. Teaching Nursing. Addison-Wesley, Menlo Park, CA.

DfES, 2005. NVQ: Department for Education and Skills website. Online. Available: <http://www.dfes.gov.uk/nvq/what.shtml> (accessed May 2005).

Duffy, K., 2004. Failing Students Report. Nursing and Midwifery Council, London, Online. Available: <http://www.nmc-uk.org> (accessed December 2005).

Edwards, C., 2003. The involvement of service users in the assessment of diploma in social work students on practice placements. Soc. Work. Educ. 22 (4), 341–349.

Elliott, J., 1991. Action Research for Educational Change. Open University Press, Milton Keynes.

Elliott, T., Fraser, T., Garrard, D., et al., 2005. Practice learning and assessment on BSc (Hons) social work: service user conversations. Soc. Work. Educ. 24 (4), 451–466.

Ewan, C., White, R., 1996. Teaching Nursing: A Self-instructional Handbook, second ed. Chapman & Hall, London.

Fahy, K., Lumby, T., 1988. Clinical assessment in a college program. Aust. J. Adv. Nurs. 5 (4), 5–9.

Fero, L.J., O'Donnell, J.M., Zullo, T.G., et al., 2010. Critical thinking skills in nursing students: comparison of simulation-based performance with metrics. J. Adv. Nurs. 66 (10), 2182–2193.

Fielding, N.G., Fielding, J.L., 1986. Linking Data. Sage, Beverly Hills, CA.

Fish, D., Twinn, S., 1997. Quality Clinical Supervision in the Health Care Professions. Butterworth-Heinemann, Oxford.

Fletcher, S., 1991. NVQs Standards and Competence. A Practical Guide for Employers, Managers and Trainers. Kogan Page, London.

Forker, J.E., McDonald, M.E., 1996. Methodologic trends in the healthcare professions: Computer adaptive and computer simulation testing. Nurse. Educ. 21 (4), 13–14.

Fotheringham, D., 2010. Triangulation for the assessment of clinical nursing skills: A review of theory, use and methodology. Int. J. Nurs. Stud. 47, 386–391.

Fraser, D., 2000. Action research to improve the pre-registration midwifery curriculum. Part 3: Can fitness for practice be guaranteed? Midwifery 16, 287–294.

Gerrish, K., McManus, M., Ashworth, P., 1997. Levels of Achievement: A Review of the Assessment of Practice. The English National Board for Nursing, Midwifery and Health Visiting, London.

Gibbs, G., 1988. Learning by Doing: A Guide to Teaching Learning Methods. Further Education Unit, London.

Gipps, C.V., 1994. Beyond Testing: Towards a Theory of Educational Assessment. The Falmer Press, London.

Gomez, D.A., Lobodzinski, S., Hartwell West, C.D., 1998. Evaluating clinical performance. In: Billings, D.M., Halstead, J.A. (Eds.), Teaching in Nursing: A Guide for Faculty WB Saunders, Philadelphia, pp. 407–422.

Gonczi, A., Hager, P., Athanasou, J., 1993. The Development of Competency-Based Assessment Strategies for the Professions. National Office of Overseas Skills Recognition, Research Paper No. 8. Australian Government Publishing Service, Canberra.

Govaerts, M.J.B., Schuwirth, L.W.T., Pin, A., et al., 2001. Objective assessment is needed to ensure competence. Br. J. Midwifery. 9 (3), 156–161.

Hager, P., Gonczi, A., 1996. Professions and competencies. In: Edwards, R., Hanson, A., Raggatt, P. (Eds.), Boundaries of Adult Learning Routledge, London, pp. 246–260.

Harden, R., Stevenson, M., Downie, W.W., et al., 1975. Assessment of clinical competence using objective structured examination. Br. Med. J. 1, 447–451.

Harden, R.M., Gleeson, F.A., 1979. Assessment of clinical competence using an objective structured clinical examination. Med. Educ. 13, 41–54.

Harlen, W. (Ed.), 1994. Enhancing Quality in Assessment. BERA Policy Task Group on Assessment Paul Chapman Publishers, London.

Hoban, J.D., Casbergue, J.P., 1978. Simulation: A technique for instruction and evaluation. In Ford, C.W. (Ed.), Clinical Education for the Allied Health Professions. Mosby, St Louis, pp. 145–157.

Hodges, B., 2003. OSCE! Variations on a theme by Harden. Med. Educ. 37, 1134–1140.

Humphris, G.M., Kaney, S., 2001. Examiner fatigue in communication skills objective structured clinical examinations. Med. Educ. 35, 444–449.

Jarvis, P., Gibson, S., 1997. The Teacher Practitioner and Mentor in Nursing, Midwifery and Health Visiting, second ed. Stanley Thornes, Cheltenham.

Jevis, A., Tilki, M., 2011. Why are nurse mentors failing to fail student nurses who do not meet clinical performance standards? Br. J. Nurs. 20 (9), 582–587.

Jones, D., Stephens, J., Innes, W., et al., 2009. Service user and carer involvement in physiotherapy practice, education and research: getting involved for a change. N. Z. Aust. J. Physiother. 37 (1), 29–35.

Ladyshewsky, R., 1999. Simulated patients and assessment. Med. Teach. 21 (3), 266–269.

Lankshear, A., Nicklin, P., 2000. Methods of assessment. In: Nicklin, P., Kenworthy, N. (Eds.), Teaching and Assessing in Nursing Practice, 3rd edn. Baillière Tindall, London, pp. 119–138.

Luhanga, F., Yonge, O.J., Myrick, F., 2008. Failure to assign failing grades: issues with grading the unsafe student. Int. J. Nurs. Educ. Scholarsh. 5 (1), 1–14. Article 8.

Medley, C.F., Horne, C., 2005. Using simulation technology for undergraduate nursing education. J. Nurs. Educ. 44 (1), 31–34.

Meechan, R., Jones, H., Valler-Jones, T., 2011. Do medicines OSCEs improve drug administration ability? Br. J. Nurs. 20 (12), 728–731.

Minton, D., 1997. Teaching Skills in Further and Adult Education, revised ed. Macmillan, Basingstoke.

Moriaty, J., MacIntyre, G., Manthorpe, J., et al., 2010. My expectations remain the same. The student has to be competent to practise: Practice assessor perspectives on the new social work degree qualification in England. Br. J. Soc. Work. 40, 583–601.

Neary, M., 2001. Responsive assessment: Assessing student nurses' clinical competence. Nurse. Educ. Today. 21, 3–17.

Newble, D., 2004. Techniques for measuring clinical competence: objective structured clinical examinations. Med. Educ. 38, 199–203.

Nicol, M., Freeth, D., 1998. Assessment of clinical skills: A new approach to an old problem. Nurse. Educ. Today. 18, 601–609.

Nursing and Midwifery Council, 2005. Consultation on Proposals Arising From a Review of Fitness for Practice at the Point of Registration. NMC, London, Online. Available: <http://www.nmc-uk.org> (accessed December 2005).

Nursing and Midwifery Council, 2007. Standards for Medicines Management. NMC, London, Online. Available: <http://www.nmc-uk.org/Publications/Standards/> (accessed November 2011).

Nursing and Midwifery Council, 2008. Standards to Support Learning and Assessment in Practice, second ed. NMC, London, Online. Available: <http://www.nmc-uk.org/Publications/Standards> (accessed August 2011).

Nursing and Midwifery Council, 2010. Standards for Pre-registration Nursing Education. NMC, London, Online. Available: <http://standards.nmc-uk.org/Pages/Welcome.aspx> (accessed November 2011).

Oliver, R., Endersby, C., 1994. Teaching and Assessing Nurses: A Handbook for Preceptors. Baillière Tindall, London.

Papinczak, T., Young, L., Groves, M., et al., 2007. An analysis of peer, self, and tutor assessment in problem-based tutorials. Med. Teach. 29, e122–e132.

Perrott, E., 1982. Effective Teaching. Longman, London.

Phillips, T., Schostak, J., Tyler, J., 2000. Practice and Assessment in Nursing and Midwifery: Doing it for Real. The English National Board for Nursing, Midwifery and Health Visiting, London.

Polit, D.F., Beck, C.T., Hungler, B.P., 2010. Essentials of Nursing Research: Appraising Evidence for Nursing Practice, seventh ed. Lippincott Williams & Wilkins, London.

Quinn, F.M., 2000. The Principles and Practice of Nurse Education, fourth ed. Chapman & Hall, London.

Redfern, S., Norman, I., 1999a. Quality of nursing care perceived by patients and their nurses: An application of the critical incident technique. Part I. J. Clin. Nurs. 8, 407–413.

Redfern, S., Norman, I., 1999b. Quality of nursing care perceived by patients and their nurses: an application of the critical incident technique. Part II. J. Clin. Nurs. 8, 414–421.

Redfern, S., Norman, I., Calman, L., et al., 2002. Assessing competence to practise in nursing: a review of the literature. Res. Pap. Educ. 17 (1), 51–77.

Redfern, S.J., 1994. Validity through triangulation. Nurse. Res. 2 (2), 41–56.

Rentschler, DD, Eaton, J., Cappiello, J., et al., 2007. Evaluation of undergraduate students using objective structured clinical evaluation. J. Nurs. Educ. 46 (3), 135–139.

Repper, J., Breeze, J., 2007. A review of the literature on user and carer involvement in the training and education of health professionals. Int. J. Nurs. Stud. 44, 511–519.

Rethans, J.J., Sturmans, F., Drop, R., et al., 1991. Does competence of general practitioners predict their performance? Comparisons between examination settings and actual practice. Br. Med. J. 303, 1377–1380.

Rhodes, C.A., 2012. User involvement in health and social care education: a concept analysis. Nurse Education Today, 32, 185–189.

Rogers, C., 1983. Freedom to Learn for the 80`s. Charles E. Merrill, Columbus, Ohio.

Rowntree, D., 1987. Assessing Students: How Shall We Know Them?, second ed. Kogan Page, London.

Schön, D., 1987. Educating the Reflective Practitioner. Jossey-Bass, San Francisco.

Shepherd, C.K., McCunnis, M., Brown, L., 2010. Investigating the use of simulation as a teaching strategy. Nurs. Stand. 24 (35), 42–48.

Skills for Health, 2005. National Occupational Standards and National Workforce Competences. Online. Available: <http://www.skillsforhealth.org.uk/frameworks.php> (accessed December 2005).

Stengelhofen, J., 1993. Teaching Students in Clinical Settings. Chapman & Hall, London.

Stoker, D., 1994. Assessment in learning: (iii) Methods of assessment. Nurs. Times. 90 (13 Section 7iii), i–viii.

Stuart, C.C., 1997. Reflective journals as a teaching/learning strategy. Br. J. Midwifery. 5 (7), 434–438.

Swanwick, M., 1994. Observation as a research method. Nurse. Res. 2 (2), 5–12.

Toohey, S., 2002. Assessment of students` personal development as part of preparation for professional work – is it desirable and is it feasible? Assess. Eval. High. Educ. 27 (6), 529–538.

Verhoeven, B.H., Hamers, J.G.H.C., Schepbier, A.J.J.A., et al., 2000. The effect on reliability of adding a separate written assessment component to an objective structured clinical examination. Med. Educ. 34, 525–529.

Walsh, M., Hill Bailey, P., Koren, I., 2009. Objective structured clinical evaluation of clinical competence: an integrative review. J. Adv. Nurs. 65 (8), 1584–1595.

Westwood-Timms, J., 1995. Critical incident scenarios. MIDIRS. Midwifery. Dig. 5 (3), 268–270.

Weinrott, M., Jones, R., 1984. Overt versus covert assessment of observer reliability. Child. Dev. 55 (3), 1125–1137.

While, A.E., 1994. Competence versus performance: Which is more important? J. Adv. Nurs. 20, 525–531.

Wotton, K., Davis, J., Button, D., et al., 2010. Third year undergraduate nursing students` perceptions of high-fidelity simulation. J. Nurs. Educ. 49 (11), 632–639.

Chapter | 5 |

Conducting defensible and fair assessments

INTRODUCTION

Generally, in pre-registration health care education students spend up to 50% of the course time in clinical practice. Learners' lived experience in authentic practice contexts and their competence in dealing with the care situations they face should therefore form the basis of assessment (Gopee 2008, Phillips et al 2000). Competency-based assessment in the professions therefore needs to be based on realistic, complex workplace problems to generate the range of evidence of competence required to make valid and reliable assessments (Masters & McCurry 1990). This can be done by the careful selection and combination of methods of assessment that will best assess the particular component of competence (e.g. using observation to assess psychomotor skills and questioning to assess cognitive skills).

It is not possible or desirable to assess everything a person might need to know or be able to do. Assessment of clinical practice is inevitably based on a sample of the student's performance in assessment tasks perceived to be relevant. An inference of competence is then made from the student's performance on the set of arranged tasks. Competence is a construct that is not directly observable; rather, it is inferred from performance. Most typical assessments involve making inferences (e.g. tests of knowledge usually sample only a fraction of the required knowledge). On the basis of that score, an inference is made as to whether or not a student knows enough to be assessed as satisfactory (Rowntree 1987). Grades and degree classifications are made on that basis; hence assessment of clinical practice, in common with other types of assessment, involves inference – and inferences are subject to error (Gonczi et al 1993). This is perhaps one major weakness of most, if not all, of our assessment systems.

As I see it, two major expectations are made of practice educators. First, they are required to make professional judgements in interpreting what the minimum acceptable levels of competence with respect to professional standards. These judgements are frequently made within the role relationship of that of a mentor cum assessor to a student – this role relationship may very well influence assessment judgements. The reader is directed to a discussion of the issues and dilemma of the mentor–assessor interface in Chapter 2. Secondly, assessment evidence obtained through the methods used requires to be 'subjectively scored'. Reliability, and perhaps even validity, may be compromised. Students may then be assessed unfairly or incorrect assessment decisions are made – and what could be worse than passing a student who has not achieved the goal of professional health care education, which is to be 'fit for purpose' and 'fit for practice'.

Our assessments need to be defensible to the public and fair in that they distinguish between good and under performers correctly (Schuwirth et al 2002). Assessments are relied upon to make some quite specific, but also far-ranging, judgements about students' future competence as registered practitioners. In deciding whether the assessments are sufficiently robust to enable sound judgements to be made, clear criteria should be used for deciding if the assessments are both defensible and fair. A question to be asked is this: 'Do our assessments enable us to make such judgements soundly?' Deciding whether or not an assessment lives up to this task is not straightforward.

There is now an examination of those factors to be considered in order to make sound judgements in assessments. Measures to attain objective assessments and avoid subjective assessments are suggested.

THE KEY CONCEPTS OF CONDUCTING DEFENSIBLE AND FAIR ASSESSMENTS

Justice is a basic part of the functioning of a civilized society: we believe in justice not only for the accuser and the accused in criminal trials, but also for parties in any dispute. When involved with any situation when a decision about fair play has to be made, a person with a sense of justice is likely to think that the decision made to carry out a certain action is just and fair, and the other person has had fair treatment. As an assessor you have to make assessment decisions continually and these decisions about student performance must be just and fair. How can you ensure that this is so? Furthermore, assessment for certification, so-called 'high-stakes' assessment, as in professional health care education, should offer sufficient reliability and validity for public scrutiny. High-stakes assessments at national levels, as is the case with pre-registration health care education, must offer comparability (Downing 2004, Gipps 1994a). In its document *Making a Difference*, the Department of Health (1999) stated that the health service of the country needs to know that nurses and midwives, and by inference all health care professionals, are trained to broadly the same standards and have the same skills. How can we achieve these 'orders' through our assessment activities? Or are these orders too tall?

What do the words 'fair' and 'defensible' mean to you? According to the *Collins Pocket Dictionary and Thesaurus* (1993), to be fair is to act 'according to rules'. To 'defend' your position, you generally have to justify yourself with sound reasons. The next question then may be: *What are the rules of defensible and fair assessments?* Stoker & Hull (1994) state that four attributes need to be fulfilled to make assessment defensible and fair – these attributes may thus form the rules of defensible and fair assessments. Quinn & Hughes (2007) refer to these as the four 'cardinal criteria' of every effective test. The four cardinal criteria or attributes are:

- validity
- reliability
- feasibility
- discriminating power.

Validity

Gonczi et al (1993) maintain that the most important issue in competency-based assessment is that of validity. The traditional definition of validity is the extent to which a test measures what it was designed to measure. If it does not measure what it purports to measure, then its use is misleading (Gipps 1994a). There are two key issues here that are important to the assessment of clinical practice: *how* measurements are made and *what* measurements are made. The use of the strategy of triangulation will help ensure that a more complete picture of the student's competence is obtained, thereby enhancing validity. The reader is referred to Chapter 4 for a discussion of the use of appropriate methods of assessment and the strategy of triangulation to achieve validity of assessment. Valid assessment in clinical practice depends on methods of assessment used that are appropriate to the attribute of the competence being assessed (e.g. valid assessments of psychomotor skills are unlikely to be provided by the use of questioning). In health care education, what we purport to measure must be that of 'the ability to actually care for patients' (Gerrish et al 1997:70). Assessment for accountability purposes, as in health care professions, should aim for high validity, as health care professionals must be fit for the purpose of caring for patients and clients. We therefore have to be clear about *what* we want to measure. Rowntree (1987) tells us to 'articulate as clearly as possible the criteria by which we assess, the aims and objectives we espouse, what qualities we look for in students'.

When assessing in clinical practice, validity is inferred. It is difficult to measure validity (Gonczi et al 1993). The way to infer validity is to collect evidence of the different types of validity that matter to us in clinical practice. The types of validity to be discussed here are:

- content validity
- face validity
- predictive validity
- construct validity
- concurrent validity.

Content validity

This concerns the coverage of appropriate and necessary content (Gipps 1994a). Newble (2004:38) states that content validity is the 'most fundamental requirement in ensuring the quality of a competency test'. The following questions can be asked in association with this concept:

- Has the assessment sampled adequately the content of the course? In the case of pre-registration health care students, has the assessment sampled adequately the NMC and HCPC standards of proficiency? Newble (2004) and Crossley et al (2002) recommend using a 'blueprint', and Fraser et al (1997) an 'assessment matrix', for adequate sampling. This is a way of including the sample of items to be included in the assessment. The simplest form is a two-dimensional matrix with one axis representing the generic competencies such as history taking, communication skills, management skills and care-planning skills. The other axis represents the problems or conditions or clinical tasks or types of patients/clients on which the competencies will be demonstrated. A sample of practice representing a valid selection from each dimension can then be identified.

- Has the assessment sampled across the range of context for a particular competency? Ability to perform in one situation is a very poor predictor of performance in another, even similar, situation; wide sampling across a competency is therefore required to achieve an adequate level of content validity and reliability (Newble 2004).
- Is the item being assessed within the content of the course?
- Does the item being assessed require to be assessed at this stage of the student's training?

It is of course necessary to have knowledge of the content and structure of the course of students being assessed in order to achieve content validity.

Face validity

This is the extent to which an assessment appears to be testing what we want students to be able to do. Gerrish et al (1997) point out that many pre-registration nursing programmes require students to produce written evidence of the achievement in practice, but that this does not necessarily indicate their ability to actually care for patients (i.e. this form of testing for clinical competence lacks face validity). Another example of a test lacking in face validity comes from Wolf (1995), who gives the example of the use of multiple-choice tests of the type often used to license professionals in the USA. For example, in the case of a physician after qualification, the multiple-choice questions that have to be taken do not test the physician's competence to practise (McGaghie 1991, in Wolf 1995). Masters & McCurry (1990) believe that face validity is likely to be enhanced by making set tasks resemble those encountered in day-to-day practice in a profession. During the clinical practice of students, careful planning of learning experiences will help students participate in the day-to-day activities of their profession to facilitate the achievement of face validity.

Predictive validity

This relates to whether the assessment predicts accurately or well some future performance (Gipps 1994a). Rowntree (1987:189) gives this warning about predictive validity:

Predicting how a person will turn out in the future, on the basis of what we know about him now, is hazardous. Even if he retains the ability, he may no longer have the disposition.

In the health care professions, it is important to try to predict students' competence in the future so that, as a minimum, at the point of qualification, they are competent to practise. Whether they remain competent in the future is of course beyond our control. What can be done in attempts to achieve predictive validity? The use of continuous assessment may help here. The constant and regular supervision, guidance and feedback given to students will reinforce learning and hence their development and achievements. Keeping an evidence log, as shown in Figure 7.5, will assist in keeping track of the progress of students and the types of experiences they are having. Ensuring that students have a range of clinical experiences, with repetitions if necessary, will help them acquire the skills to practise with confidence and perhaps predictability. Stoker (1994:v) says that:

If a learner can do it once, it's an event; twice may be a coincidence; three times may show that a consistent pattern is emerging.

If there is consistency of performance, there is a higher chance of predictive validity in assessment as 'the best indicator of future performance is past performance' (Wolf 1995:44). Correspondingly, the best predictor measure will be to incorporate and assess those future behaviours that are of interest.

Construct validity

Constructs are the qualities, abilities and traits that explain aspects of human behaviour; these cannot be observed directly (Rowntree 1987). Honesty, maturity, kindness and intelligence are some examples of constructs. Construct validity is the extent to which assessment reveals the construct being assessed. We are required to make value judgements about certain aspects of the student's behaviour or personality. Rowntree (1987:84) asks whether we are deluding ourselves when we make those judgements. 'Is what we see (or not see) in students a figment of our imagination – a fabrication of the mind of the beholder to some extent?' To what extent do our personal constructs influence construct validity? Abstract concepts such as attitudes and values are notoriously difficult to measure (Nolan & Behi 1995, Ashworth & Morrison 1991). Again, the use of continuous assessment may be helpful here. Working with and assessing the student over a period of time in conjunction with other practitioners, and utilizing a range of care-giving situations, will give the practice educator more opportunities to assess the student's attitudes and values, thus making assessment in this area of learning more accurate. It will also allow students more opportunities to demonstrate the attitudes and values they hold. For example, imagine you are trying to assess a student's attitudes to the elderly and you work with him/her on one occasion with one elderly person. Your student appears to have difficulty demonstrating sensitivity to the needs of the patient, even though questioning reveals that he/she is theoretically well aware of those needs. Do you then assume that the student's attitudes towards the elderly are not good? No, of course you don't. Your student's performance on that occasion might be due to a number of factors; for example, she may find it particularly difficult to relate to that individual patient, or she may simply be very tired or is distracted by some pressing problems.

Concurrent validity

This is concerned with whether an assessment in an aspect of performance correlates with, or gives substantially the same results as, another assessment in a related area of performance (Gipps 1994a, Davis 1986). In other words, does the assessment predict performance in related areas? How far can we generalize from the ability to perform one task to an ability to perform other tasks in the same domain? For example, if you are working with a student who is able to assess and give immediate nursing care to asthmatic patients in relation to their dyspnoea – that of nursing them at rest in a comfortably supported and upright position – can you conclude from the student's care of these patients that the student is able to assess and give the necessary immediate nursing care to patients with dyspnoea from other causes? I would suggest that you could, because the principle of care is the same for all patients with dyspnoea. Your assessment has concurrent validity. Consider this other example: there is assessment evidence to say that the student is able to give intramuscular injections safely into the gluteus muscle. Can you assume that the student is able to give intramuscular injections safely into other sites of the body? I would suggest that you could not make this assumption because, even though the principles of giving an intramuscular injection remain the same, there are different dangers associated with the use of these alternative sites.

To achieve concurrent validity, the assessor needs to be aware of the range of context of practice (see Ch. 6) to achieve competence in an area of care so that the required experiences can be arranged. Specifying the range in the assessment plan is therefore necessary to achieve concurrent validity. In other words, the number of tasks should be increased to ensure comprehensive coverage of the domain to improve generalizability (Linn 1993).

There are two final points to make about validity. First, the more measures there are in agreement, and the more closely they agree, the more likely it is that they do actually measure what they claim to (Crossley et al 2002). Secondly, a general principle underlying validity in

competency-based assessment is that the narrower the base of evidence for the inference of competence, the less generalizable it will be to the performance of other tasks (Gonczi et al 1993). Generalizability is a particular problem for performance assessment, as direct assessments of complex performance do not generalize well from one task to another (Gipps 1994a). This is because competent performance is heavily task-dependent.

Reliability

Reliability is concerned with the degree to which a result reflects all possible measurements of the same aspect of competence or performance (Gipps 1994a). In other words, how accurately does the test measure the performance or attainment it is designed to measure? In a review article on the reliability of assessment in medical education, Downing (2004) noted that the level of acceptable reliability depended on the purpose, use and consequences of the assessment. If the stakes of the particular assessment were high, such as certification examinations in medicine, a high level of reliability was recommended; whereas for formative, classroom-type assessments, a moderate level of reliability was deemed acceptable.

A test or assessment is said to be reliable if it gives similar results when used on separate occasions and with different assessors. Evaluating reliability requires a clear statement of the range of circumstances that the result is supposed to represent (Crossley et al 2002). The assessment of the history taking skills of a particular student from a particular patient today may be reproducible but it does not necessarily reflect the assessment of any assessor or the history taking skills of that student with any patient or on any day.

There are two underlying reliability questions: Would an assessment produce the same or similar results on more than one occasion? Or if done by other assessors? There are several key issues here:

- consistency of student performance
- consistency of interpretation
- consistency, and therefore agreement of interpretation, between assessors
- consistency of context.

Clinical performance is made up of complex behaviours. Their valid assessment depends on subjective judgements based on specific instances of practice. This threatens reliability. It is a fact that the core of any assessment is the judgement of the assessor – any form of assessment involves activity and judgement on the part of the assessor (Wolf 1995). For judgement to be valid and reliable, all assessors are presumed to be able to:

feel, understand and judge in much the same way when confronted with the work of a particular student. It is [also] presumed that they would notice and value the same skills and qualities and would broadly agree in their assessments (Rowntree 1987:191).

Furthermore, the assessor is 'construed as the "neutral" value-free "gatherer of evidence" and it is this evidence that is subjected to the "objective" assessment of the same [assessor]' (Cowburn et al 2000). There is abundant evidence that attests to the falsity of these assumptions (see, for example, Gipps 1994a, Rowntree 1987). The unreliability of assessment first became an issue when it was noticed that the mark awarded for a student essay depended on who marked it. The following excerpt is rather amusing and illustrates the unreliability of assessment. Ben Wood (1921, cited in Rowntree, 1987) tells how one of the six college professors grading a set of history papers wrote out, for his own satisfaction, what he considered to be a model paper for the set of questions. By some mischance this paper got among those being marked. It was unsuspectingly graded and deemed unworthy of a pass mark! According to standard precautions, this paper was duly marked by the other professors to double-check its grade and was given marks ranging from 40 to 90.

Factors that can affect the reliability of assessment in the clinical setting can be grouped under the three headings of *student factors*, *environmental factors* and *assessor factors* (Stoker & Hull 1994). Each set of factors is now considered in turn.

Student factors

As stated above, to achieve reliability, student performance has to be consistent. Can students perform with consistency all the time? Obviously not – there are many human factors that militate against being the 'perfect all-singing all-dancing' student. Those physical and emotional factors that may affect performance could be poor health, fatigue, lack of interest in the placement and therefore motivation to learn, anxiety and lack of confidence about giving patient care and personal problems affecting concentration at work. Physical disabilities such as mobility problems and any speech impediments may affect learning. The presence of other students in the clinical area may be supportive and positive for each other, thereby enhancing learning, or it may be detract from learning if students are negative.

Another group of factors that students have no control over, such as their gender and racial background, may also affect the way they are assessed. In mainstream education it has been shown that when markers can infer gender or racial group from the pupil's name, stereotypes come into play that affect marks awarded. For example, both male and female markers rated the same paper more highly when it was attributed to John T McKay than to Joan T McKay (Gipps 1994a). Even when names are

not attached to scripts, surface effects such as neatness can affect marking. Now try Activity 5.1.

ACTIVITY 5.1

Make a list of those student factors that you have encountered, either personally or from a colleague's experience, that have affected assessments either positively or negatively.

A group of practice educators came up with the following list of factors that they thought might have affected the way they view the students and potentially their assessment of the students:

- Physical appearance, such as dress code, body piercing, tattoos and dyed hair.
- Age of the student in relationship to themselves – the younger practice educator may feel threatened by the older practice student and the mature practice educator wishing to 'mother' a younger student.
- Social class of the student – more may be expected of the student from a higher socioeconomic background as these students are 'associated with higher intelligence'. Conversely, less may be expected from the student from a lower socioeconomic background.
- Accent of the student – students speaking with the 'Queen's English' accent are accorded a higher intelligence and assessed accordingly.

Environmental factors

There are particular problems that are the direct consequences of assessing in the clinical setting. These problems will contribute to assessments being unreliable if they are not recognized and managed:

- There is an inherently high variability in the context of clinical assessment; patients/clients or situations cannot be standardized and therefore cannot produce identical situations in which students can be assessed. The conditions for learning and practice can be highly inconsistent, which will impact directly on the consistency of performance of the student and the assessment.
- The work environment is often very busy. Phillips et al (2000) found that there were a large number of clinical environments where the level of staffing is such that all available time is given to coping with the demands of patient care. Practice educators are simply too busy as carers. Over the years, the workload of practice educators has increased whilst resource and support have not (Beskine 2009), There is, therefore, insufficient time for reliable evidence collection.

- There are many distractions that may interfere with the student's and the practice educator's concentration. A preoccupation with something that has happened, concern with jobs still to be done and the busyness and noise on a ward are examples of distractions that will affect learning and assessment activities.
- The learning climate of the working environment should also be considered. The support and encouragement given to learners contribute to their confidence, which will enable them to participate more effectively in the learning and assessment process (Neary 2000).

As can be seen, there are many environmental factors that may contribute to the unreliability of assessments. Phillips et al (2000) recommend that time should be prioritized for assessment-only activity, so that there is more time for reliable evidence collection. The NMC (2008:34) has reinforced this in its *Standards to Support Learning and Assessment in Practice* by stating that 'sign-off mentors must have time allocated to reflect, give feedback and keep records of student achievements in their final period of practice learning. This will be the equivalent of an hour per student per week'. Additionally, the workload of practice educators needs to reflect the demands of being a mentor as time is needed to be able to explain, question, assess performance and provide feedback to the student in a meaningful way (NMC 2008:30).

The length of time spent on each clinical placement should also be sufficiently long (a minimum of 4 weeks is recommended) to enable continuity of practice educator/student contact. Longer placements will also provide more opportunities for the student to engage in a range of care situations, thereby giving the student more opportunities to achieve consistent performance.

Assessor factors

As with factors attributed to the student and the environment, there are many factors attributed to the assessor that can detract from the reliability of assessment. The research evidence that is available on assessors' behaviour emphasizes the very active role that their own concepts and interpretations play when making judgements and final assessment decisions (Lewis et al 2008, Cowburn et al 2000, Wolf 1995). These concepts and interpretations are likely to be influenced by the assessors' own competence and standards of practice. In a study to determine the inter- and intra-rater reliability of one form of clinical assessment used for physiotherapy students, Lewis et al (2008) found that individual practice educators often awarded their own students the highest or equal highest mark when compared with other raters. The conclusion was that each practice educator appeared to mark the assessment task according to his or her own individual clinical practice.

Wolf explains that assessors do not simply 'match' students' performance to assessment criteria in a mechanistic fashion. On the contrary, they draw on an internalized, holistic set of concepts about how, and how far, they can take account of the context of the situation, what students should 'get out' of an assessment and how much allowance they can make by offsetting lapses and weaknesses with strengths from other areas of performance and so on. Making allowances is particularly apparent when assessing students performing difficult and complex tasks. In short, assessors make what Wolf describes as judgemental aggregation, which is to 'compensate, make allowances, interpret, explain away' (Wolf 1995:71). The more experienced the assessor, the more they will have internalized a model of competence that in turn affects the degrees of judgemental aggregation. People are often unaware of the degree to which they are operating in this way. Conversely, the inexperienced practitioner/assessor does not make as much compensation or as many allowances – there is a tendency to expect every performance criterion to be achieved.

One claim made with competency-based assessment is that, because the assessment criteria are so clearly defined in such detail, assessors are required to make far less in the way of complex judgements. Fletcher (1991:66) stated that 'individual performance … is judged against explicit standards … and individuals know exactly what they are aiming to achieve'. There is evidence to say that this is far from the truth (Wolf 1995). The inherent variability of the contexts and complexity of clinical practice in which competence is displayed and assessed means that assessors have to make complex judgements and constant major decisions. They must also determine how to take account of the conditions of practice when judging whether a piece of evidence fits a defined criterion. It is not clear that judgements, in particular complex judgements, are derived from specified assessment criteria. Wolf (1995:69) states:

> *The key judgements have far more to do with whether someone has actually performed up to the assessor's standards than with the individual performance criteria at all. And whether or not one assessor applies standards that are the same as another's will also, in a case like this, have rather little to do with the focus on competence and outcomes.*

An example of the above situation comes from a study by Hayter (1973) where 31 nurse educators viewed a film of students in three clinical situations. The educators were instructed to assess only the students' ability to care for a patient in shock. They were required to assign and justify the letter grade awarded (A for best performance to F for worst performance). Only 27 of the 155 reasons for the grades related to the care of the patient in shock. Some reasons for below-average grades were: 'seemed very cold

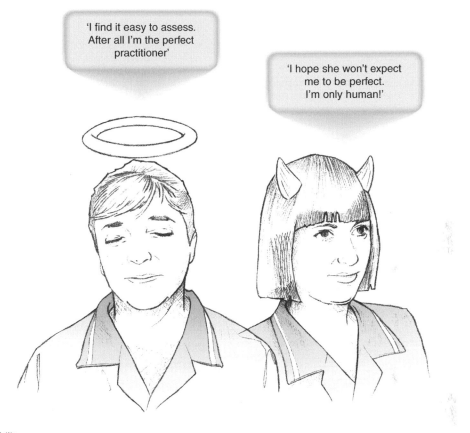

Figure 5.1 Reliability.

and distant', 'did not seem sure of herself' and 'she was clumsy when taking the pulse'. The grades awarded in one clinical situation were: A – 1 student, B – 10 students, C – 16 students, D – 3 students, and F – 1 student. These grades were also typical of the grades awarded in the other two situations.

Up to now the discussion has been on how the assessor's judgement is influenced by personal concepts and expectations, which are likely to be based on the person's standards and model of competence. Another set of factors that can influence the assessor's judgement and detract from reliability of assessment even more is our personal biases. We all carry prejudices of some kind, many of which we are not even aware of. If we are biased either in favour of or against the student – based on prior knowledge of the student's work or prejudices or stereotypes we might hold about the student – our assessment of the student is likely to be influenced. If this prior knowledge of the student or some personal aspect about the student that we like influences us to make a more favourable assessment, it is known as the *halo* effect. If the student's performance is underrated because our knowledge of that student's poor past performance has

influenced that judgement, it is known as the *horn* effect (Philp 1983). I once knew a student who shaved his head bald, chewed gum frequently and had several visible tattoos. Coincidentally, he failed the placement but that is another story! I'm sure you have other similar stories.

Assessors should also consider the influence that their presence may have over students. A student who is being observed may become nervous. Conversely, the student may become much more attentive to the task and attend to detail more than she/he normally would. If the latter situation is the result of a positive and constructive relationship between the assessor and the student, it is known as the *Hawthorne effect* – 'the tendency for persons to perform as expected because of special attention' (Sullivan & Decker 1988). This inconsistent performance on the part of the student may affect reliability of assessment if the assessor overlooks the student's usual lower standards when the student is working with others.

The point is not that assessors cannot assess to an acceptably common standard: they can, but the process is complex and judgemental. Furthermore, each set of factors influencing reliability – student, environmental, assessor – does not operate on its own to affect reliability;

rather, they all have an impact on each other. The conclusion to be drawn from this is that the reliability of assessment is threatened even more. An awareness of those factors that may influence the reliability of assessment will help the assessor in overcoming difficulties contributing to unreliable assessments. Problems of reliability reinforce the use of one recommended aspect of assessment practice in that summative assessment should consider a broad range of evidence of competence from several sources (Bedford et al 1993).

There is much call (see, for example, Huybrecht et al 2011, Gopee 2008, NMC 2008, Phillips et al 2000, Gerrish et al 1997, Bedford et al 1993) for the training of practice educators to include developing their competence in collecting evidence and analysing data. It is also recommended that there should be discussions around how best to make valid and reliable assessment decisions in a busy work environment.

Try Activity 5.2. This activity is to help you consider those factors in your work environment that may contribute to unreliable assessments.

ACTIVITY 5.2

During your next spell of duty, identify an item you assess in others, e.g. feeding a patient or a similar simple item. Complete the following:

The following item was assessed:

The assessment of this item was/was not reliable because:

Remember to ask the following questions about reliability:

- Would I interpret the student's performance of a particular skill in the same way if I saw it again?
- Would I interpret another student's performance of the same skill in the same way? What quality assurance measures are in place to ensure consistency of approach (Gipps 1994b)?
- Would other assessors agree with my interpretations of the student's performance? What quality control measures are in place to ensure that outcomes are judged in a comparable way (Gipps 1994b)?
- How consistent is the student's performance?
- Has there been an adequate sample across the range of context?

Feasibility

If we were given a task to do but had not been given the time or resources to complete the task, we would say that it is unfair because it had not been feasible to complete the task, and perhaps even complain bitterly! Likewise, in assessment, it is only a fair assessment if it is feasible in terms of:

- allowing sufficient time for students to practise and demonstrate competence
- there are sufficient resources in terms of, for example, opportunities for students to learn and demonstrate that they have developed the abilities and skills
- assessors have had enough time and opportunities to work with and assess students.

Try Activity 5.3.

ACTIVITY 5.3

Make a list of any restrictions that you think your clinical environment may place on what is feasible in terms of assessment. Can anything be done to reduce/remove these restrictions?

Time constraint is likely to be one major restriction – the result of students' perceived 'short' placement or your workload or differing shifts with your student. All these factors could result in students not having enough time to practise, or you not being able to spend enough time with students to perform a fair assessment.

Generally, a student's length of placement in a clinical area cannot be altered as these periods have already been determined in the curriculum. Prior planning of clinical experiences – for example, by agreeing a learning contract/action plan with the student – will maximize the potential of clinical time. The use of alternative assessment methods and strategies other than observing the student in practice yourself can make the assessment fairer. These strategies are discussed in Chapter 4.

Remember to ask the following questions about feasibility:

- Has the student been given enough time to practise?
- Has the student been given enough learning opportunities?
- Has enough time been spent assessing the student, either by you or another assessor?

Discriminating power

An assessment that has discriminating power is one that:

- reflects the different levels of ability in those for whom it is used (Stoker & Hull 1994)
- decides clearly between those students who are of a certain standard and those who are not (Davis 1986).

Most people do not possess the same level of ability, nor do they learn at the same rate. Discriminating power is important during formative assessment in order to distinguish between the different levels of performance to assist in identifying those areas that require further development. Validity is highly important so that those areas of learning to be improved can be identified (Gipps 1994b). During summative assessments it is necessary to be able to identify whether the student has attained the required level of competence and thus achieved the standard of training required at that stage of the course. An adequate level of reliability is needed in terms of consistency of performance (Gipps 1994b).

So far as the health care professions are concerned, there should be a basic level of measure for many professional activities – that of *safety* (Davis 1986). For example, where asepsis is concerned there cannot be a standard that is 'fairly safe'! An aseptic technique is either safe or not safe. On the other hand, some professional activities do not come into this category – empathy is an example. There is a difficulty in attempting to decide what is and what is not acceptable behaviour over a wide range of variables such as can be encountered with measuring the ability to show empathy.

Remember to ask the following questions about discriminating power:

- Has my assessment identified the correct level of ability of the student?
- Has my assessment identified the correct standard to be achieved?

Readers are directed to the sections on 'Criteria for assessing development in the novice, advanced beginner and competent levels of performance' and 'Making assessment decisions' in Chapter 7 for discussions on how to determine whether a student is competent or not at a particular level.

CONCLUSION

All assessments must balance rigour (validity, reliability and discriminating power) against feasibility. Validity is traditionally considered to be more important than reliability: a highly reliable test is of little use if it is not valid. However, according to classical test theory a test cannot be valid if it does not have a basic level of reliability (Gipps 1994a). Validity and reliability are in constant tension – what is needed is an appropriate balance between the two. Gipps goes on to say that generalizability bridges validity and reliability – inferences of competence are based on a sample of performance and we have to generalize from this sample in conferring fitness for purpose and fitness for practice. In performance assessment, increasing the number of tasks assessed is the most effective way of enhancing generalizability. In order to generalize with any confidence, we need to ensure that what we want to assess is carefully defined to achieve validity and the assessment itself is reliable. To generalize without achieving validity and reliability would be unsafe.

The situation surrounding conducting and achieving fair assessments is complex. Gipps & Murphy (1994) say that the notion of a fair test is simplistic. The biggest challenge to fairness faced by assessors and students during clinical practice is the context: we cannot assume identical clinical experiences for all. However, by paying attention to what we know about factors that affect the fairness of assessment we can begin to work towards assessments that are defensible and fair.

KEY POINTS FOR REFLECTION

To be fair is to act 'according to rules'. To 'defend' your position, you generally have to justify yourself with sound reasons.

Four cardinal criteria or attributes guide achievement of defensible and fair assessments. These are validity, reliability, feasibility and discriminating power.

1. **Validity** is the extent to which a test measures what it was designed to measure.
   - *Content validity:* concerns the coverage of appropriate and necessary content.
   - *Face validity:* is the extent to which an assessment appears to be testing what we want students to be able to do.
   - *Predictive validity:* relates to whether the assessment predicts accurately or well some future performance.
   - *Construct validity:* is the extent to which our assessment reveals the construct we are measuring.
   - *Concurrent validity:* is concerned with whether an assessment in an aspect of performance correlates with, or gives substantially the same results as,

another assessment in a related area of performance.

2. **Reliability** is concerned with the degree to which a result reflects all possible measurements of the same aspect of competence or performance. A test or assessment is said to be reliable if it gives similar results when used on separate occasions and with different assessors. Reliability can be adversely affected by factors present in the student, the environment and the assessor. These can act subjectively to make assessments unreliable.

3. **Feasibility** is about providing sufficient time and resources to enable the achievement of competencies.

4. An assessment that has **discriminating power** is one that reflects the different levels of ability in those for whom it is used and it decides clearly between those students who are of a certain standard and those who are not.

All assessments must balance rigour (validity, reliability and discriminating power) against feasibility.

REFERENCES

Ashworth, P., Morrison, P., 1991. Problems of competence-based education. Nurse Educ. Today 11, 256–260.

Bedford, H., Phillips, T., Robinson, J., et al., 1993. Assessment of Competencies in Nursing and Midwifery Education and Training. The English National Board for Nursing, Midwifery and Health Visiting, London.

Beskine, D., 2009. Mentoring students: establishing effective working relationships. Nurs. Stand. 23 (30), 35–40.

Collins Pocket Dictionary, Thesaurus 1993, reprinted 1995). Glasgow: Harper Collins.

Cowburn, M., Nelson, P., Williams, J., 2000. Assessment of social work students: standpoint and strong objectivity. Soc. Work Educ. 19 (6), 627–637.

Crossley, J., Humphris, G., Jolly, B., 2002. Assessing health professionals. Med. Educ. 36, 800–804.

Davis, M., 1986. Managing Care (Pack 11): Assessing Nurses. South Bank Polytechnic, Distance Learning Centre, London.

Department of Health, 1999. Making a Difference. Department of Health, London.

Downing, S., 2004. Reliability: on the reproducibility of assessment data. Med. Educ. 38, 1006–1012.

Fletcher, S., 1991. NVQs standards and competence. A Practical Guide for Employers, Managers and Trainers. Kogan Page, London.

Fraser, D., Murphy, R., Worth-Butler, M., 1997. An Outcome Evaluation of the Effectiveness of Pre-registration Midwifery Programmes of Education. The English National Board for Nursing, Midwifery and Health Visiting, London.

Gerrish, K., McManus, M., Ashworth, P., 1997. Levels of Achievement: A Review of the Assessment of Practice. The English National Board for Nursing, Midwifery and Health Visiting, London.

Gipps, C.V., 1994a. Beyond Testing: Towards a Theory of Educational Assessment. The Falmer Press, London.

Gipps, C., 1994b. Quality in teacher assessment. In: Harlen, W. (Ed.), Enhancing Quality in Assessment Paul Chapman Publishers, London, pp. 71–86. BERA Policy Task Group on Assessment.

Gipps, C., Murphy, P., 1994. Assessment, Achievement and Equity. Open University Press, Buckingham.

Gonczi, A., Hager, P., Athanasou, J., 1993. The Development of Competency-Based Assessment Strategies for the Professions. Australian Government Publishing Service, Canberra, National Office of Overseas Skills Recognition, Research Paper No. 8.

Gopee, N., 2008. Assessing student nurses' clinical skills: The ethical competence of mentors. Int. J. Ther. Rehabil. 15 (9), 401–407.

Hater, J., 1973. An approach to laboratory evaluation. J. Nurs. Educ. 12, 17–22.

Sabine Huybrecht, S., Loeckx, W., Quaeyhaegens, Y., et al., 2011. Mentoring in nursing education: Perceived characteristics of mentors and the consequences of mentorship. Nurse Educ. Today 31, 274–278.

Lewis, L.K., Stiller, K., Hardy, F., 2008. A clinical assessment tool used for physiotherapy students-Is it reliable? Physiother. Theory. Pract. 24 (2), 121–134.

Linn, R.L., 1993. Educational assessment: expanded expectations and challenges. Educ. Eval. Policy Anal. 15: 1.

McGaghie, W.C., 1991. Professional competence evaluation. Educ. Res. 20 (1), 3.

Masters, G.N., McCurry, D., 1990. Competency-Based Assessment in the Professions. Australian Government Publishing Service, Canberra, National Office of Overseas Skills Recognition, Research Paper No. 2.

Neary, M., 2000. Teaching, Assessing and Evaluation for Clinical Competence. Stanley Thornes, Cheltenham.

Newble, D., 2004. Techniques for measuring clinical competence: Objective structured clinical examinations. Med. Educ. 38, 199–203.

Nolan, M., Behi, R., 1995. Validity: A concept at the heart of research. Br. J. Nurs. 4 (9), 530–533.

Nursing and Midwifery Council, 2008. Standards to Support Learning and Assessment in Practice, second ed. NMC, London, Online. Available: <http://www.nmc-uk.org/Publications/Standards> (Accessed August 2011).

Phillips, T., Schostak, J., Tyler, J., 2000. Practice and Assessment in Nursing and Midwifery: Doing it for Real. The English National Board for Nursing, Midwifery and Health Visiting, London.

Philp, T., 1983. Making Performance Appraisal Work. McGraw-Hill, Maidenhead.

Quinn, F.M., Hughes, S.Z., 2007. Principles and Practice of Nurse Education, fifth ed. Nelson Thornes, Cheltenham.

Rowntree, D., 1987. Assessing Students: How Shall We Know Them, second ed. Kogan Page, London.

Schuwirth, L.W.T., Southgate, L., Page, G.G., et al., 2002. When enough is enough: A conceptual basis for fair and defensible practice performance assessment. Med. Educ. 36, 925–930.

Stoker, D., 1994. Assessment in learning: (i) Understanding assessment issues. Nurs. Times 90, i–viii. 11, Section 7i.

Stoker, D., Hull, C., 1994. Assessment inlearning: (ii) Assessment and learning outcomes. Nurs. Times 90, i–viii. 12, Section 7ii.

Sullivan, E.J., Decker, P.J., 1988. Effective Management in Nursing, second ed. Addison-Wesley, Menlo Park, California.

Wolf, A., 1995. Competence-Based Assessment. Open University Press, Buckingham.

Wood, B.D., 1921. Measurement of college work. Educ. Adm. Superv. Vol. VII.

Chapter | 6 |

Assessment as a process to support learning

INTRODUCTION

It is discussed in Chapter 2 that assessors of students on health care courses have both professional responsibility and accountability to ensure that students they assess achieve safe and competent standards of clinical practice. These onerous tasks of assessing and conferring safety and competence are based on inferences made on a sample of the student's performance. Such inferences are subject to error (Gonczi et al 1993, Rowntree 1987). Procedures need to be in place to ensure that the kind and amount of assessment evidence gathered are sufficient to make a safe inference and that the assessment is managed to ensure reasonable reliability to accompany greater validity. In other words, a carefully planned and managed assessment strategy is required so that the goal of professional education, which is to achieve fitness for purpose and practice, is fulfilled through the assessment processes. It would perhaps be a truism to say that students do not just achieve this 'fitness'; rather, their learning requires facilitation as they work alongside practitioners during clinical placements. This implies that assessment has another key function besides that of obtaining evidence of competence: having a constructive focus where the aim is to help rather than sentence the individual (Gipps 1994). An important message from Crooks (1988) is that assessment appears to be one of the most potent forces influencing education, and it can have positive as well as negative effects. It is therefore necessary to plan and manage clinical assessment so that the powerful effects of assessment can be harnessed and directed positively onto learning about clinical practice.

The continuous assessment process will be explored as the key assessment strategy to facilitate assessment as a learning process. Integral to the continuous assessment of clinical practice are the strategies of using the learning contract, with its concomitant assessment plan, formative assessment and summative assessment. These are examined with respect to the successful management of the continuous assessment of practice in order to realize the positive impact of assessment.

CONTINUOUS ASSESSMENT OF CLINICAL PRACTICE

This section starts with an activity (Activity 6.1). The assumption made here is that not all of our experiences of being assessed are positive ones!

ACTIVITY 6.1

Recall an occasion as a learner when you felt you
were assessed unfairly. What were the circumstances
surrounding that assessment?

You may have thought that the assessment was unfair
because:

- you were not given sufficient learning opportunities
  to develop and prove yourself
- you were unaware of incorrect practices
- your opinions of your progress were not considered
- your assessor did not know you well enough to make
  the assessment decision
- you did not have enough time to practise.

Nicklin & Kenworthy (1995) and Rowntree (1987)
believe that assessments give students opportunities to
demonstrate the learning that has taken place. Assessments
should thus have a constructive focus (Gipps 1994)
whereby students are given the support, supervision and
opportunities to demonstrate learning. Glaser (1990:480)
emphasizes the importance of placing assessment in the
service of learning, saying that assessments should:

*… display to the learner models of performance that
can be emulated and also indicate the assistance,
experiences, and forms of practice required by learners
as they move toward more competent performance.*

In health care, practical assessments of a student's learning are context bound. Each patient or client cared for has
different health care needs, which means that the student
has to learn different aspects of care and different ways of
responding constantly. An 'accurate estimate' of total learning can be made fairly only over a period of time, after a
student has had continuous supervision and sufficient
learning opportunities to provide the range of clinical
experiences required to develop competence. In the UK,
the impetus for the use of continuous assessment of theory
and practice in nursing and midwifery education can be
directly attributed to the perceived injustices of the final
'one-off' assessment, where factors such as anxiety and
ill health may adversely affect the competence demonstrated on the day of the assessment. The result may not
be representative of the overall abilities demonstrated by
the student. Within early guidelines for continuous assessment, the English National Board for Nursing, Midwifery
and Health Visiting stated (ENB 1986) that:

*Assessment should be a cumulative process, relating to
learner progress as well as achievement, and be more
closely integrated with learning (rather than separated
from it) and with development of the individual
student. [original emphases]*

In later (1997) guidelines for continuous assessment
the ENB stated:

*The assessment of learning of theory and practice
is a continuous process culminating in a judgement
of achievement. Formative processes guide student
learning and summative assessment measures
integration of subject disciplines and the application of
theories in practice.*

The position of the ENB in 1986 and 1997 on continuous assessment calls then for the use of formative and
summative assessments, with the formative assessments
feeding into, and informing, the summative assessment.
The use of the continuous assessment of practice requires
assessments to take place continually with periodic discussion, feedback, educational counselling and documentation throughout the student's placement. Good
continuous assessment demands substantial time and
effort. This allows students' performances to be monitored continuously during their day-to-day activities in
clinical practice. Student efforts have to be steady and
regular throughout (Rowntree 1987). Over the duration
of the programme then, 'a series of progressively updated
measurements of a student's achievement and progress'
are formally maintained in the student's portfolio/ongo-
ing record of achievement (NMC 2010, 2009, ENB 1996).
Such measurements are made against given learning
outcomes. The reference by the ENB in 1986 that 'assessment should be a cumulative process' means that every
effort made by the student is assessed, and these series
of assessments obtained through the continuous assessment process contribute to the summative assessment
(see below); a final 'end-of-the placement' assessment
is generally dispensed with (Rowntree 1987). The use of
continuous assessment allows the quality and quantity of
information about the student to be increased. In the case
of pre-registration nursing and midwifery education, the
requirement for students to spend a minimum of 40% of
their time with their practice educators (NMC 2008) will
facilitate the collection of a more comprehensive range
of assessment evidence. The more we know about a student's abilities the more likely it is that our assessment
will be accurate. Continuous assessment of clinical practice has the following advantages:

- Practitioners who are responsible for student learning
  can assess progress as it takes place.
- The context-bound nature of practical assessments
  is reduced as the learner is assessed over the varied
  circumstances of different patients/clients cared for.
- The learner receives continual and accurate feedback
  on performance and can identify areas where
  improvement is required. The practice educator's
  personal knowledge of the learner and understanding
  of the context of the performance are significant
  advantages in providing valid feedback.

- Areas for development and improvement can be planned jointly by the practice educator and the student.
- The student is likely to feel supported and encouraged, as any learning and achievement will be seen as contributing to the summative assessment. Rowntree (1987) reports that students in higher education who have experienced continuous assessment believe it to be less stressful than the 'all-or-nothing' final assessment. However, White et al (1994) found that student nurses in their study felt continuous assessment during clinical practice to be stressful, saying that they were under scrutiny at all times and consequently had to exhibit best behaviours always. And is that such an onerous requirement, remembering that the behaviours of health care professionals towards their patients and clients and colleagues should be of an acceptable standard at all times?

FORMATIVE ASSESSMENT

Both formative and summative assessments influence learning (Boud 2000). Summative assessment provides an 'authoritative statement of ... what counts ... and directs students attention to those matters' (Boud 2000:155). It tells students what to learn. The influence of formative assessment is no less profound. It provides the fine-tuning mechanism for *what* is learnt and *how* it is learnt. It should guide students in how to learn what they need to learn. It should also tell them the progress they are making. Formative assessment is founded on the principle of maximizing learning; assessment information about the student's knowledge, understanding and skills are used to feed back into the teaching/learning process (Gipps 1994).

In clinical practice, formative assessment refers to assessment taking place during learning activities and throughout the placement. It is conducted while the event to be assessed is occurring and focuses on identifying student learning and progress (Reilly & Oermann 1990). It focuses on parts of learning. The practice educator determines whether to re-explain, arrange further practice or move to the next stage. The assertion is that formative assessment can, and will, aid learning (Torrance & Pryor 1998). For this to take place, it is crucial that formative assessment becomes a process whereby both 'feedback' and 'feedforward' occur. Within this, practice educator–learner interaction becomes an important part of the process: it goes beyond the communication of assessment results, judgements of progress and provision of additional instructions. The practice educator and learner collaborate actively to produce a best performance (Torrance & Pryor 1998). An important role for the practice educator is to assist the learner in comprehending and engaging with new ideas and problems. The process of assessment itself is seen as having an impact on the learner as well as on the result of the assessment.

Student self-assessment in formative assessment

Engage students in self-assessment. It is important to allow students to assess their own learning. Facilitate, and allow students to vocalize their perceptions of their achievements, ability and level of competency so that learning can start from, and build on, what the student already knows and can already do. From educational psychology, Ausubel (1968:163) stated strongly that:

> *If I had to reduce all educational psychology to one principle, it would be this: the most important single factor influencing learning is what the student already knows. Ascertain this and teach him [sic] accordingly.*

Some educationalists believe that assessment is truly formative only if it involves the student directly (Sadler 1989, Torrance & Pryor 1998). Self-assessment helps students feel that they own the learning and can thus control the way they meet their learning needs (Stoker 1994). It is linked with motivation, monitoring one's own learning and becoming an independent learner (Gipps 1994). This is reinforced by Rowntree (1987:65) who says that a 'pupil does not really know what he [sic] has learned until he has organized it and explained it to someone else'. Self-assessment facilitates this process. Additionally, Chambers (1998) says that self-assessment is an efficient and effective learning tool in that students are required to identify their own strengths and weaknesses. Students may need to be facilitated to be realistic so that they do not over- or underestimate their ability and capabilities.

Students have an important role to play in planning their own learning and assessment. If they are to become competent assessors of their own work, they need sustained experience in ways of questioning and improving the quality of their work, and supported experience in assessing their work. The ability to self-assess one's competence and achievements accurately is not a natural gift, but a skill that can be learned and improved upon with practice (Mattheos et al 2004). Feedback is crucial in helping students develop accurate self-assessment skills. Sadler (1989) argues that if students are to be able to compare actual performance with a standard, and subsequently act to close that gap, they must possess some of the same evaluative skills as their assessor. Writers such as Yorke (2003) and Boud (2000) stated that assessors should focus on the quality of feedback given, which in turn will enable students to develop and strengthen their skills of self-assessment. There is a discussion below of how to manage feedback constructively.

Students are often well placed to assess their own learning and to regulate their own work appropriately. They will thus be able to indicate the amount and nature of clinical experiences they have had and recognize what clinical experiences they need in order to achieve competence. Falchikov & Boud (1989:395) highlight the need for students to take more responsibility for their own learning: 'life-long learning requires that individuals be able not only to work independently, but also to assess their own performance and progress'. One key aim of self-assessment should be to shift the student's focus from 'how good am I?' to 'how can I get better?' (Mattheos et al 2004:385). This ability will help students develop awareness of their own standards of practice. It is therefore important to handle student self-assessment well and in a positive, constructive way rather than in a negative norm-referenced way, as this can be demotivating (Gipps 1994). By listening to students the practice educator will learn what students consider their own learning needs to be. What is known about how adults learn says that adults learn best when they can see the relevance of what they are learning (Jarvis & Gibson 1997, Knowles 1990). The practice educator should therefore respond to the student's expressed learning needs. It may be necessary to probe more deeply so that the self-assessment helps students monitor their own learning to help them become independent learners (Gipps 1994). Finally, practice educators should encourage students to consider what they want feedback on, as this will help the latter to develop self-awareness of personal and professional development (Bailey 1998).

Opportunities and time should be made available to engage in the essential process of formative assessment with learners to provide them with targeted and evidence-based feedback, so that action plans for further learning and development of competence can be made. Adequate documentation of progress can thus be made. Duffy (2004) warns that the omission of formative assessment with opportunities for student self-assessment leads to inadequate documentation of progress, and is a potential cause for the student's inability to achieve the required level of competence.

In clinical practice, how does the formative assessment process discussed above fit into the teaching/learning and working cycles of the practice educator and the learner? These issues will be taken up in subsequent sections.

FEEDBACK IN ASSESSMENT

In academic settings, feedback is commentary about a learner's performance that aims to provide the learner with insight into performance, with the aim of improving that performance (Billings et al 2010, Clynes & Raftery 2008). It is an interactive process. Feedback may be categorized into two broad groups: constructive/corrective/negative and reinforcing/positive (Clynes & Raftery 2008).

The crucial role of feedback in learning cannot be emphasized enough, with Rowntree (1987:27) stating that it is the 'lifeblood of learning'. Torrance & Pryor (1998) emphasize the importance of identifying not just what learners have achieved but also what they might achieve and what they are now ready to achieve. Butler (1988) has shown that feedback comments alone had more effect on students' subsequent learning than comparable situations where marks alone or feedback and marks were given. The award of grades or simply confirming correct responses or performance has little effect on subsequent performance (Crooks 1988) as such feedback is very non-specific. It does not tell the student what has been done to merit such a grade or response, or what could be done to earn a better grade or to improve performance. Rowntree (1987) considers that such non-specific feedback becomes increasingly useless to the student as the size and diversity of performance being assessed increases during the placement. This factor is important for the practice educator to consider, as students are required to engage in, and learn through, a diverse range of clinical activities. Specific and detailed feedback, with descriptions of what actually occurred, is required on a myriad of activities and situations that the student will have taken part in. Examples from the student's practice should be used to illustrate points being made in the feedback. This should be clear to the student and offered in terms of specific standards achieved or not achieved.

Formative assessment processes, then, require quality feedback of the kind and detail that tells learners what to do in order to improve; such quality feedback is more effective as students know explicitly and reliably what they are expected to do. This is because the mere provision of feedback is insufficient for optimal learning. What students need in order to make any improvement is to have knowledge of the desired standard or goal, to be able to compare their own performance with the desired performance and, subsequently, to explore options for improving practice and take part in the appropriate activities to close the gaps – *they need to know in some detail what to do, and what they can do, in order to improve.* Feedback will then help the student to grow, boost confidence, and increase motivation and self-esteem (Clynes & Raftery 2008). There is detailed discussion of how to manage constructive feedback sessions in Chapter 7.

SUMMATIVE ASSESSMENT

Whereas formative assessments take place throughout the student's clinical placement, summative assessments usually take place at the end of the placement, where the aggregate of learning is represented. Summative assessment focuses on the whole and is used to provide information about how much students have learned and to what extent learning outcomes have been met. There is a judgement of achievement. In the event of negative outcomes, nothing can now be done to remedy the situation.

The competency-based assessment system allows only two judgements of competence: competent or not yet competent (Wolf 1995:22). Wolf goes on to say:

> … *either the person has consistently demonstrated workplace performance which meets the specified standards or they are not yet able to do so – 'competent' or 'not yet competent'.*

This has to be the position of the assessment of clinical practice in the professions, as the main purpose of assessment is for accountability purposes. The specified competencies (in the UK these are referred to as standards for pre-registration nursing and midwifery students, and pre-registration health care courses regulated by the Health and Care Professions Council) for each clinical placement must be achieved at the summative assessment in order to progress in the training. Students who are not yet competent at progression points (HCPC 2011, NMC 2010, 2009) are generally not allowed to progress further in their training until they have successfully achieved competence.

Two positions are taken with formative assessment in this discussion: first, it is a facilitative process that aims to guide and maximize learning; secondly, it serves to provide a series of assessments so that a summative assessment can be compiled from them. Rowntree (1987) suggests that final 'end-of-the-placement' assessments may be dispensed with altogether if a satisfactory summative assessment can be compiled from the series of formative assessments. However, Harlen et al (1992) maintain that summative assessments should be separated into two types: 'summing-up' and 'checking-up'. In the former, information collected over a period of time is simply 'summed' at intervals to assess how students are getting on. This collection of pieces of assessment evidence from formative assessments is kept in the student's portfolio of learning in order to preserve the richness of the data. The summing-up provides a picture of current achievements. 'Checking-up' is when summative assessment is done through the use of assessment tasks specifically devised for the purpose of assessing competence at a particular time. For example, at the end of the placement, on summing-up the evidence of competence of a learner in relationship to admitting a client to the ward, the assessor requires some more evidence of competence. In this example, checking-up can be in the form of observing the learner admit a client or simulating the activity. In your clinical area you may identify competencies that are crucial for the safe delivery of care and choose to use 'checking-up' as a matter of course when assessing the learner summatively.

Having examined formative and summative assessments, and the continuous assessment process in general, the next section will examine how to engage in and use the process of continuous assessment.

ENGAGING IN THE PROCESS OF CONTINUOUS ASSESSMENT

The three little words 'assessment takes time' was probably written with much feeling and understanding by Phillips et al (2000:150) after their intensive investigation of the assessment of clinical practice in pre-registration nursing and midwifery education. Assessment does indeed take time. I would contend that good assessment takes even more time. Time has to be allocated for 'assessment-only' activity to enable assessors to engage in the process of continuous assessment so that assessments serve the intended purposes. Recently, the NMC (2008) recommended that consideration is given to the practice educator's workload to enable more meaningful conduct of assessment activities. The assessment activities to be undertaken within the continuous assessment process may be represented in Figure 6.1.

It can be seen from Figure 6.1 that one of the central assessment activity is that of student–practice educator meetings. Bedford et al (1993) found that these valuable meetings do not function as effectively as they might because they are hurriedly carried out. If students feel that they pose an additional burden in a busy clinical area, the quality and quantity of learning is extremely negatively affected (Phillips et al 2000). Protected, that is timetabled, time should be prioritized and allocated for 'assessment-only activities' (NMC 2008, Phillips et al 2000, Bedford et al 1993). Professional responsibility and accountability for learners require us to ensure that learning takes place, and allocating and spending time with learners is part of that contract we enter into with learners in our care. Readers are directed to Chapter 8 in the section 'Staff commitment to teaching and learning' for some suggestions on how to support student learning and assessment activities.

The first meeting/interview

This first formalized meeting/interview is important for students: they will be feeling anxious in a new place of work (Phillips et al 2000) and unsure about what to expect from their practice educator they may be meeting for the first time. When asked about their first day on clinical placement, most students in Phillips et al's study (2000:72), provided, as their first word descriptor, 'scary', 'frightening', 'terrified' and 'anxious'. Students will also be feeling, for example, uncertain about how the ward functions, whether they will fit in and be accepted and

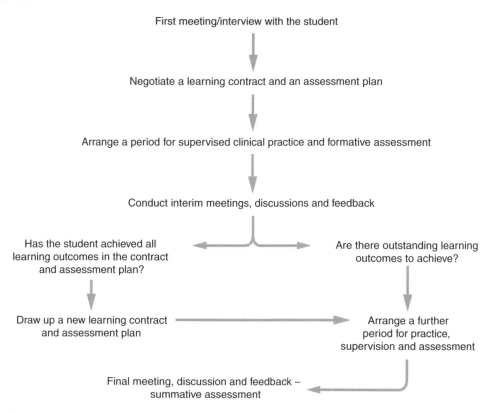

First meeting/interview with the student

↓

Negotiate a learning contract and an assessment plan

↓

Arrange a period for supervised clinical practice and formative assessment

↓

Conduct interim meetings, discussions and feedback

← →

Has the student achieved all learning outcomes in the contract and assessment plan?   Are there outstanding learning outcomes to achieve?

↓   ↓

Draw up a new learning contract and assessment plan   →   Arrange a further period for practice, supervision and assessment

Final meeting, discussion and feedback – summative assessment   ←

Figure 6.1 The process of continuous assessment of clinical practice.

what they are going to learn, particularly if the student has never worked in that area of speciality. The student will thus be looking for support and guidance from the practice educator. Anxiety can be a barrier to learning (Rogers 1983). The first meeting/interview gives the practice educator an ideal opportunity to start forming a facilitative relationship with the student and introducing the student to, for example, the clinical area, its routine, the learning opportunities available and the members of staff. What we know about what helps learners in a new clinical area tells us that 'beginners' feel more secure if their practice can be guided by the structure of a specified routine (Benner et al 1996). Practice educators in Fraser et al's study (1997) found that these meetings gave them valuable insight into a student's understanding of the clinical setting and their aspirations during the placement. Their 'readiness to learn' (Knowles 1990) can thus be determined.

Vygotsky (1930, in Spouse 1998) introduced the concept of 'zone of proximal development' (ZPD) to describe the range of activities in which learners are capable of engaging. The ZPD comprises a two-stage theory of development whereby a learner who is intellectually ready to move to the next stage could be assisted to reach this potential through support and guidance from a more

experienced other. Having an accurate assessment of a learner's level of capability is crucial in assisting a learner to develop a higher level of competence. Work in educational psychology tells us that, for effective learning and development to take place, the task must be matched to the student's current level of understanding, and pitched at that level to provide practice in the first instance, and subsequently a slightly higher level in order to extend and develop the student's skills (Bigge 1982). If the new task is too easy, the student can become bored; if too difficult, the student can become demotivated. By matching the learning tasks to the student's level, the learning contract/assessment plan is individualized and the emphasis on assessment is placed on the student's progress and learning.

The first meeting/interview with the student should be done as soon as possible – preferably within the first 2 days of the commencement of the placement. This is important to enable the practice educator and the student to draw up a learning contract that contains an assessment plan. This plan for learning and assessment should utilize the information from the student self-assessment to contribute to the identification of learning needs. It should also consider the student's ZPD to maximize learning and professional development.

As soon as the learning contract and assessment plan are negotiated and agreed, the direction that both the practice educator and student require for the teaching/ learning and assessment processes to commence is provided. It is recognized that students appreciate the development of an initial plan and think that this is good practice (Fraser et al 1997).

Try Activity 6.2.

ACTIVITY 6.2

Make a list of the points you would discuss with your student during the first meeting/interview. Why have you included these points?

In Chapter 2, it was discussed that one of your responsibilities as practice educator is to be familiar with the structure, organization and content of the programme of students you are assessing. This will allow you to have cognizance of the learning outcomes that your student will be required to achieve during the placement. The first meeting/interview allows you to evaluate what prior learning has taken place to inform and guide subsequent plans for learning. Phillips et al (2000) found that students on new placements often had to endure being treated as though they knew nothing – previous learning and accomplishments were ignored. Apart from this being disabling and demotivating, it can lead the practice educator to shape learning experiences inappropriately. Phillips et al (2000), very rightly in my view, contend that all students know something and some know a great deal.

The points to discuss with the student should include the following:

- find out and attempt to allay any anxieties
- confirm the student's stage of training and current module of study to ascertain course learning outcomes
- discuss any personal learning outcomes the student may have planned
- jointly examine and discuss the student's portfolio of learning to ascertain prior learning and progress
- ask about any written assignments or projects that have to be prepared
- discuss the learning opportunities the placement can provide to generate assessment evidence to enable achievement of competencies and learning outcomes
- discuss arrangements to supervise and support the student in your absence
- discuss the ward's routine and care philosophy.

The outcomes to aim for after the first meeting/ interview may be represented in Figure 6.2. This meeting/ interview should culminate in the mutual drawing up of the learning contract and assessment plan. The next section examines the learning contract, which also contains the assessment plan.

THE LEARNING CONTRACT AND THE ASSESSMENT PLAN

The use of learning contracts can be made integral to the continuous assessment process, as both the formative and summative assessment components of this process can

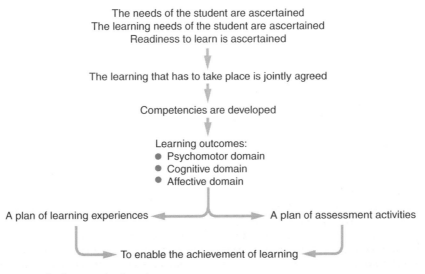

Figure 6.2 The outcomes of a first meeting/interview.

be fulfilled. As discussed above, the intention of formative and summative assessment processes is to guide learning. Careful negotiation and planning of a learning contract will result in a framework to guide the teaching, learning and assessment requirements of the student. This framework will also provide the direction for teaching and assessing activities, including the management of feedback, for the practice educator. This framework should not be seen as something that fixes students to a certain course of action. It should be seen as a statement of intent that gives structure to learning activities to facilitate the fulfilment of educational learning outcomes and the development of professional competence.

In the clinical setting, the learning contract approach involves an individual student negotiating with, and entering into an agreement with, a practice educator to pursue certain goals of a course of training. Commonly, in a pre-registration programme, these goals are to achieve the competencies of the training programme. Post-registered practitioners may enter into contracts with their preceptors or managers to develop further their competence, roles and expertise. As the purpose of these kinds of learning is to develop and/or improve one's competence to perform as a professional, the needs and expectations of the profession must be taken into account. How the

learning is to be assessed is usually determined by the necessity to produce practitioners who are 'fit for purpose' and 'fit for practice' (United Kingdom Central Council for Nursing, Midwifery and Health Visiting (UKCC) 1999). Learners frequently have no choice in what they have to learn and how they are assessed. Furthermore, in the clinical setting, although there are many resources for learning, these are not unlimited. Constraints may also be imposed by timing of the availability of some resources. For example, certain clinical experiences, such as rarely occurring clinical events, do not manifest to order so that the student can learn and be assessed.

The above-imposed structures on learning and assessment frequently conflict with an adult learner's need to be self-directing and having the 'freedom to learn' (Rogers 1983). They may also stifle a learner's creativity and motivation to learn and, according to Knowles (1986), may induce resistance, apathy or withdrawal. The use of learning contracts could be one way of reconciling the requirements imposed by the above structures and the learner's internal need of having 'freedom to learn'. Chan & Chien (2000), Neary (1998) and Tompkins & McGraw (1988) found this reconciliation possible within the constraints of the curriculum – they used learning contracts in the clinical setting, which successfully increased individualized

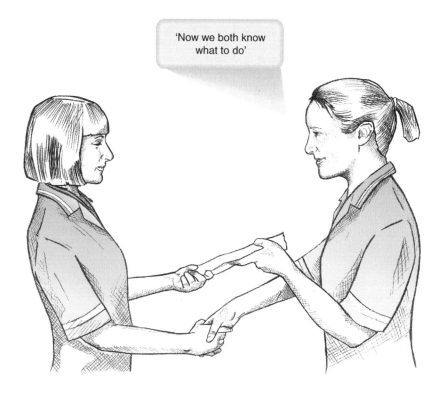

Figure 6.3 Have you contracted with your student?

learning and student autonomy. Interactions for planning and feedback activities between the clinical instructor and the student also improved – this finding confirmed Knowles' (1986) belief that learning contracts provide the means through which the planning of learning experiences can become a mutual undertaking between the student and the practice educator. In the nursing literature, Bailey & Tuohy (2009), Chan & Chien (2000), Neary (1998), McAllister (1996), Donaldson (1992), and Tompkins & McGraw (1988), for example, report other benefits of using the learning contract in the clinical setting. Knowles (1986) reported the disadvantages and benefits of contracting based on the experiences of a number of teachers in higher education. It is not the intention here to enter into a debate of the advantages and disadvantages of using learning contracts. The reader is therefore directed to the work of these authors for a further discussion of the advantages and disadvantages of using learning contracts.

The elements of a learning contract

The core that underpins any learning contract is made up of learning objectives, learning activities to be completed, strategies and resources for learning and both learner and practice educator evaluation of outcomes. Specific elements can be developed from this core to suit individual and institutional practices as well as fulfil the learning needs of students in a complex and an area rich with learning opportunities such as the clinical setting. For the purposes of competency-based assessment in the clinical setting, the elements given in Box 6.1 are suggested as the framework for the development of a learning contract. A discussion of these elements and how to develop them now follows.

Planning a learning contract

An understanding of the format of the learning contract and the process of contract learning is important for the

successful implementation and their use. Students must be well prepared for contract learning for this form of learning to succeed – preparation is crucial and should not be omitted (Knowles 1986). Personal discussion with students and practice educators tells me that the planning, developing and writing of a learning contract is not a straightforward affair. Authors such as McAllister (1996) and Donaldson (1992) report that contract formats can be confusing to use.

Using the elements of a contract as shown in Box 6.1 as the basis for planning, the sequence of steps given in Box 6.2 is proposed for planning and developing a learning contract/assessment plan for competence-based assessment in the clinical setting.

There is now a discussion of the rationale underpinning each element of the contract and how each element can be developed and used for learning and assessment activities.

Box 6.1 **The elements of a learning contract for competency-based assessment**

1. Clear statements of the aim and learning outcomes
2. State the level of performance to be achieved
3. Define the range of context for clinical practice to enable the achievement of the aim and learning outcomes
4. Specify the resources and learning activities
5. Develop an assessment plan
6. Identify the roles and responsibilities of both the learner and the practice educator
7. Decide a time frame – set review date(s) and a target date
8. Signatures

Box 6.2 **The steps to the construction of a learning contract/assessment plan**

Step 1
At the initial interview/meeting:
- Facilitate student self-assessment.
- Identify prior learning and clinical experiences the student had engaged in.
- Examine student portfolio.

Step 2
- Identify and jointly agree learning needs and competencies to be achieved.
- For each competency, identify the knowledge outcomes, performance outcomes and attitudes and values to be developed.

Step 3
- Identify the range and context of practice for each competency.
- Identify resources and learning activities such as clinical experiences that are required to enable the student to achieve each competency.

Step 4
- Consider how evidence of learning can be generated and evaluated.
- Decide most appropriate assessment methods to assess learning.
- Map methods against clinical activities and other learning activities.

Step 5
- Agree the roles and responsibilities of both to achieve the leaning contract/assessment. plan

Step 6
- Set and agree review and target dates.

1. Statements of the aim and learning outcomes

Once the learning needs and expectations are outlined from the perspective of the student and the practice educator, both will be in a position to define and describe what needs to be achieved. These require to be developed into statements that can provide the direction for learning and assessment strategies. The statements can then act as the criteria against which student progress can be measured. In its document *Fitness for Practice*, the UKCC (1999:38) recommends that:

> *Students, assessors and mentors should know what is expected of them through specified practice outcomes which form part of a formal learning contract.*

In a pre-registration programme, the learning, of necessity, needs to be related to the achievement of the statutory professional competencies. In the case of midwifery and nursing students and students in professions regulated by the Health and Care Professions Council (HCPC) in the UK, these competencies are laid down by the HCPC (2011) and the NMC (2010, 2009). In terms of statements of the aim and learning outcomes for competency-based assessment, the following aspects should be addressed:

- Define the element of competency to be achieved.
- Define the attributes that underlie the successful performance of the competency.

For the purposes of this discussion, the example is used of a student nurse or student midwife who has identified the need to learn about caring for clients and others at times of loss and death. Elements of competence are the tasks within the wider function described by a 'unit of competence', which represents a wide work function. This **element of competency** may be written thus: *to be able to care for clients and others at times of imminent death, death and loss.*

Professionals are competent as a result of the possession of a set of relevant attributes such as knowledge, understanding, skills, personal traits, attitudes and values. The attributes that underlie the successful performance of the element of competency to be able to care for clients and others at times of imminent death, death and loss need specifying so that they serve as the criteria for the assessment of successful performance of this element of competency. These criteria are the standards in competency-based assessment. Performance is judged against these pre-specified standards. It is suggested here that these standards are specified under the three domains of learning:

- the cognitive domain – *knowledge outcomes*
- the psychomotor domain – *performance outcomes*
- the affective domain – *attitudes and values to be developed.*

Thus the standards, which are not intended to be an exhaustive list, for the above element of competency may be grouped under these headings, as follows.

Knowledge outcomes

- Discuss the stages of the grieving process and the individual's needs during each stage.
- Describe the policies and guidelines relating to care of clients and others at times of loss and death.
- Discuss recent research in this area and recommendations for practice.

Performance outcomes

- Support clients, significant others and friends of clients during their initial adjustment to knowledge of the client's condition.
- Support clients during the critical period before death.
- Comfort and support significant others and friends of clients who have suffered loss.
- Comfort and support significant others and friends of clients who have died.
- Debrief and support colleagues as necessary.
- Use the appropriate verbal and non-verbal communication skills.
- Perform the necessary care of the dead person.

Attitudes and values

- Be empathetic towards grieving clients, significant others and friends of clients.
- Be empathetic towards colleagues.
- Possess the appropriate respect for clients from diverse cultural and religious backgrounds.
- Show the appropriate respect for the dead person.

Bedford et al (1993) found that documentation of this nature is most likely to promote reflective discussion of practice and integrate theory with practice. This research team also found that defining and documenting the competency statement, knowledge and performance outcomes and the attitudes and values enabled the practice educator to use them as measures against later analysis of student achievement of competence. This is perhaps the most persuasive argument for using standards in the assessment of clinical practice – standards define what are meant by quality care practices and quality practitioners. When standards and other requirements of good performance (see section 2 below) are made clear before tasks are attempted, misdirected efforts and undue anxiety can be avoided.

2. State the level of performance to be achieved

A statement of the level of performance tries to make clear the degree of proficiency expected of the learner. The specified level of performance required is an important component of any learning contract because it is the measure used for the summative assessment of the element of competence. The specified level of performance also guides the development of the learner. Generally, in a 3-year pre-registration programme, there are three levels of performance to be achieved: level 1, performance to be achieved by first year students; level 2, performance to be achieved by second year students; and level 3, performance to be achieved by third year students. Standards of performance to be reached in assessment should be clearly specified to students – they should be high, but attainable (Gipps 1994).

Bedford et al (1993) found that clinical assessors frequently experienced difficulty in ensuring that students were advised and assessed at the appropriate level. Specifying the criteria for a level of performance is a thorny issue (Phillips et al 2000, Gerrish et al 1997). The reader is directed to a discussion of this issue in Chapter 3. As I see it, one possible way around this problem is to specify the level of performance and then match this with the amount of supervision/support needed, the level of practice that

can be expected of the student and the conditions of competent practice for the specified performance level. This eclectic framework to assess clinical practice is shown in Table 6.1. The reader is referred to Chapter 7, where there is a discussion of the theoretical basis of this format, and how to monitor and assess the progress of students using this framework.

3. Define the range of context for clinical practice to enable effective performance of the element of competence

The range of context for clinical practice identifies the various care-giving situations that the student is expected to be able to carry out in order to achieve the element of competence in a specified clinical setting. These different care-giving events will provide the student with the opportunities to achieve the knowledge and performance outcomes and develop the appropriate attitudes and values specified in the learning contract. Here, there is room for negotiation and the exercise of autonomy

Table 6.1 Matching the levels of performance to levels of supervision and practice and conditions of competent practice

Level of performance	Level of supervision/ support	Level of practice	Conditions of practice for the achievement of clinical competencies	
			Competence achieved	**Competence not achieved**
Level 1	Direct to close supervision	Observes, participates, assists in	Performs with few prompts	Requires detailed and explicit instructions
			Can explain the rationale underpinning practice	Cannot explain the rationale underpinning practice
Level 2	Close to minimal supervision	Active participation Planning most activities and leading some	Performance is smooth and complete	Performance lacks completeness
			Does not require prompting in practised activities	Requires prompting in practised activities
			Can explain the rationale underpinning practice and discuss pertinent research	Cannot explain the rationale underpinning practice
Level 3	Minimal to indirect supervision	Active participation Planning all activities and leading most	Does not require prompting	Requires prompting
			Is organized and efficient	Unable to organize care
			Critiques evidence-based practice and its implementation	Does not consider evidence-based practice

111

by the student. If the student has already had particular clinical experiences that fulfil the requirements of any of the range statements (see Ch. 3), then these specific clinical experiences may not be required.

An example of the range statements for the element of competence – *to be able to care for clients and others at times of imminent death, death and loss* – is given below. The following range statements assume that the clinical setting is that of a medical unit:

- the imminent death of patients who have suffered a protracted illness
- the imminent death of patients with a sudden acute illness
- the imminent death of patients with different cultural and religious needs
- patients who have died.

In the midwifery setting, range statements may include:

- women who require the termination of their pregnancy for an abnormal fetus
- women who have experienced an intrauterine death
- women who have experienced a neonatal death
- women whose babies are in the special care baby unit
- women whose babies are acutely ill in the neonatal intensive care unit
- women who give up their babies for adoption.

It can be seen that the range statement serves to indicate the range of clinical situations to which the element of competence applies. It ensures that the element of competence has been learned and can be demonstrated in a range of contexts. Jessup (1991) warns that, although range statements can act to broaden the range of contexts in which mastery can be assumed, specifying the range can also be limiting.

Notwithstanding the possible disadvantage of specifying the range, there are sound educational reasons for doing so. What is now known of cognitive processes indicates that there is a close connection between skills and knowledge, and the context in which they are learned and practised. Eraut (2004) and Gipps (1994) suggest that we cannot teach a skill component in one setting and expect it to be applied automatically in another. This means, in turn, that a competence cannot be assessed with validity in a context very different from the context in which it has been taught and practised. In mainstream education, Koretz et al (1991 in Gipps 1994) found that high performance on a regularly used test did not generalize to another test for which students had not been specifically prepared. The conclusion that can be drawn from this is that teaching to perform for a particular test invalidates the test results as indicators of more general learning.

In their work with young people in the Youth Training Scheme, Wolf et al (1990) found that the transferability of complex problem-solving skills was limited. Trainees were given training on problem-solving tasks either within their own occupational group only or in a range of occupational groups; a control group was given no training at all. Both groups that received training showed improved performance over the group that did not, and the group that had received training in a variety of contexts performed better outside their occupational area than did the group that had training within their own occupational area. The authors concluded that varied training encouraged generalized learning (i.e. generalized skills do not develop from context-specific learning). Experiences with performance-based licensure examinations in medicine confirm the need for a large number of tasks in order to achieve acceptable levels of generalizability (Linn 1993). In his review of the generalizability of performance from one task to another, Linn (1993:12-13) concluded that:

> … *low levels of generalisability across tasks limit the validity of inferences about performance for a domain and pose serious problems regarding comparability and fairness to individuals which are judged against performance standards based on a small number, and perhaps different set, of tasks.*

Generalizability is a particular problem in performance assessment because performance is heavily context dependent – direct assessment of complex performance does not generalize well from one task to another. Linn (1993) recommends that, in performance assessment, increasing the number of tasks on the assessment is the most effective way of enhancing generalizability. Students must therefore be given new problems to solve or be asked to apply the concepts in different contexts of care to assess whether they can transfer and apply skills and knowledge. Increasing the number of tasks assessed clearly increases the resources required, such as time and expense. This is, however, justified by the need to achieve more valid assessment, so that health care professionals are the safe and competent practitioners we desire. Wolf (1995:43, 49) suggests the use of this guiding principle in assessment:

> … *the best predictor of future performance is past performance … [therefore] … assessments should be as close as possible to the outcomes one is interested in … you will get the best results if you sample directly the item you are interested in.*

The specification of a range of contexts will enable this important guiding principle to be put in place. Assessments will then have more validity.

4. Specify the resources, learning activities and learning opportunities

Resources required may be both material and human. These need to be identified and their use planned. Material resources, which should be available, up to date and directly relevant to the desired learning outcomes, could include equipment and care-giving aids, textbooks, journal articles, resources from the Internet, teaching aids, videos and self-directed learning programmes. There should be a discussion of how these resources can be best utilized to contribute to the achievement of learning outcomes. Learning activities around material resources may include reading text material, viewing a video and learning to use a piece of equipment. The practice educator should arrange to provide the necessary instructions.

When identifying human resources, the name, designation, availability and contact details of the person, usually another professional, should be specified. There should be a discussion of how the person can contribute to the learning so that the student is better prepared to utilize the expertise of that person. Learning activities here may include observing and working with the person, followed by discussions, or simply asking questions and talking to the person. In the example of the element of competence used so far – *to be able to care for clients and others at times of imminent death, death and loss* – human resources and learning activities could include observing the hospital chaplain, observing and working with the bereavement counsellor, and so on.

Some learning opportunities, such as direct participation in certain clinical experiences, may not be identified ahead of time. It should, however, be made clear to students those specific types of clients/patients whose care they need to participate in. The student will then be in a better position to negotiate with other team members they need to work with when they are looking after such clients/patients.

The reader is directed to the discussion on identifying and utilizing resources and learning opportunities in the clinical environment in Chapter 8.

5. Develop a learning and assessment plan

There should be a clear plan of how the learning and assessment of the element of competence are to proceed over a specified period. Both the student and practice educator should agree the following:

1. How learning and assessment will be managed, e.g. making firm arrangements:
   a. to look after certain clients/patients
   b. to work together on specified shifts
   c. to spend time together to review progress on specified occasions.
2. What evidence of learning should be collected.
3. How the evidence will be generated and collected.
4. What will be accepted as evidence that learning outcomes are achieved.

Students should be allowed to exercise choice and autonomy, where feasible, when decisions are made about how evidence is to be generated and provided. The student may negotiate to do written pieces of work, or present information verbally to peers, to support the achievement of specific learning outcomes, in particular the knowledge outcomes. The student must know

at the outset how the assessment will be done (e.g. if a written piece of work is used, a description of what must be included is identified). If an oral presentation is to be given, the student must know how long the presentation will last and how it will be evaluated.

Evidence of having taken part in care may be collected in a written format in the form of an *evidence log*. It is suggested that the student has the responsibility for maintaining this log. Within an evidence log, the student records details of clinical activities undertaken that will act as evidence of achievement of learning outcomes in the learning contract. Questioning and reflective discussions of these records will provide evidence of the underpinning knowledge and understanding of care delivered. The reader is directed to the section on *recording evidence* in Chapter 7 for a further discussion of the use of evidence logs.

Within a scheme of the continuous assessment of clinical practice, the student will generally work alongside the practice educator so that the practice educator is facilitating learning, at the same time assessing learning and progress, as they work together. The practice educator will be gathering evidence of learning that should be discussed with the student during feedback sessions. In the absence of the allocated practice educator, firm arrangements should be made for the student to work with another practitioner. The learning contract should be explained to the other practitioner so that continuity of supervision and support is maintained, and the validity and reliability of the assessment is enhanced.

6. Identify the roles and responsibilities of both the learner and the practice educator

A written learning contract signals a commitment from both the student and the practice educator. In contract learning, the student and practice educator work together to achieve the specified outcomes. Tompkins & McGraw (1988) emphasized the importance of recognizing that contracting does not mean that the student learns *independently*; rather, an *interdependent* relationship develops between the student and the practice educator. Within this interdependent relationship, the roles and responsibilities of each party should be made clear.

While one key aim of using learning contracts is to promote student autonomy and responsibility by encouraging self-directed learning, this may be intimidating for some students. McAllister (1996) found that some students did not enjoy the freedom and control when they were working through their learning contracts. Both Chan & Chien (2000) and McAllister (1996) discussed the uncertainties and anxieties students felt when contract learning was an unfamiliar learning strategy. However, levels of anxiety diminished quickly as students learned how to manage their own learning. Students' active participation in the development of the contract and agreement to the work to be done in order to achieve are helpful in reducing anxiety.

The practice educator needs to assess the level of readiness and ability of the student to deal with the demands of using learning contracts as advanced learning skills are required. These advanced learning skills include self-direction, critical self-appraisal, the ability to participate actively in the learning activities provided and in the management of their learning and to seek help, guidance and feedback when appropriate (Refshauge & Higgs 2000).

Knowles (1986:43) suggested that, in contract learning, 'the role of the instructor shifts from that of a didactic transmitter of content and controller of learners to that of a facilitator of self-directed learning and content resource'. In the case of the practice educator in the clinical setting, it is suggested here that the role shifts from someone who has the responsibility for making sure that learning experiences take place, and indeed controls the clinical experiences that students have, to that of someone whom students approach to negotiate the types of clinical and other learning experiences they require to achieve the outcomes in the contract. McAllister (1996) observed that practice educators still need to be aware that, even though power is more evenly distributed, they should not abrogate all control and responsibility – new and deep-level learning still need to be promoted. Neary (1998) suggests that what students want to learn can be developed only if the practice educator, through facilitation, directs and gives clear guidelines on expected outcomes of learning. Vygotsky's (1930, in Spouse 1998) theory of the zone of proximal development (ZPD) states that the potential of a learner to progress to the second stage of development could be capitalized upon if support and guidance from a more experienced other is available.

Stenhouse (1975, in Mazhindu 1990) made the contentious point that the quality of the facilitator is either the main weakness or the greatest strength of the learning contract. There is no doubt that the success of contract learning depends not only on the student's own enthusiasm and commitment to the agreement but also on the enthusiasm, commitment and ability of the practice educator as facilitator. The practice educator needs to assist the student with making a successful transition to this form of learning, if required, and also to help the student sustain the interest and commitment to the contract. One key strategy in maintaining student motivation in contract learning is to provide opportunities for success and to give regular immediate formative and summative feedback (Neary 1998).

Students must also make a shift in their perceptions of their roles as learners. A traditional learner role is that of dependency. Students are perceived, and perceive themselves to be, dependent on the teacher for planning and evaluating their learning, and are more or less dependent and passive recipients of transmitted content. In contract learning, the role of the student shifts from that of 'more or less passive receiver of transmitted information and submissive executor of the instructor's directives, to that of initiative-taking planner and executor of strategies and resources for achieving mutually agreed [outcomes]'

(Knowles 1986:44). As an adult learner, the student should also make use of learning opportunities and resources identified in support of the learning contract. It must be pointed out here that the practice educator/assessor of nursing and midwifery students in the UK (NMC 2008) is ultimately accountable and responsible for student learning and so must accept the ultimate responsibility for the quality of the learning and for ensuring that the requirements of the contract have been met. Some roles and responsibilities of the practice educator could be to:

- act as a resource and share ideas and recommend learning resources
- identify and negotiate learning opportunities for the student
- support and encourage the student
- assess and evaluate the student's work, giving regular constructive feedback
- provide stimulating learning experiences.

Some roles and responsibilities of the student could be to:

- seek out and make use of learning opportunities and resources
- make a study of relevant literature and evidence-base to increase underpinning knowledge and understanding
- take the initiative to seek guidance and feedback regularly
- participate in assessment and evaluation through self-evaluation.

7. Agreement on a time frame – set review date(s) and a target date

Setting a target date allows the student and practice educator to pace the learning and provides the student with a goalpost. It is important to meet at specified intervals to determine progress, make changes to the contract and provide help if needed. The student should be left with the responsibility of seeking guidance and feedback outside of these scheduled times if required. The frequency varies with the type of contract, the level of the student and the ability of the student for self-direction and discipline. The highly motivated, self-directing and self-disciplined student may require little help and therefore fewer occasions for formal review and feedback. The student who is less motivated or has difficulty in maintaining self-discipline will require more frequent meetings to verify understanding, check progress and to provide encouragement and motivation.

It is useful to identify some specific outcomes from the learning contract to work towards during a specified period so that these can be evaluated at each review meeting. This will provide the direction and the goals for learning for that period. Learning is then divided into chunks and is likely to be more manageable and achievable. Opportunities for success are provided: these will act as extrinsic motivators to encourage the student to set sights that are progressively higher (Neary 1998). At these review meetings, the student should participate actively through self-assessment and by the seeking of feedback about performance and learning. The following points may be useful for the review of progress:

- Review the learning contract. Discuss how far the activities that the student has participated in have contributed to the achievement of the learning outcomes and the range.
- Discuss any difficulties that the student may be experiencing.
- Discuss and plan future learning activities.
- Amend the learning contract if necessary – few learning contracts ever go to plan.

If the learning outcomes and the range have been achieved before the target date, a new learning contract should be drawn up. If the actual clinical experience cannot be provided towards the end of the contracted period, plans should be made to use simulation in the place of naturalistic observation as the alternative method of assessment.

8. Signatures

It is suggested that both the student and practice educator sign the contract, as this strengthens the commitment of both participants.

The following checklist of questions may be helpful when you are reviewing the completed contract that has been drawn up:

- Are the identified learning opportunities relevant to the needs of the learner?
- Do the selected learning opportunities utilize normal clinical events?
- Have arrangements been made to use continuous assessment to monitor progress?
- Has the learner been involved in discussing and agreeing the contract?
- Does the contract specify the level of performance, knowledge and performance outcomes?
- Do knowledge and performance outcomes illustrate a link between theory and practice?
- Do knowledge and performance outcomes reflect evidence-based practice?
- Are the roles and responsibilities of you and the learner clearly identified?

PERIOD OF SUPERVISED CLINICAL PRACTICE AND FORMATIVE ASSESSMENT

The learning contract and assessment plan formulated will provide the practice educator and the student with the framework for teaching, learning and assessment. The period of supervised clinical practice and formative

assessment can now proceed more meaningfully, and with the intent that is required in order to help the student achieve the learning during the precious time spent on clinical placements. During this period the student is learning under supervision and working towards achieving the competencies that the training requires. This learning may occur as a result of interacting with patients/ clients, giving patient/client care and being taught by yourself and other staff members. With reference to the learning outcomes and range of context identified in the contract above, it is clear what types and nature of learning experiences are required. Arrangements should be made so that the student and the practice educator work together and with other members of the team as necessary to enable the student to engage in the necessary clinical experiences. Working with other team members will also provide assessment evidence that can be attributed as 'testimony of others'.

During the formative assessment period, assessment activities are informal; you may observe activities, evaluate care given, give feedback, pose questions or discuss care given in a planned systematic or ad hoc way. The information obtained may be partial or fragmentary in the early days and will not allow you to make a firm evaluation of the student's competence. But repeated assessments of this sort, over a period of time and in a range of contexts, will allow you to build up a solid and broadly based assessment of your student's attainment. This will increase the validity and reliability of assessment.

Phillips et al (2000) found that where practice educators are able to work with students for only short intermittent and ad hoc stretches they are not able to collect reliable assessment evidence. This in turn reduces the validity of the assessment. They recommend that there should be a minimum time prioritized for assessment-only activities involving working and observing alongside the learner as part of a specified minimum overall learner entitlement. It is an NMC (2008) requirement that the practice educator directly observes and supports the student for at least 40% of the student's placement learning time (nominally 15 hours in a working week).

The formative assessments that take place as you work with the learner and give feedback on performance are generally ad hoc and informal. However, there need to be occasions when formative assessments are more formalized to enable you and the student to review and reflect on experiences, identify learning that has taken place and plan further experiences. It is recommended that these formative assessment sessions be documented. Remember that the aim of formative assessments is to motivate your student and maximize learning. These formalized sessions should be planned, and dates specified in the learning contract. The NMC (2008) and Bedford et al (1993) recommend allocating protected time for these discussions. The number of formal meeting/discussion sessions you hold altogether during the student's placement would be dependent on the length of the placement and the progress the student is making. There should be at least one formalized meeting/discussion session. As a guide, try to hold a formal meeting/discussion session at least every 2 weeks so that you can formally review with your student the progress that is made and identify any difficulties at an earlier rather than a later stage of the placement. Work on learning tells us that shorter units of work with linked assessment are more motivating for many students (Gipps 1994).

At the end of each interim meeting/discussion session, you and your student should jointly decide to what extent the competencies and learning outcomes in the learning contract/assessment plan have been achieved. As indicated in Figure 6.1, if all learning outcomes in the learning contract/assessment plan have been achieved, a new learning contract/assessment plan will be drawn up and a further period for practice and assessment arranged. Likewise, if the student requires more clinical experience to enable the outstanding learning outcomes to be achieved in the existing assessment plan and contract, a further period for practice and assessment will also need to be arranged. It is important to record in writing the discussion that has taken place, as this record should be filed in the student's portfolio for future reference. The student's assessment of practice record is completed as required (e.g. signing those competencies that have been achieved). This will serve to motivate the student.

THE FINAL MEETING/DISCUSSION SESSION AND SUMMATIVE ASSESSMENT

The final meeting/discussion session to perform the summative assessment is done at the end of the placement. As a guide, this meeting should be done during the last week of the student's placement, preferably on the last day. During this final meeting/discussion session, additional time should be allocated to review and analyse fully the evidence of competence. It is important to record the discussion and complete the student's assessment of practice record to be filed in the student's portfolio, so that it can be available to the student for future reference and to other practice educators in subsequent placements. Time should also be spent in preparing the student for future placements. As the supervising practice educator, you can see any changes in the student that provide specific information for fostering future development. Through your guidance learning can be influenced. Glaser (1990) makes the case that assessment must be used in support of learning rather than just to indicate current or past achievement. Assessment must be looked at not only in terms of outcomes measurement but also in terms of the learning process. The NMC (2008:34) requires the final

assessment of proficiency to draw on evidence of assessment over a sustained period of time to check to see if competence has been achieved and maintained previously, as well as demonstrated in the current placement.

Suggestions on how you might conduct these meeting/discussion sessions, the summative assessment meeting, analyse assessment evidence and give feedback more effectively are made in Chapter 7.

CONCLUSION

It is acknowledged that outcome measurement in the health care professions is important in order to achieve fitness for practice and fitness for purpose. This chapter has considered that assessment should not be looked at just in terms of outcome measurement but also as part of the learning process. One of the oldest and most robust findings of educational research is that assessment is the major influence on what gets learned (Eraut 2004). Assessment should be, and can be, facilitative and constructive and should never be used as a punitive tool. It should be used to identify what students have learned, what they have not learned and where they are having difficulty. In this way, it supports the teaching–learning process; this form of assessment is known as formative assessment. Assessment in the caring professions also needs to be used for accountability purposes to confer competence and certificate students; this form of assessment is known as summative assessment.

The continuous assessment of practice allows the practice educator to work closely with, supervise and assess the student in the everyday working environment. Assessments that take place in these 'natural' surroundings are more likely to reflect the real abilities of the student. There has been much emphasis that assessments should be of this nature so that they are 'authentic' (Govaerts et al 2001, Gipps 1994) – authentic assessments allow us to test those performances at which we want students to be good. It is important to plan assessments carefully so that these time-consuming assessment activities result in high quality assessment.

If we could work with students all the time they are in clinical practice, we would be in a very good position to tell whether they are any good. As a general rule, however, we make judgements on rather small amounts of evidence (Wolf 1995), which is why it is important that assessments should be as well designed as possible. Wolf reminds us that the prime responsibility for assessment planning lies with the assessor. This is particularly the case with assessments in professional education that confer professional qualifications; for example, a nursing, midwifery or physiotherapy qualification is taken to guarantee safe and competent practice for the public that these professions serve.

KEY POINTS FOR REFLECTION

Assessment should be a cumulative process, relating to learner *progress* as well as *achievement*, and be more closely integrated with learning (rather than separated from it) and with development of the individual student. One of the oldest and most robust findings of educational research is that assessment is the major influence on what gets learned (Eraut 2004).

Formative assessment processes guide and maximize student learning and takes place throughout the placement. Both the practice educator and learner collaborate actively to produce a best performance where 'feedback' and 'feedforward' take place. This also requires students to engage in self-assessment.

Feedback is an essential learning activity. The only way to tell if there is learning consequent to feedback is for students to make some kind of response to complete the feedback loop (Sadler 1989). Unless students are able to use feedback to produce improved work (e.g. to improve upon a similar/same aspect of care), neither they nor those giving feedback will know that it has been effective.

Summative assessment measures achievement at the end of the placement. It focuses on the whole and is used to provide information about how much students have learned and the extent to which learning outcomes have been met.

The assessment of clinical practice should be a continuous process that culminates in a judgement of achievement. In summary, the stages of the continuous assessment process are as follows:

1. Arrange and conduct the first meeting/interview. Be clear about what you want to include in the learning contract and the assessment plan.
2. Arrange clinical experiences to enable your student to practise and achieve the assessment plan and the learning outcomes in the contract. During this period, arrange to work with and assess your student in practice.
3. Arrange and conduct interim meeting/discussion sessions – formalized formative assessments – throughout the placement. Facilitate self-evaluation by the student. Complete assessment documentation.
4. Arrange and conduct the final meeting/discussion session – summative assessment. Complete assessment documentation.

The use of learning contracts can be made integral to the continuous assessment process. Careful negotiation and planning of a learning contract will result in a framework to guide the teaching, learning and assessment requirements of the student. This framework will also provide the direction for teaching and assessing activities for the practice educator.

REFERENCES

Ausubel, D.P., 1968. Educational Psychology: A Cognitive View. Holt, Rinehart & Winston, New York.

Bailey, J., 1998. The supervisor's story: from expert to novice. In: Johns, C., Freshwater, D. (Eds.), Transforming Nursing through Reflective Practice Blackwell Science, London, pp. 194–205.

Bailey, M.E., Tuohy, D., 2009. Student nurses' experiences of using a learning contract as a method of assessment. Nurse Educ. Today 29, 758–762.

Bedford, H., Phillips, T., Robinson, J., et al., 1993. Assessment of Competencies in Nursing and Midwifery Education and Training. The English National Board for Nursing, Midwifery and Health Visiting, London.

Benner, P., Tanner, C.A., Chesla, C.A., 1996. Expertise in Nursing Practice. Springer, New York.

Bigge, M.L., 1982. Learning Theories for Teachers, fourth ed. Harper & Row, London.

Billings, D.M., Kowalski, K., Cleary, M.L., et al., 2010. Giving feedback to learners in clinical and academic settings: practical considerations. J. Contin. Educ. Nurs. 41 (4), 153–154.

Boud, D., 2000. Sustainable assessment: Rethinking assessment for the learning society. Stud. Contin. Educ. 22 (2), 151–167.

Butler, R., 1988. Enhancing and undermining intrinsic motivation: The effects of task-involving and ego-involving evaluation on interest and involvement. Br. J. Educ. Psychol. 58, 1–14.

Chambers, M., 1998. Some issues of assessment of clinical practice: A review of the literature. J. Clin. Nurs. 7 (3), 201–208.

Chan, S.W., Chien, W., 2000. Implementing contract learning in a clinical context: report on a study. J. Adv. Nurs. 31 (2), 298–305.

Clynes, M.P., Raftery, S.E.C., 2008. Feedback: An essential element of student learning in clinical practice. Nurse Educ. Pract. 8, 405–411.

Crooks, T.J., 1988. The impact of classroom evaluation practices on students. Rev. Educ. Res. 58 (4), 438–481.

Donaldson, I., 1992. The use of learning contracts in the clinical area. Nurse Educ. Today 12, 431–436.

Duffy, K., 2004. Failing Students Report. Nursing and Midwifery Council, London, Online. Available: http://www.nmc-uk.org/nmc/main/publications/mentor_study.pdf (accessed December 2005 August 2011.

English National Board, 1986. Guidelines to Preparing Continuous Assessment. The English National Board for Nursing, Midwifery and

Health Visiting, London, Circular 1986 (16) ERBD.

English National Board, 1996. Regulations and Guidelines for the Approval of Institutions and Courses. The English National Board for Nursing, Midwifery and Health Visiting, London, Section 5 – Regulations and Guidelines Relating to Assessment.

English National Board, 1997. Standards for Approval of Higher Education Institutions and Programmes. The English National Board for Nursing, Midwifery and Health Visiting, London.

Eraut, M., 2004. A wider perspective on assessment. Med. Educ. 38, 800–804.

Falchikov, N., Boud, D., 1989. Student self-assessment in higher education: a meta-analysis. Rev. Educ. Res. 59 (4), 395–430.

Fraser, D., Murphy, R., Worth-Butler, M., 1997. An Outcome Evaluation of the Effectiveness of Pre-registration Midwifery Programmes of Education. The English National Board for Nursing, Midwifery and Health Visiting, London.

Gerrish, K., McManus, M., Ashworth, P., 1997. Levels of Achievement: A Review of the Assessment of Practice. The English National Board for Nursing, Midwifery and Health Visiting, London.

Gipps, C.V., 1994. Beyond Testing: Towards a Theory of Educational Assessment. The Falmer Press, London.

Glaser, R., 1990. Toward new models for assessment. Int. J. Educ. Res. 14 (5), 475–483.

Gonczi, A., Hager, P., Athanasou, J., 1993. The Development of Competency-Based Assessment Strategies for the Professions. Australian Government Publishing Service, Canberra, National Office of Overseas Skills Recognition, Research Paper No. 8.

Govaerts, M.J.B., Schuwirth, L.W.T., Pin, A., et al., 2001. Objective assessment is needed to ensure competence. Br. J. Midwifery 9 (3), 156–161.

Harlen, W., Gipps, C., Broadbent, P., et al., 1992. Assessment and the improvement of education. Curriculum J. 3, 3.

Health and Care Professions Council 2011 Standards of proficiency. Online. Available: <http://www.

hcpc-uk.org/aboutregistration/standards/standardsofproficiency/> (accessed October 2012).

Jarvis, P., Gibson, S., 1997. The Teacher Practitioner and Mentor in Nursing, Midwifery, Health Visiting and the Social Services, second ed. Stanley Thornes, Cheltenham.

Jessup, G., 1991. Outcomes: NVQs and the Emerging Model of Education and Training. The Falmer Press, London.

Knowles, M., 1990. The Adult Learner: A Neglected Species, fourth edn. Gulf, Houston.

Knowles, M.S., 1986. Using Learning Contracts. Jossey-Bass, San Francisco.

Koretz D., Linn R., Dunbar S. et al 1991 The effects of high stakes testing on achievement: preliminary findings about generalization across tests. Paper presented to the AERA/NCME, April, Chicago.

Linn, R.L., 1993. Educational assessment: expanded expectations and challenges. Educ. Eval. Policy Anal. 15 (1), 1–16.

McAllister, M., 1996. Learning contracts: an Australian experience. Nurse Educ. Today 16, 199–205.

Mattheos, N.M.C., Nattestad, A., Falk-Nilsson, E., et al., 2004. The interactive examination: assessing students' self-assessment ability. Med. Educ. 38 (4), 378–389.

Mazhindu, G.N., 1990. Contract learning reconsidered: a critical examination of implications for application in nurse education. J. Adv. Nurs. 15, 101–109.

Neary, M., 1998. Contract assignments and change in teaching, learning and assessment strategies. Educ. Prac. Theory 20 (1), 43–58.

Nicklin, P.J., Kenworthy, N., 1995. Teaching and Assessing in Clinical Practice, second ed. Baillière Tindall, London.

Nursing and Midwifery Council, 2008. Standards to Support Learning and Assessment in Practice, second ed. NMC, London, Online. Available: <http://www.nmc-uk.org/Publications/Standards> (accessed August 2011).

Nursing and Midwifery Council, 2009. Standards of Pre-registration Midwifery Education. NMC, London, Online. Available: <http://www.nmc-uk.org/Publications/Standards/> (accessed August 2011).

Nursing and Midwifery Council, 2010. Standards of Pre-registration Nursing Education. NMC, London, Online. Available: <http://www.nmc-uk.org/Publications/Standards/> (accessed August 2011).

Phillips, T., Schostak, J., Tyler, J., 2000. Practice and Assessment in Nursing and Midwifery: Doing it for Real. The English National Board for Nursing, Midwifery and Health Visiting, London.

Refshauge, K., Higgs, J., 2000. Teaching clinical reasoning. In: Higgs, J., Jones, M. (Eds.), Clinical Reasoning in the Health Care Professions, second edn. Butterworth-Heinemann, Oxford, pp. 141–147.

Reilly, D.E., Oermann, M.H., 1990. Behavioural Objectives: Evaluation in Nursing. National League for Nursing, New York.

Rogers, C., 1983. Freedom to Learn for the 80's. Charles E. Merrill, Columbus, Ohio.

Rowntree, D., 1987. Assessing Students: How Shall We Know Them, second ed. Kogan Page, London.

Sadler, R., 1989. Specifying and promulgating achievement standards. Instr. Sci. 18, 119–144.

Spouse, J., 1998. Scaffolding student learning in clinical practice. Nurse Educ. Today 18, 259–266.

Stenhouse, L., 1975. An Introduction to Curriculum Research and Development. Heinemann, London.

Stoker, D., 1994. Assessment in learning: (i) Understanding assessment issues. Nurs. Times 90, i–viii. 11, Section 7i.

Tompkins, C., McGraw, M.-J., 1988. The negotiated learning contract. In: Boud, D. (Ed.), Developing Student Autonomy in Learning, second ed. Kogan Page, London, pp. 172–191.

Torrance, H., Pryor, J., 1998. Investigating Formative Assessment. Open University Press, Buckingham.

UKCC, 1999. Fitness for Practice. United Kingdom Central Council for Nursing, Midwifery and Health Visiting, London.

White, E., Riley, E., Davies, S., et al., 1994. A Detailed Study of the Relationship between Teaching, Support, Supervision and Role Modelling in Clinical Areas within the Context of P2000 Courses. The English National

Board for Nursing, Midwifery and Health Visiting, London.

Wolf, A., 1995. Competence-Based Assessment. Open University Press, Buckingham.

Wolf, A., Kelson, M., Silver, R., 1990. Learning in Context: Patterns of Skills Transfer and Training Implications. The Training Agency, Sheffield.

Yorke, M., 2003. Formative assessment in higher education: moves towards theory and the enhancement of pedagogic practice. High. Educ. 45 (4), 477–501.

Chapter | 7 |

Monitoring progress, managing feedback and making assessment decisions

INTRODUCTION

Monitoring progress, managing feedback and making assessment decisions are interrelated activities that are integral to the continuous assessment of practice. These activities are central to and essential in helping students learn through their practice to develop clinical competence. Using the continuous assessment process enables the monitoring of progress continually and the giving of feedback informally and constantly as the learner works alongside the practice educator – even over one working shift, feedback is an activity that occurs many times. There are, however, specific times when formal feedback should be given based on a more detailed examination of progress. As discussed in Chapter 6, when pre-scheduled and pre-planned 'formal' formative and summative assessments are conducted, time and opportunities are available to discuss progress with the student, formally give feedback and make assessment decisions based on the analysis of assessment evidence. The practice educator is in a 'unique position in being able to provide precise feedback to individual students on all aspects of practical professional development' (Stengelhofen 1993:153). However, if assessment is to be a true learning process, the student should be an equal partner in these activities – progress is monitored jointly through the formative assessment process set up, and the student participates actively during feedback and assessment decision-making sessions. It is important that these activities occur, not only to maintain the integrity of the assessment process itself but also to meet the rights of the student as a learner. Torrance & Pryor (1998) believe that assessment is truly formative only if it involves the student directly in self-assessment.

MANAGING FEEDBACK

'Managing feedback' is used in this chapter to signify the activity of holding constructive discussions with the student about clinical experiences that the student and the practice educator have been involved in. Feedback can take place informally as the practice educator works alongside the student, or more formally during pre-arranged feedback sessions. Rowntree (1987:24) considers that this essential learning activity is the 'life-blood of learning'. There is research evidence that suggests that this 'life-blood' is not well sustained – feedback is either not done well or as frequently as needed or, worse still, not at all (Figure 7.1) (Fitzgerald et al 2010, Clynes & Raftery 2008, Neary 2000, Fish & Twinn 1997, Bedford et al 1993). Bedford et al (1993:107) quoted one practice educator on assessment feedback:

> … *I shy away from having to give criticism anyway. I'll always go to great lengths not to give criticism, so I'm not a good assessor from that point of view as I'll always highlight the positive aspects and I'll tend … not to go into too many details if a student isn't doing terribly well in certain areas.*

As noted in Chapter 6, it is knowledge of the results of performance provided by detailed factual constructive feedback that enables students 'to monitor strengths and weaknesses of their performances, so that aspects associated with success or high quality can be recognized and reinforced, and unsatisfactory aspects can be modified or improved' (Sadler 1989:120). Feedback therefore contributes directly to learning through the process of formative assessment.

Constructive feedback not only has an impact on the teaching/learning process but also gives messages to students about their effectiveness and worth – their self-esteem (Gipps 1994). Feedback therefore has an indirect effect on learning by how the academic self-esteem of the student is affected. Coopersmith (1967 in, Gipps 1994:132) defined self-esteem as:

> … *the evaluation which the individual makes and customarily maintains with regard to himself – it expresses an attitude of approval or disapproval and indicates the extent to which an individual believes himself to be capable, significant, successful and worthy.*

A major determinant of self-esteem is feedback from significant others. Consequently, students look to, and

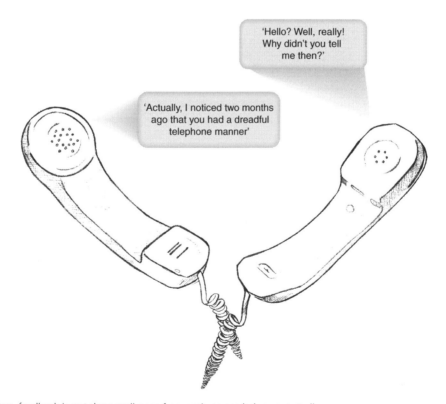

Figure 7.1 Often, feedback is not done well or as frequently as needed, or not at all.

indeed expect and welcome, constructive feedback from significant others such as their teachers and assessors (Embo et al 2010, Neary 2000, Phillips et al 2000, Gipps 1994, Bedford et al 1993). Other authors found that students view good clinical experiences to include receiving constructive feedback (Kotzabassaki et al 1997, Bedford et al 1993, Neville & French 1991). What we know about the effects of assessment on motivation tells us that students give up trying if they do not see themselves as capable of success. If they feel relatively worthless and ineffectual they will reduce their effort or give up altogether when work is difficult (Child 1997). On the other hand, people who hold positive self-perceptions usually try harder and persist longer when faced with difficult or challenging tasks.

There are therefore many challenges for the practice educator on how to manage feedback so that it has a positive impact on learning and, more importantly, on the self-esteem of the student.

Managing feedback sessions

The following framework is suggested for managing feedback sessions:

- timing of the feedback session
- format of the session
- involving the student in self-assessment
- using some 'rules of thumb' for managing constructive feedback.

Timing of the feedback session

Feedback will have maximal motivational impact on learning if it takes place while it is still recent and therefore still relevant: points and issues raised are therefore more meaningful and alive (Bailey 1998, Gipps 1994); furthermore, the event and its details are fresh and accessible to memory and not distorted with time (Jones 1995). In the clinical setting, if appropriate, this could take place as a running commentary whilst the learner is performing, or as soon as possible after the event. These are used to offer feedback on aspects of practice that are observed by the practice educator. Such opportunistic feedback will thus be situation specific, which ensures that important elements are included. In addition, this lends itself to discussions and demonstrations of how theory is related to practice.

Prompt and timely feedback gives the learner the opportunity to act upon feedback as soon as possible to improve future performance. A quote from a first-year student nurse in Neary's (2001:8) study illustrates this point:

I was nervous because [practice educator] worked with me all week and right away she told me where

I was going wrong. She responded quickly by helping me to understand what I needed to learn. [Practice educator] did not waste any time in telling me how and what to do. I like that, I know where I need to improve ... I can respond to this level of feedback. I feel more confident now; I can get on with the job.

The practice educator who works alongside the student should take advantage of this unique position in being able to offer accurate and timely feedback on all aspects of learning: opportunistic feedback is a vital element of the clinical learning experience.

Feedback sessions after the event will be more beneficial if the practice educator takes the responsibility for making time available and arranging a suitable venue (Gomez et al 1998). It will not be conducive for engaging in constructive feedback if either the practice educator or the student is still preoccupied with activities on the ward or after a busy clinical shift. The session could then prove to be counterproductive. It is important to remember that feedback must be timely to give the student enough time and opportunities to improve.

Format of the session

The format can be oral or written or both. Students usually look for both. Fish & Twinn (1997) believe that written notes are essential in providing continuity in the monitoring of progress. When written notes are kept, the valuable details of the situation are not forgotten, which increases the potential for learning (Bailey 1998). Within the continuous assessment process of pre-registration of health care students, written records of sessions reviewing progress are generally required. Constructive feedback sessions may be used to review progress formally and written records kept of these sessions.

Involving the student in self-assessment

The importance of asking for the student's self-assessment before giving feedback cannot be underestimated as it provides the practice educator valuable insight into the student's own perceptions of performance and learning that had taken place. The process of delivering constructive feedback is considerably easier when personal practice limitations are identified by the student. There is more detailed discussion on student self-assessment in the sections on formative assessment in Chapter 6, and the section 'Discussion with the student' below.

Using some 'rules of thumb' for managing constructive feedback

It is essential that constructive feedback is managed systematically and with discipline. The following rules of thumb for the management of constructive feedback are based upon and extended from the work of Bailey (1998), Fish & Twinn (1997) and Paul (1988):

- Prepare for the session remembering that feedback should not occur in a vacuum but on the basis of explicit aims or objectives of the placement (Billings 2010). When you need to engage in constructive feedback with another person, it generally means that there is some aspect of the person's performance or behaviour that you perceive is a problem and that you wish the person to correct (Paul 1988). You need to think carefully about what you want the outcome to be; this means that you need to be able to specify exactly what you want the other person to do or to stop doing. If you cannot do this, do not attempt the session as it means that you are not clear enough about what the problem is. You then run the risk of ending up making generalized statements, which frequently offend.
- Keep your appointment with the student and give him/her your undivided time, attention and interest – do not look at your watch constantly. Allocate sufficient time.
- Use a quiet venue and maintain privacy. Be careful not to be interrupted or distracted.
- Do not tackle too many things at once – try to foster a sense of progress. Gipps (1994) says that the most effective forms of feedback are those that focus students' attention on their progress in mastering the required performance. This emphasis tends to enhance self-efficacy and encourages effort attribution.
- Always try to make the session a learning situation for the student. Be positive as a first step. Just as important as identifying areas of weakness is identifying areas of relative strength. Temper negative comments with praise – the so-called 'praise sandwich' (Hinchliff 2004). Rowntree (1987:45) quoted the pioneering chemist Sir Humphrey Davy, who wrote of 'the love of praise that never, never dies'. Students tend to remember the negative rather than the positive – good points therefore need reinforcing. Help the student to see negative comments as points for growth.
- Use evidence from episodes of practice in as objective a way as possible. Stick to facts and present them in as neutral a way as possible. Use any written evidence from the student's portfolio to provoke discussion.
- Avoid generalizing and making subjective comments. A statement such as 'you were brilliant' may be pleasant to hear, but does not give any detail to be useful as a source of learning. Try to pinpoint what the student did that led you to use the label 'brilliant'. Praise effort and strategic behaviours and focus students on learning goals; this will lead to higher achievement than praising ability or intelligence, which can result in a learned-helplessness orientation

(Nicol & McFarlane-Dick 2005). However, the praise must fit the achievement; overzealous praise may cause embarrassment or be considered insincere.
- Do not compare with other students.
- Above all, remember that criticism is usually counterproductive.
- Be clear about your role – that of being an assessor giving constructive feedback on practice. It is your responsibility to *establish communication, clarify any problems* and either *get a commitment for change* or *offer a solution* (Paul 1988).

Establish communication (Figure 7.2)

- Use positive and warm non-verbal communication. Smile. Make eye contact. Do not be confrontational.
- Listen to the student. Get the comments and ideas from the student. Asking makes the student feel valued and is better than telling. You may become aware of facts and circumstances that you were not aware of; these may cause you to change your mind about the problem or the nature of the problem.
- Work *with* the student not *on* her or him. Avoid a power struggle. Do not take control of the situation.
- Giving negative feedback or leading the student to focus on the things that did not work is also important and should not be avoided. It is tempting to avoid unsatisfactory work, but performance will not improve without knowledge of what was wrong. Remember that there will come a time when it may be too late to give negative feedback.
- Use open-ended questions and give reasons for your questions and comments.
- Encourage frankness and share worries and uncertainties – we are all learners. Remember that feedback works best when a climate of trust exists between the giver and receiver.

Clarify Any Problems

- Always take account of as many dimensions of the practice situation as possible. Try not to be biased by your own strong reaction or views about any individual part of the situation as this might colour the feedback session.
- If the student counterattacks, do not rise! Try to see it from the student's point of view – take account of the student's prior experiences, interpretations and perceptions of what has happened. Explore and clarify what the student is saying.
- Be prepared to see that your own and perhaps different value-base and skills are only of indirect importance. You are not trying to cast the student into a mould of yourself but rather, within professional parameters, to help the student be more fully herself or himself.

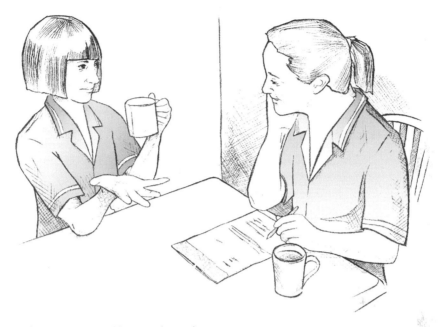

SMILE, LISTEN,
COMMUNICATE,
CLARIFY, COMMIT

Figure 7.2 Smile, make eye contact and listen to the student.

- Once you have a clear picture, state the problem in specific terms. Focus on *behaviour* and *facts* and not on *opinions*, *personalities* and *generalities* (Paul 1988). For example, instead of saying 'I wish you'd do something about the way you respond to patients, you do not seem to care', state the facts and behaviours: 'Yesterday, I noticed that Mrs Bell had to press her buzzer three times over 15 minutes before you got up from the nurses' station to respond to her. Today, when you were talking to Mr Hunt you did not make any eye contact and I thought you gave an abrupt answer when he asked you a question. You were also frowning all the time.'

Get a commitment for change or offer a solution

- Ask the student how performance can be improved. The only way to tell if there is learning consequent to feedback is for students to make some kind of response to complete the feedback loop (Sadler 1989). Unless students are able to use feedback to produce improved work (to improve upon a similar/ same aspect of care), neither they nor those giving feedback will know that it has been effective.

- You may need to show how performance can be improved. Be specific: offer alternatives. Avoid suggesting that there are simple right answers. Suggest a small new target that will lead to success.
- Make sure the student understands what is expected by asking the student to say what she/he will aim for and what first steps will be taken. Without this commitment, there is the possibility that nothing will happen.
- You may wish to make a written agreement with the student in the form of an action plan. Within this, set clear targets for the next period of supervised practice.

Readers are directed to the training package by Paul (1988) for some more information on how to give and receive constructive criticism.

MONITORING PROGRESS

Monitoring the progress of students is an essential part of the continuous assessment process. Progress can be monitored most accurately if there is continuity of supervision by the same practice educator. The same practice educator is better placed for keeping abreast of the clinical activities the student has had and will therefore know the amount of learning the student has achieved and how the competence of the student is developing. Monitoring progress is an ongoing assessment activity and takes place throughout the duration of the student's placement. Monitoring in this context, and not 'policing', is viewed as a process to help student learning, development and progression. We need to keep track of whether the student is developing competence and achieving the statutory competencies for professional practice. We therefore need to consider carefully what the student is learning, the clinical activities the student has been participating in and how further learning can be facilitated. When monitoring the progress of the student it is important to consider the prior clinical experiences of the student, the competencies and learning outcomes that the student needs to achieve during the placement and the stage of training the student is at. Curriculum documents will frequently state the expected level of performance at a specified stage of training.

When monitoring progress, the role and responsibilities of the practice educator centre on answering these key questions:

- What has the student done and learned so far? How will I know?
- Is the student having any difficulties? How will I know?
- What can be done to facilitate further learning and development?

To obtain answers to these questions, the assessment activities shown in Figure 7.3 are suggested.

Observation of practice for developing levels of competence

In Chapter 4 there is a detailed discussion of how observation may be used as a method of assessment to obtain direct evidence of the ability to perform care activities. When monitoring the progress of students during observation of their practice, the practice educator needs to gather evidence of:

- continuing safe and accurate performance of care activities with increasing speed and dexterity as the student engages in more clinical experiences and gains confidence
- the development in the level of a student's competence from the outset of a placement and at its conclusion (Bedford et al 1993).

What we know about the nature of expertise tells us that there are well-defined characteristics, across domains, that differentiate the performances of experts from novices (Benner et al 1996, Glaser 1990, Benner 1984). Glaser (1990:477) sums up the situation thus:

As proficiency develops, knowledge becomes increasingly integrated, new forms of cognitive skills emerge, access to knowledge is swift, and the efficiency of performance is heightened.

Glaser puts forward the case that, with growing proficiency, the changes in a person's cognitive ability and psychomotor performance can define criteria by which competence can be assessed. The Dreyfus model (in Benner 1984) considers that, in the acquisition and development of a skill, a learner passes through five levels of proficiency: novice, advanced beginner, competent, proficient and expert. As a learner passes through these levels, there are corresponding changes in three general aspects of performance. First, there is a move away from reliance on rules and principles to the use of past experience to guide practice. Secondly, the learner begins to see a situation less and less as a combination of equally relevant bits and more and more as a complete whole in which only certain parts are relevant. Thirdly, the learner becomes an involved performer and engages in the situation.

Benner et al (1996) and Benner (1984) applied the Dreyfus model to the study of *skills* acquisition in the practice of qualified nurses. They are careful in stating

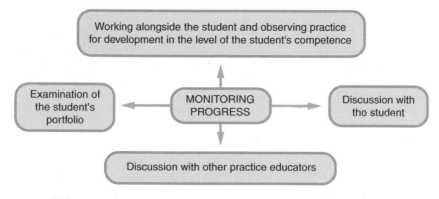

Figure 7.3 Assessment activities to monitor progress.

that skills in the nursing context refer exclusively to skilled nursing interventions and clinical judgement skills in actual clinical situations and not to psychomotor skills or to other skills learnt in the laboratory setting. For the purposes of this discussion, a summary of the performance characteristics from the work of Benner et al (1996) and Benner (1984) at the levels of development of the novice, advanced beginner and competent will be made here. Although these characteristics are derived from the performance of qualified nurses, it is my view that they can be extrapolated to the developing performance of pre-registration students. Following this exposition, the characteristics of the knowledge base with increasing proficiency described by Glaser (1990) are summarized.

The novice

- Students enter a new clinical area as novices with no experience of the situations in which they are expected to perform.
- They must be given rules and explicit detailed instructions to guide their performance; procedural lists are important for successful performance.
- They focus on getting individual tasks done; novices generally do not see beyond the task at hand and may not recognize underlying problems of the patient.
- They have little understanding of how to use classroom-acquired theory to guide practice.

The advanced beginner

- The advanced beginner can demonstrate marginally acceptable performance.
- As a result of prior experiences, they are able to identify the recurring components of situations, but are unable yet to sort out what is most important.
- They cannot order information into a meaningful whole.
- Their concern for good care is almost exclusively related to physical and technological support and to completing all the ordered treatment and procedures.

Competent

Competent students have:

- increased clinical understanding and are able to focus on the clinical condition and management of the 'whole' client/patient and less on getting tasks done
- increased technical skill – performance is more fluid and coordinated and they can predict the outcomes of their performance
- more accuracy at judging the difficulty of a task
- increased ability to handle busy complex situations and they can make decisions and solve problems

- improved time management skills
- improved organizational ability – they can prioritize care and manage care for several patients
- increased awareness of the appropriateness of their actions and are able to ask questions about what they have to do to improve their level of competence.

Knowledge base

Glaser (1990) notes that, as competence in a domain grows, the person displays a knowledge base that is increasingly *coherent* and *useful*. The characteristics underpinning these descriptors are described briefly here.

The coherence of knowledge

The beginner's knowledge is spotty with superficial understanding: only fragments of information can be accessed for use. Knowledge consists of isolated definitions and superficial understandings.

As competence develops, elements of knowledge are integrated with past organizations of knowledge so that information becomes increasingly interconnected and structured: knowledge gets retrieved in larger units from memory. Proficient individuals are able to access 'chunks' rather than fragments of information from memory.

Usable knowledge

Novices generally possess theoretical knowledge without knowing the situations where that knowledge applies and how it can be used most effectively. More proficient individuals are able to assess the relevance of their knowledge and thus access relevant knowledge to inform practice. Proficient individuals are able to make inferences based on interrelated information. Experts and novices may be equally competent at recalling specific items of information, but only the more experienced are able to relate these to the conditions of practice and the goals of solving a problem.

Criteria for assessing development in the novice, advanced beginner and competent levels of performance

The following criteria for assessing the development in the level of a student's competence are based upon, and extended from, the work of Benner et al (1996), Glaser (1990), and Benner (1984). When using these criteria to assess the level of performance and monitor progress, it is important to remember that the change from the novice level to competent level is incremental (Benner et al 1996) and on a continuum. The criteria below have been developed to reflect this.

Novice level

These conditions of practice of the novice along the following continuum can be used as the criteria to monitor the progress of novice level practice.

Conditions of practice

- Requires very detailed and explicit instructions.
- Requires less detailed and explicit instructions.
- Requires some detailed and explicit instructions.
- Performs some activities with few prompts.
- Performs regularly practised activities with few prompts.
- Performs regularly practised activities in a fully integrated way.
- Beginning to assess, plan and implement care.
- Within level of practice, responds appropriately in situations requiring urgency.

It is important for each clinical area to identify those activities in which the student is expected to be able to achieve competence. The reader is directed to the discussion of 'competence' in Chapter 3.

Knowledge

- Has a grasp of theory underpinning most practices.
- Beginning to make connections between chunks of theory.
- Can explain rationale underpinning some practices.
- Can discuss pertinent research underpinning some practices.

Advanced beginner level

These conditions of practice of the advanced beginner along the following continuum can be used as the criteria to monitor the progress of advanced beginner level practice.

Conditions of practice

- Performs activities with few prompts.
- Performs regularly practised activities in a fully integrated way.
- Leads regularly practised activities with few prompts.
- Beginning to prioritize care.
- Able to assess, plan and implement care.
- Beginning to evaluate effectiveness of care.
- Beginning to involve clients in their care.
- Within level of practice, responds appropriately in situations requiring urgency.

It is important for each clinical area to identify which activities the student is expected to be able to achieve competence.

Knowledge

- Can explain rationale underpinning practice.
- Able to make connections between more complex chunks of theory.
- Can discuss pertinent research underpinning practice.
- Beginning to implement evidence-based practice.

Competent level

These conditions of practice of the competent practitioner along the following continuum can be used as the criteria to monitor the progress of competent level practice.

Conditions of practice

- Performs most activities in a fully integrated way, without prompting.
- Able to assess, plan and implement care.
- Able to prioritize care.
- Able to evaluate effectiveness of care and make changes to care plans.
- Able to plan, prioritize and manage care for a group of clients within a time span.
- Actively involves clients in their care.
- Is organized and efficient.
- Within level of practice, responds appropriately in situations requiring urgency.

Knowledge

- Critiques evidence-based research and its implementation.
- Able to make connections between complex chunks of theory.

During the early stages of a pre-registration programme, a student who is new to a clinical area is likely to start practice at the novice level, but may achieve competent practice in some aspects of care by the end of the placement. The rate of progression is dependent on many factors, such as opportunities for practice and debriefing and reflection with the practice educator, the prior experience of the student, the student as a learner and so on. In each new clinical area the 'junior' student may perform at novice level for a longer period before advancing. The 'senior' student who may have been to similar clinical areas, however, would be able to, and indeed would be expected to, move more rapidly to advanced beginner and competent level practice. The practice educator is reminded that it is a requirement of pre-registration education to prepare students to be able to apply knowledge, understanding and skills to perform to the standards required in employment when registered and practice is safe and effective. It is suggested here that the ability to perform at the competent level is the required level to enable the student to achieve the requirements of statutory training, and to enable her/him to make the transition to registered practitioner. The criteria for assessing competent level practice should thus be used when monitoring the progress and assessing the practice of students who are at the stage of being prepared for professional practice (e.g. in the last 6 months of training). This period of practice will assist the student to start to make the transition from student to registered practitioner.

Levels of supervision and support

When monitoring the progress and assessing the practice of students, it is also important to consider the amount and level of supervision/support required by the student as well as the amount and level of participation in care you expect of the student. When students are at the novice level, they should initially observe care followed by participating and assisting in giving care. When giving care, they should be supervised closely and be supported. Students at the novice level, as discussed above, will require detailed and explicit instructions initially and may not be able to explain the rationale underpinning practice. As they learn and progress in their practice, less prompting is required for practised activities and they should be able to explain the rationale underpinning these practices.

As students progress, they should be encouraged to participate more actively. This should include the joint planning of activities. They should also be allowed to lead those activities they are confident in performing. The transition from novice level practice to advanced beginner level is on a continuum. The amount of supervision required starts to decrease and practice educators may be able to 'let go' as they learn to trust the performance of the students. From performance that requires to be prompted because it lacks completeness, performance starts to become smooth and complete as students start to internalize the performance of activities. Prompting is generally not required. The rationale underpinning practice is understood.

As students move from advanced beginner level practice to competent level practice, the amount of supervision required becomes minimal, with indirect supervision only required towards the end of the training programme. Students should be taking an active role in giving care. They should be able to plan all practised activities and be leading most of them. They become organized and efficient and can carry out their own workload without having to be reminded of what to do.

Discussion with the student

Talking, questioning and listening are crucial to assessment (Phillips et al 2000) and they can be used as instruments for ongoing review of the student's progress. There is a discussion of how questioning can be used to facilitate and assess student learning during clinical practice in Chapter 4. As the practice educator and student work together, inviting the student to suggest how best to carry out care in clinical situations in which the student has been involved previously will give the practice educator opportunities to consider what the student has learnt from similar past care-giving experiences. It will also provide the practice educator with information about the student's ongoing achievement. Whenever you spend time with your student

in care activities, utilize every opportunity for discussions, using what is going on in front of you as the focus. What the student is able to articulate will indicate the amount of progress made. Subsequent discussion and questioning to explore further the quantity and quality of learning, and any difficulties the student may be having with performing particular care activities, will add to this source of evidence of student progression. In putting forward the case for using 'dialogue in assessment', Bedford et al (1993:136) note that through 'discussion about a particular event, students can demonstrate the knowledge, understanding and values that have informed their actions in the clinical area on a given occasion'. This enables the practice educator to ascertain the understanding and the values held by the student about care given. There is further discussion of using dialogue as a vehicle for pre-activity discussion and post-event reflection in Chapter 9.

Progress reviews should also include student self-assessment and constructive feedback from the practice educator. When engaging in self-assessment, students may need help in looking at themselves as they are, to judge realistically what they could become, while at the same time helping them to hold in mind the vision of how they would like to be, perhaps modelled on observations of more experienced practitioners. One aim of self-assessment should be to shift the focus from 'how good am I?' to 'how can I get better?' (Mattheos et al 2004).

Practice educators should not assume that students are able to self-assess independently (Maloney et al 1997). Srinivasan et al (2007) and Boud (1992) found that self-assessment skills require facilitation. On the other hand, students are generally aware of the standards against which to measure themselves. Woolliscroft et al (1993) suggest that accurate professional self-assessment requires individuals to be realistic about how their performance would be judged by others using valid performance-monitoring tools. Self-assessment schedules like the one devised by Woolliscroft et al (1993) can be of great value as they appear to prompt students to apply ideas to their own practice and reflect on their learning. Such schedules can be given to students prior to clinical activities and meeting sessions to discuss progress. Students can then use them to assess their own performance immediately after the clinical activity. The schedule used by Woolliscroft et al (1993) is modified and adapted for health care students and reproduced here in Box 7.1.

Such self-assessment schedules, if used throughout the placement, will help students make specific judgements about their own performance and monitor their own progress in a range of clinical activities. Those clinical activities, specified in the learning contract and assessment plan (see Ch. 6) could be the topics for self-assessment schedules.

The crucial role of constructive feedback for learning is discussed at some length in Chapter 6. Feedback sessions should be designed to help students grow in their clinical

Box 7.1 Self-assessment by students for client/patient care planning

Admission History/Interview

1. I elicit an appropriate history.
2. I am able to elicit the main problems.
3. I accurately interpret the significance of these problems.

Initial Patient Write-Ups

1. I accurately document appropriate data in my initial patient/client write-up, including all major and minor problems.

Plan of Care

1. I develop an appropriate plan of care.

Implementation of Care

1. I implement the plan of care I developed in the most appropriate ways.

Daily Patient/Client Progress

1. I am aware of my patients'/clients' daily developments.
2. I accurately document all patient developments in my daily progress notes.

Evaluation of Care

1. I am able to evaluate the effectiveness of care given.
2. I am able to modify the care plan after such evaluations.

Application of Knowledge

1. I apply my knowledge base in a well-integrated manner to patient/client problems.

Supervision Required

1. I require little direction to perform my patient care responsibilities.

Interpersonal Interactions

1. I interact with patients/clients and their families in a professional manner.
2. I interact with other members of the health care team in a professional manner.

(Modified and adapted from the questionnaire by Woolliscroft et al 1993.)

---

skills and professional competence. Beginning level students have been found to be anxious about their ability to perform basic clinical skills (Robertson et al 1997). They often fail to focus on the patient/client as they have to concentrate their attention on developing clinical skills. Robertson et al (1997) suggest that feedback for these students should be designed to prompt them to think of the client holistically and to build self-confidence to enable the shift of focus to the patient/client. Advanced level students, on the other hand, may feel confident about their

clinical skills, but anxious about becoming a fully-fledged professional in the near future (Robertson et al 1997). These students would benefit from feedback designed to promote the growth of professionalism and confidence in their professional personae to enable them to make the transition to registered practitioner.

Examination of the student's portfolio of learning

Nursing and midwifery education in the UK has a history of requiring pre-registration students to maintain portfolios of learning. In 1999, the United Kingdom Central Council for Nursing, Midwifery and Health Visiting (UKCC) recommended that 'the use of a portfolio of practice experience should be extended to demonstrate a student's fitness for practice and provide evidence of rational decision making and clinical judgement'. Currently, nursing and midwifery students (NMC 2010, 2009) are expected to maintain an ongoing achievement record. This record is to include comments from practice educators the student has worked with and must be passed from one placement to the next to enable judgments to be made on the student's progress. It is suggested here that the ongoing achievement record may serve as a portfolio of learning.

The following principles should guide the development of the student's portfolio (NMC 2008, UKCC 1999, ENB 1997). There should be:

1. Cumulative information about the student's achievement of outcomes and learning through reflection, demonstrating the interrelationship of theory and practice
2. Cumulative information about the outcomes of assessment of both theory and practice
3. Evidence of rational decision-making and clinical judgement
4. A record of issues raised in discussion, including causes for concern between the practice educator, the student and the personal/named lecturer as part of the formative process of development
5. A collection of the action plans or learning contracts agreed between practice educators, the student and the personal/named lecturer
6. Information on key issues from the student's experience which will inform the preparation for subsequent clinical experience. These key issues should stem from student self-assessment and constructive feedback from the practice educator.

Recording evidence

The use of different methods of assessment in order to gain a comprehensive picture of the skills, knowledge, attributes and attitudes (see Ch. 4) will clearly produce a fairly big range and different kinds of evidence. If several methods are used on a day-to-day basis, how can we possibly keep track of all the evidence that is produced? Even over a week there will be more evidence than either the learner or practice educator can remember. Memory is also dangerously selective (Jones 1995). So, unless this evidence can be recorded on a fairly frequent basis, we can lose track of the quantity and quality of learning achieved. Now try Activity 7.1.

ACTIVITY 7.1

Examine the practice assessment record of a learner you are mentoring. How does the learner record evidence of learning and achievement?

Those of you who have worked alongside National Vocational Qualification (NVQ) candidates will have

seen these learners recording details of achievement in what is known as an *evidence log*. An evidence log typically contains details of activities and achievement. Figure 7.4 is an example of the evidence log of a student learning to administer medication on the ward. This example of an evidence log compiled by a learner indicates the occasions and types of medications administered and the aspects learned. It also shows the progress the learner made. These evidence logs are usually filed with other documented evidence of learning in a portfolio. The maintenance of evidence of learning in this format will enable sufficient information of a student's ongoing achievement in practice to be available to practice educators so that professional practice requirements are addressed (NMC 2008).

The practice educator or co-practice educator may also provide written evidence logs of learning. Figure 7.5 is an example of the evidence log kept by a practice educator in the operating theatre. This evidence

16.12.98 – 11.30 hours

Today I was asked to perform a BM Stix recording, on a pleasant 72-year-old gentleman; we chatted away, while I explained the procedure to him. He was quite *au fait* with what was happening, having been diabetic for some years. Between us we chose the finger which I would be pricking. I gathered the equipment I needed, washed my hands and put on some gloves. I carried out the procedure as I have been taught. I chatted to this gentleman throughout the procedure giving reassurance. I discarded all the used equipment in the appropriate places. After washing my hands and recording the measurement, I checked that the gentleman was alright and the site was not bleeding.

21.12.98 – 13.50 hours

This afternoon I was asked by staff to perform a BM Stix measurement on a pleasant young lady; having explained to her what I was going to do, she appeared quite relaxed about it. After gathering the equipment that I needed, I washed my hands and put on gloves. After I pricked her finger, she bled a little more than usual, I asked her to press on with the cotton wool I had given her and assured her it would stop shortly, as it did, by the time I had timed the reading, which was within normal range, recorded the measurement and informed the staff nurse.

I discarded all the used equipment in the sharps bin, washed my hands, and checked once more that the lady was feeling alright, she said her finger was a little sore.

21.1.99

I gathered together the equipment that I needed to perform a BM test on a 75-year-old client. I washed my hands and put on some gloves. I then explained to him what I was going to do. I pricked his finger with an autolet pen, drew enough blood to cover the teststix and gave him some cotton wool to hold on the bleeding point.

After 1 min I wiped the end of the stick with cotton wool and waited a further minute, then recorded the result on the chart and told staff nurse what it was. I cleared away all the equipment and disposed of it in the appropriate places, and washed my hands.

I asked the gentleman if he was alright and checked that the bleeding had stopped.

Reflection

Today I perfomed a BM test on a 75-year-old gentleman. Having known this gentleman for quite some time, as he has been staying with us for a while, I felt comfortable in performing this task. He, too, I think had confidence in me. I felt bad about having to stab his finger and maybe cause him pain, but this didn't seem to bother him too much. Having completed the test, recorded the outcome and passed on the information to staff nurse, I made sure that the gentleman was alright with the procedure and the bleeding had stopped and he was comfortable.

Figure 7.4 Evidence log compiled by a learner.

Date	Clinical Activites and Teaching/Learning Support
27.10.98	Difficulty with scrub technique. Trolley setting met performance criteria. Asepsis and uses of equipment discussed using question and anwer with prompting from observer Discussed time for private study to review asepsis policy. Scrub poster and policy manual used to discuss equipment
2.11.98	Difficulty with scrub technique Trolley setting satisfactorily met performance criteria Highlighted scrub technique as major problem. Further session to be instigated
2.11.98	Practised scrub technique – applying gloves and gown
4.11.98	Practised scrub technique and applying gloves and gown. Improvement made
9.11.98	Improvement in scrub technique. Trolley setting satisfactory. Standard achieved. Further practice required. Asepsis and equipment usage discussed
13.11.98	Demonstrating competent performance. All learning outcomes achieved

Figure 7.5 Evidence log compiled by the practice educator.

log shows the areas of difficulties experienced by the learner and the facilitation of further learning, which led to progress and subsequent achievement of learning outcomes. It is of course not possible or feasible to compile evidence logs of every learning task, but crucial aspects of learning can be identified in each clinical area so that such logs of learning can be compiled. There should, however, be an accumulation of sufficient evidence for a valid assessment to be made on whether a student is competent at the point of registration (NMC 2008, Fraser et al 1997).

Using the documented evidence to monitor progress

Phillips et al (2000) found that portfolios are most often constructed as collections of evidence of practice – they provide evidence of the student's repertoire of clinical activities. The portfolio can then be used by a range of people to consider the achievement of the student. This summative function of portfolios has come to assume greater importance than its formative function of facilitating learning and development. Phillips et al (2000) warn that if the emphasis is on the portfolio's summative function there is frequently no engagement in any discussion and critique of the written evidence – this limits and narrows the usefulness of portfolios as a source of learning. In any case, most portfolios do not tell us how well prepared the student is for practice. An examination of the evidence in the portfolio is therefore only one way of assessing and monitoring progress. The portfolio needs to be complemented by other ways of assessing practice.

Potentially, portfolios are most useful for assessing theoretical understanding and intellectual capacities, such as the capacity to analyse critically the values and issues inherent in the context of the practice situations, leading to the construction of alternative ways to practise. Phillips et al (2000:110) suggest that good portfolio assessment must capture the following aspects of learning and development:

- critical analysis of the way things are currently done
- identification of the values inherent in current practice
- critical appraisal of the context of current practice
- imagination of alternative ways of practice
- imagination of alternative ways of promoting better care and core values
- envisioning strategies to make changes.

In my view, portfolios should be used as a *process* tool as well as a tool to measure achievements. The 'ongoing achievement record' kept by nursing and midwifery students is to form part of the assessment of practice document. It needs to be of sufficient detail to enable the sign off mentor to confirm proficiency at the designated point of the programme. In addition, this record must be maintained and reviewed regularly to enable discussion of strengths and areas for improvement. It thus serves as a formative and summative tool. When reviewing the progress of the student using the portfolio, the documentation within it needs to be considered in terms of:

- what the student has learnt so far
- what can be done to facilitate a greater depth and breadth of learning based on what is documented in the portfolio.

The following steps may help you review progress using the portfolio evidence.

1. Review the previous action plan or learning contract. Decide how far the activities planned have helped the student in participating in care delivery that has contributed to the achievement of the plan or contract.
2. If an evidence log is kept, discuss the nature and amount of clinical experiences the student has participated in that have contributed to the achievement of statutory competencies. (The statutory competencies are usually contained in the student's

assessment of practice document obtainable from the higher education institution of the student.)

3. If a learning journal is kept, help the student to analyse critically specific care experiences you have both shared so that the most important issues emerge in order to increase the depth and breath of learning. (See Chapters 4, 6 and 9 for guidelines on the facilitation and assessment of learning through reflection.)

4. Ask questions to help the student explain the rationale behind care, thereby enabling the student to apply theory to practice.

5. Help the student to consider how practice could change as a result of learning through the specific clinical experiences. Explore alternative practices and strategies with the student.

Discussion with other practice educators

If it is not possible for the named practice educator to work with the student on enough occasions to monitor the progress of the student with validity and reliability, it is important and only fair to the student that the practice educator seeks the views of other practitioners who have worked with the student. In the real world of the busyness of clinical practice, Phillips et al (2000) and Bedford et al (1993) found that practice educators were unable to work with students for a satisfactory length of time. This problem continues today with Myall et al (2008) reporting that whilst most students were able to work with their practice

educators for the majority of their clinical placement, others were spending less than the recommended amount of time with them. Bedford et al (1993) and Phillips et al (2000) recommend that assessment should be a team effort to obtain a stronger and wider evidence base on which formative and summative assessments may be made. This recommendation is now endorsed by the NMC (2008:32, 61). Phillips et al (2000) further recommend the following actions as part of good assessment practice:

- assessment should include discussion that occurs as part of the working day
- evidence and issues should be contributed, where possible, by all members of the team, including the assessee
- this occasion may be during a handover, a 'case' conference or some other event.

When discussing the performance and ongoing achievement of students as part of the process of monitoring progress, it is important to consider whether the quality and quantity of clinical experiences the student has had are sufficient to enable development and therefore progress. Knowledge of the length of the placement, and the stage of training the student is at, will assist practice educators in deciding how much progression, within and across each of the levels (novice, advanced beginner, competent), can be expected.

Written records (testimonies) by other practice educators will complement and strengthen records of evidence of learning kept by the student. An example of this is given in Figure 7.6.

11/09/03

I have observed Stacey undertake the preparation of an intramuscular injection. She was able to prepare the environment, understanding the importance of communicating effectively with the patient in a calm/relaxed environment. She understands the importance of informing the patient of what is being administered, offering support/reassurance.

Stacey was able to calculate the dosage of medication to be administered and drew the liquid into the syringe in a safe manner.

Stacey practised the process of administering the injection utilizing approved techniques.

11/09/03

Stacey attended a teaching session I conducted for the safe preparation and administration of depot intramuscular injections. Throughout the session Stacey demonstrated a sound knowledge of the procedure, asking appropriate questions and demonstrated correct techniques using simulation.

8/10/03

Stacey attended Clozaril Clinic. She gained an overview of the monitoring that takes place and helped with the physical observations. Stacey demonstrated an understanding of Clozapine and its effects through a question and answer session.

12/10/03

Stacy has assisted me in the administration of medication several times during her placement. She has adhered to policy guidelines ensuring safety at all times.

Figure 7.6 Evidence log compiled by the assessor.

06/09/03

I administered a depot injection using the Z track method and the safe procedure that I had previously demonstrated to my mentor.

The patient receiving the depot has the injection regularly therefore presented as quite calm and co-operative. Her mood was appropriate and she gave me good positive comments.

After the depot was given the patient stated that I had given the injection well and that I didn't hurt her.

Reflection

I gave my first depot injection today. I felt relaxed when I got all of the equipment together as I could remember what I needed from previous practice sessions. The depot I had to give was 37.5 mg Risperidal consta. I felt a little unnerved about this injection as it is different from other depots, as you have to mix the solution that is injected. It is also pre-packed.

After preparing the injection I went and got the patient. The patient that the depot was for was a patient I spend a lot of time with. The patient gave me permission to give her the injection.

I felt nervous before and during giving the injection as I was scared of hurting the patient as the needle was big and the patient was very thin.

Afterwards the patient asked me if it was my first injection as she said I was very good and it didn't hurt her. I was pleased about this but I was quite overwhelmed by the whole experience and felt a little upset.

I will be practising more depots by simulation and actually giving another three before the end of my placement to make me feel more at ease.

09/09/03

I administered a depot injection using a safe procedure which my mentor and I had discussed and practised within a simulation set up by my mentor.

After administrating the depot and safely disposing of all the equipment used my mentor and I assessed the procedure.

I felt nervous because I didn't want to hurt the patient and I didn't know how the patient would
react. I also observed that the patient presented as agitated. I used my communication skills to reassure her and make her feel at ease with the injection procedure. I also overcame my fears by communicating with the patient and with reassuring her I reassured myself. My mentor said my communication skills with the patient were excellent, taking into consideration the patient's needs and concerns. I maintained the safety for the patient, myself and mentor throughout the procedure. This involved preparing the equipment in a safe environment, ensuring the medication was correct i.e. correct dose, within the expiry date, the correct medication for the right patient. The patient was then called to the treatment room as I felt this was a safe environment. The drug was administered using the Z track method. I had maintained the comfort and dignity of the patient

11/09/03

I have acted out a simulation exercise of a depot injection. This is an intramuscular injection. I was able to prepare the surroundings and equipment for the injection to take place. I was given support and told what to do beforehand. I understood the importance of communicating with the patient to make them feel safe and at ease

with the injection procedure. Informing the patient of what is being administered is essential and support and reassurance was offered.

I feel that I need more practice in calculating dosages of medication even though I calculated the correct dosage for the injection on this occasion.

I drew the medication into the syringe safely and then I practised the process of giving the injection using approved techniques that I was shown. I felt nervous before I gave the injection but doing it helped me gain confidence to do the procedure again. Support was given to me throughout the exercise which helped me a lot.

12/09/03

I administered medications under the supervision of a staff nurse. At the start of giving out medications I felt a little nervous but after being supported by the staff nurse, I felt a lot more confident. I feel that I need more practice in working out the correct dosages of medication which I will do.

14/09/03

When administering my third depot injection to a male patient the Z track method was used again. This was done in a safe way that was demonstrated to my mentor previously.

I felt more at ease in giving this injection as at this stage I had given two injections before this one. I also felt that I had built up a rapport with the patient I was giving the injection to.

My mentor was quite happy with the way I gave the depot injection, stating that I am quite competent in administering depot injections.

I was pleased with the way my mentor guided me through the procedure of depot injections safely. This gave me more confidence to give the injection and let me know that I was doing the procedure correctly.

I was glad that my mentor gave me time to reflect on each depot I administered as it helped me to pick out points in the procedure that I did well, not so well and things I could have done differently.

18/10/03

I attended Clozaril Clinic in psychiatric outpatients. Clozaril is a drug used to treat schizophrenia but it can cause quite severe side effects such as making the heart beat too fast and decreasing the white blood cells. This is why the patients that take clozaril get monitored every week. In the clinic the patient gets weighed, blood pressure and pulse taken and blood is taken from them. The patient gets asked from a check list what side effects they have from the drug. The blood taken from the patient gets sent to clozaril monitoring service who check the blood and make sure that that the patient is okay to continue to take the clozaril.

I found working in Clozaril Clinic different to working on the ward. The clozaril nurse doesn't seem to get to spend much time with the patients only getting the chance to ask the patient what side effects they have.

My role in the clinic was to take the patient's blood pressure and pulse. The patient couldn't really talk about anything confidential to the clozaril nurse as the phlebotomist was there. I enjoyed it in the clinic and I am going to read up on clozaril as more and more patients are being treated by it and I will be using it as a trained nurse in the near future..

Figure 7.7 Evidence log compiled by a learner.

These testimonies strengthen the evidence of learning provided in the log kept by the student as shown in Figure 7.7.

MAKING ASSESSMENT DECISIONS

Formative assessment – is the student progressing?

As discussed above, the assessment activities of working alongside the student and observing practice, discussion with the student and examination of the student's portfolio, and discussion with other practice educators are done both informally and formally to monitor progress. During the formal sessions, which should be planned and timetabled (Phillips et al 2000), the practice educator should formally review with the student the progress made and identify any difficulties at an earlier, rather than a later, stage of the placement. The number of formal progress review meetings you hold altogether during the student's placement would be dependent on the length of the placement and the progress the student is making. There should be at least one formalized session (Bedford et al 1993). As a guide, try to hold a formal progress review session at least every 2 weeks. To decide whether the student is progressing, ask the following questions:

- Is the student achieving statutory competencies?
- Is there a demonstration of a growing level of skill and competence (see criteria in Figure 7.8)?

An important point to remember is that the level of competence of newly practitioners can vary considerably as this is dependent on the opportunities they had in training. During formative assessments, it is important to check that students are having the learning opportunities to enable the achievement of competencies.

- Is performance consistent (Maloney et al 1997)?
- Is there a demonstration of a growing understanding of the rationale underpinning practice?
- Is there a demonstration of development of the attitudes and values appropriate to professional practice?
- Is there a demonstration of a developing ability to engage in evidence-based and reflective practice?

It is important for practice educators to remember that many factors can affect a student's progress and to explore reasons for the student's difficulties. Phillips et al (2000) made the point that any judgement of a student's capabilities must take into account the circumstances in which that student is performing.

Summative assessment – should the student be passed?

All assessments involve complex decision-making as 'assessors … weigh evidence which will enable them to judge "on the balance of probabilities" or "beyond reasonable doubt"' (Gonczi 1994:33). When weighing assessment evidence of competence or incompetence, practice educators in their role as assessors must have sufficient evidence to reach a defensible conclusion that is 'responsible, reasonable and respectable', whereas 'beyond reasonable doubt' demands a greater burden of proof (Ilott & Murphy 1999:89). Here, assessors will be expected to substantiate the assessment decision of either a 'pass' or a 'fail' grade.

The summative assessment is done at the end of the placement. A final meeting/discussion session should be arranged to take place during the last week of the student's placement, preferably on the last day. Additional time should be allocated to review and analyse fully the evidence of competence. This is endorsed by the NMC (2008:34) who state that 'sign-off mentors must have time allocated to reflect, give feedback and keep records of student achievements in their final period of practice learning'.

The following questions may assist in helping you judge and analyse evidence to establish whether there is sufficient assessment evidence to confer competence. Assessors should be careful that responses to these questions are not made on the 'relative strength of student articulation of their unobserved practice' (While 1994:102).

1. Has the student achieved the statutory competencies?

Examine the student's assessment of practice document, which contain the statutory competencies. Statutory competencies have been set at the point of registration such that the student is able to fulfil the requirements of the practitioner as laid down by the statutory professional body. In order to prepare the student to practise safely and effectively so that, on registration, the student can assume the responsibilities and accountability for practice as a professional such as a nurse or a midwife or a physiotherapist, all competencies for that placement must be achieved in order to pass. In the UK, nursing and midwifery students must meet the progression criteria at each of the progression points (NMC 2010, 2009).

LEVEL 1

Competence Achieved

Close supervision required

Participates and assists in care

Performs with few prompts

Can explain the rationale underpinning practice

Competence NOT Achieved

Direct supervision required

Has difficulty participating and assisting in care

Requires detailed and explicit instructions

Cannot explain the rationale underpinning practice

LEVEL 2

Competence Achieved

Minimal supervision required

Active participation in care

Beginning to prioritize care

Planning most activities and leading some

Performance is smooth and complete

Does not require prompting

Can explain rationale underpinning practice and
  discuss pertinent research

Competence NOT Achieved

Close supervision required

Participates and assists in care

Performance lacks completeness

Requires to be prompted

Cannot explain rationale underpinning practice

LEVEL 3

Competence Achieved

Indirect supervision required

Active participation in care

Planning all activities and leading most

Does not require prompting

Is organized and efficient

Is able to prioritize care

Critiques evidence-based practice and its implementation

Competence NOT Achieved

Close supervision required

Participates and assists in care only

Requires prompting

Unable to organize care

Does not consider evidence-based practice

Figure 7.8 Criteria for assessing the achievement of clinical competence.

In recommending the use of the competence-based approach for pre-registration nursing and midwifery education, the NMC (2010, 2009) requires students, on qualification, to be able to practise safely and effectively without the need for direct supervision. If these training requirements are to be realized, only *competent* or *not competent* judgements can be made. Wolf (1995:22) states that in competence-based assessment 'either the person has consistently demonstrated workplace performance which meets the specified standards [in the competencies] or they are not yet able to do so'. Using the pre-specified levels of supervision and practice (see Ch. 6), and conditions of practice discussed earlier in this chapter, criteria are put forward to make 'competent' or 'not competent' decisions in Figure 7.8. Levels 1,

2 and 3 correspond to students during years one, two and three of the pre-registration programme respectively.

Is there sufficient performance evidence to confer competent practice? Performance evidence would have been gathered by the practice educator throughout the period of supervised practice and also generated from the testimonies provided by other members of the team. The NMC (2008:61) recommends that 'judgements are informed by feedback from colleagues and evidence from other sources leading to an assessment determining whether the student has achieved the required standard for safe and effective practice …'.

Has the student reached the required level? You may wish to review the section on 'Criteria for assessing development in the novice, advanced beginner and competent levels of performance'. Related to this is discriminating power. When making the final decision to pass or fail the student, consider carefully whether your assessment has identified the correct standard to be achieved and the correct level of ability of the student for the stage of the training. The NMC (2010:97) states explicitly that 'to pass the second progression point, normally at the end of year two, the student will need to demonstrate that they can be more independent and take more responsibility for their own learning and practice'.

2. Does the assessment evidence achieve validity of assessment?

Examine the student's portfolio. Has the learner engaged in a sufficient number and range of care situations for you to be confident that validity has been achieved? Does the student have 'the ability to actually care for patients?' (Gerrish et al 1997:70). Remember that the narrower the base of evidence for the inference of competence, the less generalizable it will be to the performance of other tasks. The reader is referred to Chapter 5 for a discussion of validity.

3. Does the assessment evidence achieve reliability of assessment?

Examine the student's portfolio. Has the learner engaged in a sufficient number and range of care situations for you to be confident that reliability has been achieved? The amount of evidence must be sufficient to ensure consistent performance to the standard required across a range of situations. To ensure reliability, evidence is needed of repeated performances; we may alternatively be able to draw upon a number of different sources of evidence. It is dubious that a single correct performance is sufficient to confer competence for assessment purposes (Gonczi et al 1993). Maatsch et al (1987 in Gonczi et al 1993) considered that assessments on five to seven cases were required for the casualty physician to achieve general competence.

4. Is there a demonstration of a sound understanding of the rationale underpinning each competency?

Knowledge and understanding underpin competent practice. Students must be able to demonstrate that they understand the rationale for care activities. It is likely that the practice educator will have assessed the student's understanding through the use of questioning throughout the period of formative assessment. This may require supplementation through further questioning when assessment evidence is being reviewed and analysed. Additionally, at level 2, can the student discuss pertinent research underpinning evidence-based practice? Further, at level 3, can the student discuss and critique pertinent research underpinning evidence-based practice?

5. Is the student developing the attitudes and values appropriate to professional practice?

The assessment of attitudes and values is not easy. Although several methods of assessment can be used to 'assess' the attitudes and values of another (see Ch. 4), it nevertheless leaves this crucial aspect of competent professional practice open to personal biases and subjectiveness. It also stands in danger of not being assessed at all (Miller 2010, Fraser 2000, Bedford et al 1993).

Many would agree with Goffman (1959, in Hodges 2003:1137) when he said that '… the "true" or "real" attitudes, beliefs and emotions of the individual can be ascertained only indirectly through his avowals or through what appears to be involuntary expressive behaviour'. A tool termed the 'professional behaviours inventory' to assess pre-specified behaviours expected of a professional exhibiting the accepted conduct of practitioner is proposed in Chapter 3. These behaviours are assumed to be underpinned by the attitudes, values and beliefs of the person. The use of such a tool is likely to assist the assessor in being more objective.

MANAGING SOME ASSESSMENT PROBLEMS

Students experiencing problems learning during clinical practice: the unsafe student

Students who experience problems learning during clinical practice are a 'cause for concern' because they are unsafe (Luhanga et al 2008, Bedford et al 1993).

Luhanga et al (2008:1) used the term 'unsafe student' to refer to students 'whose level of clinical practice is questionable regarding safety, and who exhibit marked deficits in knowledge and psychomotor skills, motivation, or interpersonal skills'. They go on to state that unsafe clinical practice is any 'act by the student that is harmful or potentially detrimental to the client, self, or other health personnel.' A grave issue in these situations is that of giving the student the 'benefit of the doubt' and 'failing to fail' these students (see, for example, Jervis & Tilki 2011, Killam et al 2010, Luhanga et al 2008, Dudek et al 2005, Scholes & Albarran 2005, Duffy 2004).

Any student who is either not progressing or failing to meet the required standard needs to be identified by assessment systems so that opportunities can be provided for that student to improve. It is suggested here that the use of the assessment activities to monitor progress discussed earlier in this chapter will help the practice educator to identify those students who require extra help and support. A number of authors (see, for example, Killam et al, 2011, Luhanga et al 2008, Scholes & Albarran 2005, Maloney et al 1997) provide some criteria for recognizing these students early. They remind us that, although some of these behaviours are exhibited by many students at some time during clinical practice, the student who is either not progressing or failing exhibits these behaviours to such a degree and extent that learning is interrupted. These behaviours are listed here:

- is inconsistent in meeting the required level of competence for expected stage of training; lacks practical skills, for example, care is not complete, bed space is untidy, patients are not left comfortable or the student may avoid direct patient contact and/or spend excessive time in distractions away from the client's/patient's bedside
- lacks caution and is not careful
- is inconsistent in clinical performance
- does not respond appropriately to constructive feedback
- appears unable to make changes in response to constructive feedback – therefore clinical skills do not improve
- exhibits poor preparation and organizational skills; if doing a handover or on a ward round may be unable to respond to questioning
- has limited interactional and poor communication skills; fails to ask questions
- may experience continual poor health, feel depressed, angry, withdrawn, sad, emotionally labile, tired or listless, high levels of anxiety
- uncommitted and unenthusiastic; may dismiss certain learning opportunities with the rationale of having done that before and not wanting repetition

- unethical behaviour, for example, failure to disclose and discuss clinical errors as this jeopardises the communication needed for safe care – when challenged is defensive with a range of excuses rather than embrace a culture of challenge and support
- has poor punctuality
- avoids working with the allocated practice educator.

How can the practice educator manage the situation when a student is either not progressing or failing? In Chapter 2 there is a discussion of the professional responsibility and accountability of the practice educator in these situations. It is acknowledged here that people are generally reluctant to pass negative judgements on fellow workers. Practice educators also experience the handling of the assessment of weak students as great challenges, both professionally and personally (Luhanga et al 2008, Duffy 2004, Ilott & Murphy 1999, Bedford et al 1993). However, the implications of poor/unsafe students 'slipping through the net' to become registered practitioners are grave as a minority of incompetent professionals can do untold damage. Appropriate management, I believe, includes using 'intelligence, sensitivity, understanding and insight' when dealing with these students, as suggested by Maloney et al (1997). It is reiterated here that the use of the strategy of triangulation to collect assessment evidence (see Ch. 4) will increase the confidence of the practice educator when dealing with these students. Although the following plan of action is offered, the practice educator should be clear of the policy laid down by the higher education institution of the student for dealing with these situations so that the correct procedure is followed:

- Arrange to have a meeting with the student as soon as possible. Explain the reason for the meeting to the student.
- Consider and discuss the evidence that has led to concern. Give honest, unambiguous feedback (Ilott & Murphy 1999). Maloney et al (1997:204) found that some students reacted positively and were relieved when their shortcomings were openly discussed with them, saying: 'It's so good not to pretend, now I feel I can say I don't know and extend my learning and increase my clinical skills'.
- Concern is documented in the assessment of practice document at an early stage, and certainly no later than the point at which formative mid-placement assessment takes place (Bedford et al 1993). The nature of the problem should be carefully, clearly and explicitly documented. Include specific examples of incidents/clinical care situations to illustrate the nature of the problem. The written word gives a visual record of problems and actions taken.
- Make sure the student understands the nature of the problem(s) – has he/she heard accurately what you are saying? The most difficult cases are those

students who are clearly not succeeding but do not recognize this. Duffy (2004) found that many students who were failing lacked insight of their weak areas of practice and therefore did not perceive any necessity for extra support. Supportive measures were then ineffective as they were not recognized as such. Students should thus be provided with the opportunity to give their own perception of their performance. Help students identify what they already know and what they need to focus on in order to learn and overcome their weaknesses. Help students identify resources they can utilize to improve knowledge and skills.

- Jointly, draw up a targeted detailed action plan. Where action plans were negotiated and monitored through reviews, Gleason (1984 in Ilott & Murphy 1999) found that 70% of students improved their grades. The good, honest, clear formative assessment motivated the students.
  - Provide a clear and unambiguous assessment plan with clear explicit goals (see Ch. 6) to retrieve the situation.
  - Set deadlines and make sure the student understands these.
  - Make arrangements to work closely with the student.
  - Arrangements should also be made for the student to work with other practice educators so that testimonies can be provided; this will increase the validity and reliability of the assessment. Furthermore, students have the right to be protected from unfair or biased assessment and should not be failed until they are judged by another assessor (Gomez et al 1998).
- Discuss the situation with the senior practitioner with overall responsibility for student learning. Following this, inform the student's personal teacher and/or the clinical link lecturer (ENB 1997). Support from the higher education institution is essential in these situations. Practice educators in Duffy's (2004) study found that more support from education staff and colleagues was required when they were supporting 'weak' students.
- It is important to establish clear and open communication between the student, practice educator and the higher education institution.
- Make arrangements to conduct a progress review in 1 week. If, despite remedial action, there is little or no improvement, make arrangements for the clinical link lecturer to be present at a tripartite meeting to discuss the situation and develop another action plan.
- A weekly progress review is advisable for as long as the student's difficulties persist.
- It is also important to keep careful notes of all discussions; there may come a time when you have to use these as evidence that you may have pointed

out the same things again and again and that the student has repeatedly failed to meet the goals you have set. It is important to remember that the report will be scrutinized by the examination board of the higher education institution. It therefore needs to be clear, accurate and well evidenced. Where students have appealed against 'fail' decisions, I have known instances when the fail decision has been overthrown by the examination board due to poor documentation and lack of substantive written evidence against the fail grade. Likewise, Fraser et al (1997) found that where there is insufficient assessment evidence the benefit of the doubt will be in the student's favour.

If, despite the actions and opportunities provided for the student to improve, improvement does not occur and standards are not achieved, failure decisions can be made with confidence, fairly and on the basis of a fully documented evidence base.

Managing the situation when a student has to be failed

There comes a time when you may have to fail a student. This is a challenging responsibility and the ability to face and deal with this situation with confidence is critical (Scholes & Albarran 2005). The arrival at this assessment decision would have been procedurally and emotionally difficult. It would also have been time consuming as you would have had to 'build up a case' to fail the student (Dudek et al 2005, Duffy 2004). It is important that failure does not come as a surprise to the student. Correct use of formative assessment processes, including feedback, would have indicated to the student those aspects of learning that were consistently not achieved. Before making this critical fail decision, you must have followed the plan of action outlined above for helping the student who is not progressing. These situations are demanding and sensitive to handle. Notwithstanding that, practice educators have professional responsibilities and accountability to make sound and accurate assessment decisions which include failing students who have not met the standards of training. The legal and ethical issues surrounding *not* failing a student who has not met the training standards and is unsafe to practise are discussed in Chapter 2. Suffice here to remind ourselves by asking the following questions dubbed the 'old test' by Scholes & Albarran (2005): Firstly, *would I want such a nurse or midwife or physiotherapist to look after me? If not, why not? And if it isn't good enough for you, why should it be good enough for clients/patients? Secondly, would you want this student when qualified to be in your team? Can you rely on this practitioner to support you when the workload is heavy or in times of crisis, or would this practitioner be a liability?*

Considerable skill and confidence are required to manage these situations effectively (Jervis & Tilki 2011, Luhanga et al 2008, Scholes & Albarran 2005, Bedford et al 1993). I would also suggest that the practice educator as assessor requires the courage and strength to fail a student – a conviction that a just assessment decision has been made will vest the practice educator with this courage. This conviction will ensue if assessment processes to ensure fair assessments are followed. The assessor, then, will have no fear that there will be reprisals for failing a student. However, it is important to remember that it is as wrong to 'fail to fail' as it is to fail unjustly (Ilott & Murphy 1999).

Consider the scenario shown in Activity 7.2. How would you deal with it?

ACTIVITY 7.2

Mark Bradshaw is the named practice educator/assessor to a student called Mary who has struggled considerably to achieve the required standard in three of the competency statements. He has been reviewing progress with her weekly. She is now approaching the end of the placement and has not achieved the required standard and, in Mark's opinion, should be failed. A fellow registered practitioner who has also worked with Mary argues strongly that Mary's practice is up to standard and she should be passed. What should Mark do?

The decision to fail a student is never an easy one to make (Jervis & Tilki 2011, Luhanga et al 2008, Dudek et al 2005, Duffy 2004, Stuart 2002, Lankshear 1990). When another practice educator/assessor disagrees with your decision, it becomes even more tricky. The starting point is perhaps to consider both your assessment evidence objectively – are both of you using the same criteria for assessment, so that assessment evidence is *reliable?* Therefore, evidence of achievement or non-achievement is based on the same criteria. The next question you may wish to consider is the *validity* of the assessment – for example, have both of you been assessing what you should be assessing? Has too much or too little been expected of the student? Other aspects of validity will also need to be considered (see Ch. 5).

Assuming that individual personal biases are not implicated and feasibility (see Ch. 5) within the assessment process has received due attention, and you still cannot agree with each other, as the named assessor you may wish to take the following action(s):

- Arrange a meeting with the senior practitioner with overall responsibility for student learning to discuss the situation.
- Arrange a meeting with your clinical link lecturer or the student's personal tutor to discuss the situation.

- Arrange a joint meeting with the senior practitioner and clinical link lecturer to discuss the situation.

The final point to remember is that, as the named assessor, you are responsible for making the final assessment decision and are accountable for passing or failing the student at the end of the period of practice placement. The grade you award should reflect the student's standard of practice in the latter part of the placement. When making the summative assessment decision, refer to the documented evidence in the student's assessment of practice document to support your decision.

Student reactions to being failed and how to manage them

Failing students may react in a number of ways (Gomez et al 1998). These behaviours need to be recognized for what they are – that is, the student's reactions to the news of failure and not a personal vendetta against the assessor. Gomez et al (1998:420) recommend giving extra time to these situations, as the student needs time to 'grieve the loss of what was, perhaps, a dream'. Students need time to process the information and should not feel rushed. Assessors should listen attentively, show concern and provide the appropriate support.

- Students may respond with *denial* – their own perception of their competence contradicts that of the assessor. They may also deny situations where their performance was observed to have been unsafe or the attitude they exhibited was inappropriate. They may make excuses for their behaviours. The conversation needs to be steered to learning outcomes not being met.
- The denial and/or anger (see below) may also be demonstrated in other ways, such as making attempts to undermine the assessor's judgement by soliciting the views of other team members behind the back of the assessor (Duffy 2004). The assessor will need to deal with these instances firmly without causing disharmony in the team. It may be useful to remember that, as the named assessor, your professional statutory body (such as the Nursing and Midwifery Council in the case of nurses and midwives, and the Health Professions Council in the case of professionals regulated by the HPC) has invested you with the responsibility and accountability for making assessment decisions. As such, you are invested with the authority to make assessment decisions as you see fit.
- Students may respond with *anger and aggression* – they may become abusive and accusing (e.g. making accusations of biases against their personal characteristics). If the assessor suspects that this situation could arise, it may be wise to have the presence of a third person, such as the personal tutor of the student. The anger should not be taken

personally. Provide guidance about feelings and focus on anger as part of the loss.

- Anger and/or denial could also be in the form of blaming others by deflecting responsibility for failure onto the staff such as saying that failure was caused by personality clashes between themselves and the staff (Duffy 2004).
- Some students may attempt to bargain for a passing grade. The assessor needs to stand firm and remain focused on the results.
- As the reality of the loss is recognized, students may respond with *sadness* – they may cry over the loss of the right to carry on with the training. For mature students with families, losing the right to train is also likely to mean loss of income. Allow them to cry before going on to discuss the reasons for the failure.
- Some students may be quite relieved. A career as a nurse or midwife or physiotherapist may not be what they want but they may not have the courage to make that decision.

Failure may be a positive experience for some students. Some learn from the experience and go on to achieve success. Maloney et al (1997) give an example of a student who learned from failure – failure for her was positive (Case study 7.1).Failure, however, is not a positive experience for many students. For some, it is a devastating experience and can appear to be a scar carried for life. In his study of the kinds of failure people remembered, Cannon (2002) found that, with few exceptions, each experience of failure was still recalled with feelings of anger and sadness. He concluded that failures are 'anxiety-raising experiences [which] are simply difficult to delete from

memory' (Cannon 2002: 76). This painful situation may be averted if lack of progress is determined early and appropriate support and help put in place. The reader is directed to the work of Maloney et al (1997) for a more comprehensive discussion of students who are either not progressing or failing.

Failure to fail

Having to fail a student causes many of us considerable anguish. At the other end of the continuum is the abuse of the power to fail, using it as a tool to exert control and punish 'difficult' or unpopular students (Wolf 1995). This complex problem of 'failure to fail' is not new and appears to be a continuing challenge for assessors of students on professional courses. In the health professions, 'failure to fail' is reported in literature relating to assessment from the fields of social work (Brandon & Davis 1979), medicine (Dudek et al 2005, Green 1991), nursing and midwifery (Jervis & Tilki 2011, Duffy 2004, Fraser et al 1997, White et al 1994, Bedford et al 1993, Lankshear 1990) and occupational therapy (Ilott & Murphy 1997). The teaching profession has the same problem (Hawe 2003). References are made to assessors giving students the benefit of the doubt in marginal situations instead of awarding a fail when it was clearly warranted. What is also of concern is that students are aware that they can get around weak areas of practice. A student in White et al's study (1994:103) said that 'it is virtually impossible to fail the practical part of the course'.

Why do assessors find it difficult to assign a fail grade? There are no straightforward answers and it would appear that professional and strong affective and personal overtones/factors influence assessors' decision-making process when confronted with having to make a fail decision. From a review of some of the literature relating to assessment in professional education, I attempt to give a summary of the main reasons for not failing students.

- Lankshear (1990) found that staff members were loath to fail students knowing that awarding a fail meant additional work for them plus having to deal with the rancour of the student. In recent years, assessors also worried about students taking out grievances against them (Jervis & Tilki 2011, Luhanga et al 2008, Dudek et al 2005).
- Ilott & Murphy (1997) explored the affective responses of assessors in fail scenarios in occupational therapy courses in the UK. Feelings reported included anxiety, guilt, distress, self-doubt, regret and relief. For some of the assessors, the emotions were so strong that a pass grade was awarded over a fail. While the failure to fail seemed the less stressful option, it often engendered its own degree of guilt and shame in the assessor.

Case study 7.1 **Learning from the experience of failure**

A university medical lecturer was surprised when approached at a social function by a confident young woman, who had recently been making her name in art design. She thanked him for helping her to make 'the most important decision of her life!' To his baffled enquiries, she told him that his 'help' had been failing her in a first-year medical subject, and taking the time to discuss her failure with her. She realized that she had in fact only done medicine because of her high university academic entrance mark and not through deep commitment. The result made her rethink her future, and decide to follow her real area of interest and skill. Thus this failure was a very effective part of her learning.

(Reproduced with the permission of Nelson Thornes Ltd from McAllister, L., et al., *Facilitating Learning in Clinical Settings*, ISBN 0 7487 3316 7, first published in 1997.)

- Ilott & Murphy (1997) also commented on the acute sense of personal failure felt by assessors when students failed, thus construing the assessment process as a reflection of their personal and/or professional worth.
- A personal dilemma for many assessors is that of feeling that failing a student is incongruent with being a health care professional whose central role is to 'care' and nurture (Luhanga et al 2008, Duffy 2004, Fraser et al 1997, Ilott & Murphy 1997, Stengelhofen 1993).
- Where assessors lacked confidence in assessing, had poor preparation for their role, did not know the student very well or where they did not have sufficient documented assessment evidence, the benefit of the doubt was more likely to be given (Jervis & Tilki 2011, Luhanga et al 2008, Duffy 2004, Fraser et al 1997, Bedford et al 1993).
- Students manipulate assessors or the system to avoid failure (Duffy 2004, Fraser et al 1997, White et al 1994).
- Duffy (2004) also found that mentors need more support from colleagues and education staff to fail incompetent students. A lack of support from colleagues, managers and lecturing staff made it more difficult to make fail decisions, with assessors even experiencing considerable pressure to pass students (Jervis & Tilki 2011, Green 1991).
- It is difficult to fail students in their third year as assessors do not want to be responsible for ending students' careers so late in a programme (Duffy 2004, Phillips et al 2000). Equally difficult is failing first year students as there is the held notion that problems will resolve as students progress through the course (Luhanga et al 2008, Duffy 2004).
- Assessors were reluctant to assign a failing grade based on poor attitude or unprofessional behaviours (Jervis & Tilki 2011, Luhanga et al 2008, Duffy 2004). This is contributed to by the lack of assessment tools for assessing the affective domain.

An awareness of those factors that contribute to 'failure to fail' may be a first step to understanding why we experience difficulties when dealing with a failing student, and may thus end up passing a student when a fail is clearly warranted. It may also help us to identify the support we need when dealing with these difficult situations.

CONCLUSION

When working with learners it is important to be able to indicate to them the progress they are making. Progress during clinical practice needs to be tracked carefully and feedback given so that learners may be able to learn and develop further. A discussion of the four assessment activities – working alongside the student and observing practice for development in the level of the student's competence, discussion with the student, examination of the student's portfolio and discussion with other practice educator – shows how they can be used to monitor the progress of learners. Based upon what we know about the nature of expertise (Benner et al 1996, Glaser 1990, Benner 1984), a model that outlines the performance characteristics of novice, advanced beginner and competent practice is proposed here to monitor and assist with progression during clinical practice.

Monitoring progress is not about policing the learner. It is very much about finding out the quality and quantity of learning that has taken place and any difficulties the learner may be experiencing so that further assessment activities can be discussed and planned to further learning and development. It is inevitable that there will be instances when learners do not succeed; for these learners, early identification of difficulties and taking the appropriate remedial action may prevent failure and thus eliminate the trauma of failure for them.

If progress is carefully tracked through the four assessment activities discussed here, and done throughout the student's placement, it becomes much easier to make assessment decisions that are also more likely to be based on a valid and reliable evidence base, which means that students have a fairer deal. It also makes the task of making assessment decisions easier for the assessor – easier, as it is never easy to make fail decisions. Assigning a fail grade is something that is rarely done lightly or without misgivings. It is a formidable responsibility. Passing a student is an equally formidable responsibility. *However, do we also assign a pass grade lightly and without misgivings?* I end this chapter by leaving you to ponder this question.

KEY POINTS FOR REFLECTION

When monitoring progress, the role and responsibilities of the practice educator centre on answering these key questions:

- What has the student done and learned so far? How will I know?
- Is the student having any difficulties? How will I know?

- What can be done to facilitate further learning and development?

Answers to these questions may be obtained through the use of the assessment activities in Figure 7.3.

The period of formative assessment allows the practice educator to monitor progress. Answers to the following questions will enable the assessor to decide whether there is progress:

* Is the student achieving statutory competencies?
* Is there a demonstration of a growing level of skill and competence (see the criteria in Figure 7.8)?
* Is performance consistent?
* Is there a demonstration of a growing understanding of the rationale underpinning practice?
* Is there a demonstration of development of the attitudes and values appropriate to professional practice?
* Is there a demonstration of a developing ability to engage in evidence-based and reflective practice?

The occasion of summative assessment centres on making a 'pass' or 'fail' decision. Answers to the following questions will enable the assessor to decide whether the student should be passed:

* Has the student achieved the statutory competencies?
* Does the assessment evidence achieve validity and reliability of assessment?
* Is there a demonstration of a sound understanding of the rationale underpinning each competency?
* Is the student developing the attitudes and values appropriate to professional practice?

Students who are either not progressing or failing to meet the required standard need identification by assessment systems so that opportunities can be provided for them to improve. The following behaviours could be indicative of this:

* inconsistency in meeting the required level of competence for expected stage of training

* inconsistency in clinical performance and lacks clinical skills
* does not respond appropriately to constructive feedback
* inability to make changes in response to constructive feedback – therefore clinical skills do not improve
* exhibits poor preparation and organizational skills
* has limited interactional and poor communication skills; does not ask questions; is unable to answer questions about care
* demonstrates unethical behaviour such as not disclosing/owning up to clinical errors made
* is uncommitted and unenthusiastic
* has poor punctuality
* may experience continual poor health, or feel depressed, angry, uncommitted, withdrawn, sad, emotionally labile, tired or listless.

The following actions should be taken:

1. Document the concerns.
2. Discuss the situation with a senior practitioner and the higher education institution.
3. Discuss the concerns with the student.
4. Make sure the student understands the problems.
5. Jointly, draw up a targeted detailed action plan.

A 'fail' decision should not come as a surprise to the student. Students may react with denial, anger, aggression and sadness or may try to bargain for a pass.

The assessor is invested with the responsibility and accountability for making assessment decisions. Assigning a fail grade is something that is rarely done lightly or without misgivings. It is a formidable responsibility. Passing a student is an equally formidable responsibility.

REFERENCES

Bailey, J., 1998. The supervisor's story: from expert to novice. In: Johns, C., Freshwater, D. (Eds.), Transforming Nursing through Reflective Practice. Blackwell Science, London, pp. 194–205.

Bedford, H., Phillips, T., Robinson, J., et al., 1993. Assessment of Competencies in Nursing and Midwifery Education and Training. The English National Board for Nursing, Midwifery and Health Visiting, London.

Benner, P., 1984. From Novice to Expert: Excellence and Power in Clinical Nursing Practice. Addison-Wesley, Menlo Park, California.

Benner, P., Tanner, C.A., Chesla, C.A., 1996. Expertise in Nursing Practice. Springer, New York.

Billings, D.M., Kowalski, K., Cleary, M.L., et al., 2010. Giving feedback to learners in clinical and academic settings: practical considerations. J. Contin. Educ. Nurs. 41 (4), 153–154.

Boud, D., 1992. The use of self-assessment schedules in negotiated learning. Stud. High. Educ. 17, 185–200.

Brandon, J., Davis, M., 1979. The limits of competence in social work: The assessment of marginal students in social work education. Br. J. Soc. Work 9 (3), 295–347.

Cannon, D., 2002. Learning to fail: Learning to recover. In: Peelo, M., Wareham, T. (Eds.), Failing Students in Higher Education. The Society for Research into Higher Education and Open University Press, Buckingham, pp. 73–84.

Child, D., 1997. Psychology and the Teacher, sixth ed. Cassell, London.

Clynes, M.P., Raftery, S.E.C., 2008. Feedback: an essential element of student learning in clinical practice. Nurse. Educ. Pract. 8, 405–411.

Coopersmith, S., 1967. The Antecedents of Self-Esteem. Freeman, San Francisco.

Dudek, N.L., Marks, M.B., Regehr, G., 2005. Failure to fail: The perspectives of clinical supervisors. Acad. Med. 80 (10), 584–587.

Duffy, K., 2004. Failing Students Report. Nursing and Midwifery Council, London, Online. Available: http://www.nmc-uk.org/nmc/main/publications/mentor_study.pdf (accessed December 2005).

Embo, M.P.C., Driessen, E.W., Valcke, M., et al., 2010. Assessment and feedback to facilitate self-directed learning in clinical practice of midwifery students. Med. Teacher 32, e263–e269.

English National Board, 1997. Standards for Approval of Higher Education Institutions and Programmes. The English National Board for Nursing, Midwifery and Health Visiting, London.

Fish, D., Twinn, S., 1997. Quality Clinical Supervision in the Health Care Professions: Principled Approaches to Practice. Butterworth Heinemann, Oxford.

Fitzgerald, M., Gibson, F., Gunn, K., 2010. Contemporary issues relating to assessment of pre-registration nursing students in practice. Nurse. Educ. Pract. 10, 158–163.

Fraser, D., 2000. Action research to improve the pre-registration midwifery curriculum. Part 3: can fitness for practice be guaranteed? The challenges of designing and implementing an effective assessment in practice scheme. Midwifery 16, 287–294.

Fraser, D., Murphy, R., Worth-Butler, M., 1997. An Outcome Evaluation of the Effectiveness of Pre-registration Midwifery Programmes of Education. The English National Board for Nursing, Midwifery and Health Visiting, London.

Gerrish, K., McManus, M., Ashworth, P., 1997. Levels of Achievement: A Review of the Assessment of Practice. The English National Board for Nursing, Midwifery and Health Visiting, London.

Gipps, C.V., 1994. Beyond Testing: Towards a Theory of Educational Assessment. The Falmer Press, London.

Glaser, R., 1990. Toward new models for assessment. Int. J. Educ. Res. 14 (5), 475–483.

Gomez, D.A., Lobodzinski, S., Hartwell West, C.D., 1998. Evaluating clinical performance. In: Billings, D.M., Halstead, J.A. (Eds.), Teaching in Nursing: A Guide for Faculty. WB Saunders, Philadelphia, pp. 407–422.

Gonczi, A., 1994. Competency based assessment in the professions in Australia. Assess. High. Educ. 1 (1), 27–44.

Gonczi, A., Hager, P., Athanasou, J., 1993. The Development of Competency-Based Assessment Strategies for the Professions. National Office of Overseas Skills Recognition, Research Paper No. 8. Australian Government Publishing Service, Canberra.

Green, C., 1991 Identification of the responsibilities and perceptions of the training task held by workforce supervisors of those training within the caring professions. Project 551 prepared for the Further Education Unit, Anglia Polytechnic.

Hawe, E., 2003. It's pretty difficult to fail: the reluctance of lecturers to award a failing grade. Assess. Eval. High. Educ. 29 (4), 371–382.

Hinchliff, S., 2004. The Practitioner as Teacher, third ed. Churchill Livingstone, London.

Hodges, B., 2003. OSCE! variations on a theme by Harden. Med. Educ. 37, 1134–1140.

Ilott, I., Murphy, R., 1997. Feelings and failings in professional training: the assessor's dilemma. Assess. Eval. High. Educ. 22 (3), 307–316.

Ilott, I., Murphy, R., 1999. Success and Failure in Professional Education: Assessing the Evidence. Whurr, London.

Jervis, A., Tilki, M., 2011. Why are nurse mentors failing to fail student nurses who do not meet clinical performance standards? Br. J. Nurs. 20 (9), 582–588.

Jones, P.R., 1995. Hindsight bias in reflective practice: an empirical investigation. J. Adv. Nurs. 21, 783–788.

Killam, L.A., Montgomery, P., Luhanga, F.L., et al., 2010. Views on unsafe nursing students in clinical learning. Int. J. Nurs. Educ. Scholarsh. 7 (1), 1–17. Article 36.

Kotzabassaki, S., Panou, M., Dimou, F., et al., 1997. Nursing students' and faculty perceptions of the characteristics of 'best' and 'worst'

clinical teachers: a replication study. J. Adv. Nurs. 26, 817–824.

Lankshear, A., 1990. Failure to fail: The teacher's dilemma. Nurs. Stand. 4 (20), 35–37.

Luhanga, F., Yonge, O.J., Myrick, F., 2008. Failure to assign failing grades: Issues with grading the unsafe student. Int. J. Nurs. Educ. Scholarsh. 5 (1), 1–14. Article 8.

Maatsch, J., Juang, R.R., Downing, S.M., et al., 1987. Examiner assessments of clinical performance: what do they tell us about clinical competence? Eval. Program. Plann. 10, 13–17.

McAllister, L., 1997. An adult learning framework for clinical education. In: McAllister, L., Lincoln, M., McLeod, S. (Eds.), Facilitating Learning in Clinical Settings Stanley Thornes, Cheltenham, pp. 1–26.

Maloney, D., Carmody, D., Nemeth, E., 1997. Students experiencing problems learning in the clinical setting. In: McAllister, L., Lincoln, M., McLeod, S. (Eds.), Facilitating Learning in Clinical Settings Stanley Thornes, Cheltenham, pp. 185–213.

Mattheos, N.M.C., Nattestad, A., Falk-Nilsson, E., et al., 2004. The interactive examination: assessing students' self-assessment ability. Med. Educ. 38 (4), 378–389.

Miller, C., 2010. Literature review: Improving and enhancing performance in the affective domain of nursing students. Contemp. Nurse 35 (1), 2–17.

Myall, M., Levett-Jones, T., Lathlean, J., 2008. Mentorship in contemporary practice: The experiences of nursing students and practice mentors. J. Clin. Nurs. 17, 1834–1842.

Neary, M., 2000. Teaching, Assessing and Evaluation for Clinical Competence. Stanley Thornes, Cheltenham.

Neary, M., 2001. Responsive assessment: Assessing student nurses' clinical competence. Nurse Educ. Today 21, 3–17.

Neville, S., French, S., 1991. Clinical education: student's and clinical teacher's views. Physiotherapy 17 (5), 351–354.

Nicol D., Macfarlane-Dick D. 2005 Rethinking formative assessment in HE: a theoretical model and seven principles of good feedback practice. Online. Available: http://www.heacademy.ac.uk/assessment/ASS051D_SENLEF_model.doc (accessed September 2005).

Nursing and Midwifery Council, 2004a. Standards of Proficiency for Pre-Registration Nursing Education. Nursing and Midwifery Council, London, Online. Available: www. nmc-uk.org/nmc/main/publications/Standardsofproficiency.pdf (accessed December 2005).

Nursing and Midwifery Council, 2004b. Standards of Proficiency for Pre-Registration Midwifery Education. Nursing and Midwifery Council, London, Online. Available: http://www.nmc-uk.org/nmc/main/publications/Standardofproficiency_v2.pdf (accessed December 2005).

Nursing and Midwifery Council, 2005. Consultation on Proposals Arising from A Review of Fitness for Practice at the Point of Registration. NMC, London, Online. Available: http://www.nmc-uk.org (accessed December 2005).

Nursing and Midwifery Council, 2008. Standards to Support Learning and Assessment in Practice, second ed. NMC, London, Online. Available: http://www.nmc-uk.org/Publications/Standards (accessed August 2011).

Nursing and Midwifery Council, 2009. Standards of Pre-Registration Midwifery Education. NMC, London, Online. Available: http://www.nmc-uk.org/Publications/Standards/ (accessed August 2011).

Nursing and Midwifery Council, 2010. Standards of Pre-Registration Nursing Education. NMC, London, Online. Available: http://www.nmc-uk.org/Publications/Standards/ (accessed August 2011).

Paul, N., 1988. Constructive Criticism. Wyvern Business Training, Ely, Cambridgeshire.

Phillips, T., Schostak, J., Tyler, J., 2000. Practice and Assessment in Nursing and Midwifery: Doing it for Real. The English National Board for Nursing, Midwifery and Health Visiting, London.

Robertson, S., Rosenthal, J., Dawson, V., 1997. Using assessment to promote student learning. In: McAllister, L., Lincoln, M., McLeod, S. (Eds.), Facilitating Learning in Clinical Settings. Stanley Thornes, Cheltenham, pp. 154–184.

Rowntree, D., 1987. Assessing Students: How Shall We Know Them?, second ed. Kogan Page, London.

Sadler, R., 1989. Specifying and promulgating achievement standards. Instruct. Sci. 18, 119–144.

Scholes, J., Albarran, J., 2005. Failure to fail: Facing the consequences of inaction. Br. Assoc. Crit. Care. Nurs., Nurs. Crit. Care. 10 (3), 113–115.

Srinivasan, M., Hauer, K.E., Der-Martirosian, C., et al., 2007. Does feedback matter. Practice-based learning for medical students after a multi-institutional clinical performance examination. Med. Educ. 41, 857–865.

Stengelhofen, J., 1993. Teaching Students in Clinical Settings. Chapman & Hall, London.

Stuart, C.C., 2002. An Innovation in Midwifery Education. Proceedings from the 26th Triennial International Congress of Midwives, International Confederation of Midwives (ICM), Vienna.

Torrance, H., Pryor, J., 1998. Investigating Formative Assessment. Open University Press, Buckingham.

UKCC, 1999. Fitness for Practice. United Kingdom Central Council for Nursing, Midwifery and Health Visiting, London.

While, A.E., 1994. Competence versus performance: which is more important? J. Adv. Nurs. 20, 525–531.

White, E., Riley, E., Davies, S., et al., 1994. A Detailed Study of the Relationship between Teaching, Support, Supervision and Role Modelling in Clinical Areas within the Context of P2000 Courses. The English National Board for Nursing, Midwifery and Health Visiting, London.

Wolf, A., 1995. Competence-Based Assessment. Open University Press, Buckingham.

Woolliscroft, J.O., Tentlaken, J., Smith, J., et al., 1993. Medical students' clinical self-assessments: comparisons with external measures of performance and the students' self-assessment of overall performance and effort. Acad. Med. 68, 285–294.

Chapter | 8 |

The clinical environment as a setting for learning and professional development

INTRODUCTION

Stated simplistically, the clinical environment is where patient/client care and clinical activities take place – it is where the action is. It is the real world of health care practice. A range of health professionals interact and work together to deliver care using their 'special brand' of professional expertise, making use of available material resources where needed. The clinical environment is unpredictable, volatile and dynamic; it is frequently noisy and teems with human interactions and activities. The clinical environment is the arena where students from the health care professions learn about care and what clinical practice is all about. The practice learning of students of health care is widely acknowledged as being one of the most important aspects of their educational preparation (English National Board for Nursing, Midwifery and

Health Visiting (ENB) & Department of Health 2001). Students rate practice learning as 'the most significant, most productive, most memorable component' of their course (Kadushin 1992:11). It is during practice placements that students learn to care for patients and clients, colleagues and others they work and interact with. Qualified professionals further their learning and 'hone up' on skills and competence.

The clinical environment must therefore also be an environment where learning can take place, thus becoming an educational environment. This type of setting is one that is conducive to learning and professional development. Marton et al (1984) make the important observation that learning is a function of the relationship between the learner and the environment and is never something determined by one of these elements alone. Learners do not respond merely to tasks they are assigned; rather, they adapt to and work within the environment taken as an interrelated whole. They pay close attention to the 'hidden' as well as the 'visible' curricula (Parlett & Hamilton 1977). It is the learner's engagement with the environment that makes the particular learning experience (Boud & Walker 1990).

This chapter examines the components of the clinical learning environment and those factors that contribute to a positive learning environment. Strategies for creating this type of environment are suggested. Chapter 9 examines how the learner can interact meaningfully with this environment in order to learn through clinical experiences.

THE CLINICAL LEARNING ENVIRONMENT

The learning environment of any formal educational setting is complex. It is suggested here that the clinical environment is a formal educational setting. The practice educators are the teachers and the students are required to learn. There are norms and rules of behaviours and the practice educators and students have expectations of each other and others (Boud & Walker 1990). This complexity is captured by Parlett & Hamilton (1977:14-15), who noted that a learning environment in the formal educational setting is:

> *the social–psychological and material environment in which students and teachers work together … [it] represents a network or nexus of cultural, social, institutional, and psychological variables. These interact in complicated ways to produce, in each [clinical area], a unique pattern of circumstances, pressures, customs, opinions and work styles which suffuse the teaching and learning that occur there. The configuration of the learning milieu in any particular [clinical area] depends on the interplay of numerous different factors … there are numerous constraints … there are [also] the individual [practitioner's] characteristics … and there are student perspectives and preoccupations.*

In the nursing literature, Dunn & Burnett (1995:1166) say that the clinical learning environment is the 'interactive network of forces within the clinical setting that influence the students' clinical learning outcomes'. Orton (1981) described the clinical learning environment as a group of stable characteristics unique to that setting. These characteristics will impact on and influence the behaviour of individuals within it. The clinical environment as a formal educational setting is thus much more than the physical environment where patient/client care and other clinical activities take place; it is inclusive of the material resources within it, the formal requirements, the culture, procedures, practices and standards of particular clinical areas, the expectations and interactions of all the people who are in it, as well as the personal characteristics of individuals who are part of this environment. The richness of the clinical environment provides a rich texture for learning during clinical practice. This setting provides the context and events within which the student operates and learns (Boud & Walker 1990). However, it also acts as a distraction and competes for the student's attention.

The environment for teaching and learning in the community opens another world for students. Although they do not have to work within the constraints of a hospital environment, students have to learn a different set of factors that influence practice. Professional carers are visitors in the client's own home – caring and teaching/learning activities are carried out in the client's domain. The client's lifestyle, values and health priorities could challenge the student's value systems. Students need to learn to respond sensitively in these situations as they learn about the complex forces that influence health care (White & Ewan 1991).

You may wish to try Activity 8.1.

ACTIVITY 8.1

Think about the clinical area where you work. This can be a ward, your community 'beat', an outpatients clinic, day care, operation theatre, casualty and so on.

1. Make a list of all the people who you think influence the learning ethos of the environment. How do they exert this influence?
2. What other factors influence your clinical environment as a learning environment?

This chapter examines the components of the clinical learning environment and their associated factors that contribute to a positive learning environment.

It is necessary to take into account several components and factors and the interaction between these when considering the clinical environment as an educational environment. These components and factors can be grouped into the following categories:

1. The people:
   a. the leader of the team
   b. the members of the team
   c. the students
   d. the practice educators.
2. Learning opportunities and experiences 'provided by':
   a. patient/client care
   b. other clinical activities.
3. Staff commitment to teaching and learning:
   a. support and supervision of learners
   b. continuing professional development.
4. Material resources.

The people

The leader of the team

In nursing much of the work that explored the direct influences of the leader of the team on the learning environment was done in the 1980s in the UK. Until the mid-1980s in the UK, one of the key roles of the ward sister was to teach, supervise and assess student nurses. The ward sister was the only person who was directly responsible for student learning during clinical practice. The ward sister as the leader of the ward team was seen to be the single most important person in creating the learning climate (Jacka & Lewin 1987, Fretwell 1982, Ogier 1982, Orton 1981, Pembrey 1980). A positive learning climate is characterized by a democratic non-hierarchical structure and teamwork and good communication are displayed. The conclusion that can be drawn from the work of these researchers is that, for learning to occur, the clinical area has to be managed by a leader who is in touch with the needs and abilities of her team. The leader should also have the ability to create an atmosphere conducive to learning, a point that is developed below. Ogier (1989:37) has perhaps captured these messages in the following succinct statement: 'facilitating learning cannot be divorced from competent management and humane leadership'.

The reality today is that the team leader as ward manager has a wider diversity of roles to fulfil. This has resulted in removing the ward manager from much, if any, direct patient and student contact. Nevertheless, the importance of the ward manager's indirect influences on the learning climate should not be underestimated. The positive attitude of the ward manager towards students has been found to be important in influencing the circumstances for a positive ward learning culture (Saarikoski & Leino-Kilpi 2002, Dunn & Hansford 1997). With the support of a ward manager who is committed to the training and development of students and staff, team members are more likely to be motivated in their role of practice educator to students, and to the development of the clinical environment into an educational environment.

The members of the team

Each member of the team can contribute to an environment that fosters learning. The NMC (2008a) expects nurses and midwives who are practice educators to create an environment conducive to learning. Orton (1981) found that in wards that were highly rated by students there was a combination of teamwork, consultation and an awareness of the needs of others. In these wards, students' and patients' physical and emotional needs were amply met. A ward team that is committed not only to delivering a high standard of patient/client care but also to learning and assessing activities will contribute much to the creation of an educational climate. In a later study, Fraser (1994 in Gilmore 1999) also found that, where the ward culture was positive, there was good teamwork. Students and staff used terms such as 'friendly', 'happy', 'involving', 'teaching' and 'explaining to students'. Such a ward culture was perceived to be as important as or more important than individual practitioners in helping students learn.

Interprofessional learning and collaboration Remember also that members of the multi-professional team make up the team even though they are not as visible as nurses and midwives in the clinical area. The multi-professional team's philosophy of patient/client care and their attitudes towards learning and students will also greatly influence the learning environment. It is important that they contribute to the educational environment so that not only do all

members of the team learn with and from each other, but also a spirit of teamwork may be created for the benefit of the patient/client.

The delivery of high-quality health care requires partnership by practitioners within and between professions (Lait et al 2011), and students must 'learn to learn and practise collaboratively and interdependently' (Taylor 1997:5). Taylor goes on to say that 'the complexity of a post-modern society means that problems presented to practitioners and structures to respond to them requires responses which go beyond those traditional, rigid professional boundaries'(Taylor 1997: 5). Students should therefore gain, where possible, experience as part of a multi-professional team so that they learn to function as an effective team member (Lait et al 2011, ENB & Department of Health 2001). Now you may wish to try Activity 8.2.

ACTIVITY 8.2

How do you help your students fit into the team?
  What opportunities are available in your setting to help students fit into the team?
  What opportunities are available to enable students to work and learn with members of the multi-professional team?

The health care team is a complex one. Students need to learn to relate and work with the team members: this is demanding, as it is not easy for students to feel valued as good team members (Stengelhofen 1993). In particular, new students may feel anxious even with the simple act of speaking with a professional, especially when that person is viewed as a senior member of the team. Practice educators should ensure that students have opportunities to experience teamwork through observing different members of the team at work and working as a member of the team. The following ideas, based upon and extended from the work of Lait et al (2011) and Stengelhofen (1993), are offered to help students fit into the team and to learn about multi-professional team working:

1. Ensure that students have opportunities to fit into their own professional team – the 'home team'. Initially, this can be done informally by introducing the student to these team members. Students should be invited to attend staff meetings, journal clubs, training days, seminars, social events and so on. Arrangements can also be made to enable students to observe the team members – this need not involve any teaching. In preparation for the observational activity, students should be briefed on those specific aspects of the job role that are pertinent to the student's learning and development at the time. It is important that students demonstrate the ability to

fit into the 'home team' before they are expected to become a member of the multi-professional team.

2. *Meeting members of the multi-professional team.* Introducing students to members of the multi-professional team informally – in the corridor, during coffee and meal breaks and in the staff room – can help others recognize new students. Later on, students can be gradually introduced to the work of these team members by making arrangements for students to observe them providing care for patients and being involved in situations that do not make any professional demands on the student, such as attending a team meeting and case discussion. These activities will increase the student's understanding of the roles of the multi-professional team and also give students opportunities to interact with these professionals.

3. *Meeting, working and learning with students from other professions.* If your setting has students from the other professions, explore opportunities for these students to meet and perhaps work together (e.g. discussing a patient/client they have looked after). These sessions will require to be facilitated to ensure that learning is collaborative (Holland 2002). Each student will be able to contribute to the discussion of care given, viewed from the perspectives of that particular professional group. Students will also be able to learn about the roles of some of the other professionals in this way. Respect for each other's professional roles is likely to be engendered. Students are thus engaging in interprofessional learning as they will be learning from and about each other to improve collaboration and the quality of care (Barr et al 2005, in Lait et al 2011). This strategy sows the seed for good team working, as students who have such positive experiences of the multi-professional team are likely to carry this into their professional practice.

4. *Working with members of the multi-professional team.* Plan graded steps to team involvement. As students' confidence increases they can be placed in situations where they are required to work alongside a member of the multi-professional team. In the first instance, be careful to involve the student with professionals who are patient and cooperative. The student should gradually become independent in interacting with all team members and develop the confidence to participate in care.

5. *Learning actively from members of the multi-professional team.* Encourage students to talk to these team members to gather information or discuss management of specific patients/clients who have required multi-professional input. The practice educator can assist the student to draw up the aims for the meeting and, subsequently, hold a debriefing session on the conduct and outcome of the meeting. Students will then be able to learn about the contribution that each professional makes to the care of that patient/client. This type of experience will make interprofessional collaborative care real for students. Lait et al (2011) cited the example of a physiotherapy student who participated in the care of a patient with traumatic brain injury. The student interacted with and interviewed the nine types of professionals involved in the care of this patient to understand their contributions.

6. *Explore ways information is communicated within the multi-professional team.* As well as the use of formal letters, written reports and documentation in the patient/client's case notes, discuss other ways that communication takes place within the team, such as chats over coffee, telephone calls, during ward rounds and verbal reports.

The students

Students bring their own personalities, dispositions, hopes and aspirations, past experiences and backgrounds, and also worries and anxieties, to the clinical setting. For many beginning students, the impact of the clinical environment can be strong (Lefevre 2005, White & Ewan 1991). They have to deal with the unpleasant experiences such as sights, smells and cries of pain and difficult problems such as the abusive or disturbed patient/client. Many will not have done shift work, or been on their feet for long hours. Students who come from an affluent and comfortable home background may have to learn to cope with the realities of social and economic differences, particularly when in the community setting.

Unlike permanent members of the team, students are more likely to feel like a visitor or short-stay resident (Parlett & Dearden 1977). And if they are not made to feel welcomed or, worse, if they are made to feel a burden (Phillips et al 2000), their plans, hopes and aspirations can be thwarted, and any worries and anxieties compounded by an uncongenial environment. Learning is likely to be affected negatively in this type of environment. Learning plans may be abandoned (Boud & Walker 1990).

White & Ewan (1991) think that the differences between learning in the classroom and in the clinical setting are profound – in the classroom setting, students can 'hide' behind the mantle of the group, which shields them from the close attention of the teacher. In the clinical setting, students are visible as they work closely with their practice educators and members of the team. Patients and clients may be observing their performance. They can feel threatened and vulnerable, as their performance and behaviours are visible and open to the scrutiny of a range of people. It is important to recognize the differing needs of recent school leavers and mature students with, and without, health care experience. Learners also have different learning styles – these need to be utilized to maximize student learning (McAllister 1997).

Each student forms part of the educational environment, enriching it with his/her personal contribution (Boud & Walker 1990). On entry into the environment, students create interactions that become learning experiences for themselves and others. Lincoln et al (1997) believe that students who have chosen to become health care professionals tend to be committed to the ethos of caring and curing. Clinical practice provides the opportunity for students to experience their desires to care and help and to put into practice the theory they have learned – they will be learning how to care and to develop the competencies required of a professional.

Stengelhofen (1993:48) points out that it is unfortunate if a student is not seen as a student member of the department or team. They should be viewed as valuable student members of the team with specific clinical learning needs, rather than as valuable members of the team with the emphasis on 'getting the work done' and in providing a service contribution (Melia 1987). A clinical environment that is an educational environment will be able to support students so that they achieve their personal and professional goals in the best possible ways. This seems to be in the hands of practice educators – Eraut et al (1995) report that qualified clinical staff exercises a major influence on the quality of pre-registration programmes.

Students become professionals through the process of 'professional socialization', which takes place predominantly in the clinical setting (McKenna et al 2010, Lincoln et al 1997, McAllister 1997, Melia 1987). They need to acquire that 'set of values, attitudes, knowledge and skills which are displayed within the culture of a profession by practising professionals' (Lincoln et al 1997:75). From their review of the literature on the components of professionalism, Lincoln et al identified the following four components:

- technical competence
- professional interpersonal skills, encompassing communication skills, values and attitudes of the professional
- knowledge of professional standards of conduct
- ethical competence, which is essentially about moral obligation to those for whom professionals care.

It is suggested here that the patient/client care practices of a clinical environment will significantly influence the professional socialization of a student. A clinical environment that is also an educational environment needs to espouse a philosophy of care, reflected in practice, which will enable students to develop into professionals who can truly meet the needs of society for care and caring. The ENB & Department of Health (2001) recommend that the philosophy of care should be in the form of a written statement. High standards of care need to be modelled. As discussed earlier, Orton (1981) found that wards that were highly rated by students amply met the physical and emotional needs of patients. There are other studies that have also found that students value high standards of care being modelled (Saarikoski & Leino-Kilpi 2002, Kotzabassaki et al 1997, White et al 1994) White & Ewan (1991) make the point that simply setting a good example for students to follow is not enough. Students must be encouraged to be active in experiencing, discussing and evaluating professional behaviours and care in order to extract personal meaning.

The practice educators

It has long been accepted that using the 'apprenticeship' system in nursing and midwifery training is educationally unsound (Fretwell 1982, Ogier 1982, Pembrey 1980). What is known about learning in the workplace tells us that learning is ineffective if students are placed in practice environments as part of the workforce where supervision is inadequate and active facilitation of learning does not take place (Spouse 2003, 1998, Jacka & Lewin 1987, Melia 1987). Within the apprenticeship system, the clinical environment for students was in effect a working environment and not an educational environment. Project 2000 (UKCC 1986) challenged the ways that students were expected to learn during clinical practice. As a consequence, students currently undertaking pre-registration nursing and midwifery programmes enjoy supernumerary status. The NMC (2008) makes it a mandatory requirement for all students on approved educational programmes to be supervised by a practitioner who is capable of supporting learning and assessment in practice, making judgements on fitness for practice to enter the register or to record a specialist practice qualification. These practitioners are accountable to the NMC for such judgements. The fulfilment of these responsibilities is not so easy and straightforward and frequently causes dilemmas for the practitioner who is both mentor and assessor to the student (Bray & Nettleton 2007, Neary 1997b, Holloway 1985). However, the ethical and legal implications of mentoring, supervising and assessing students have to be considered: these are discussed in Chapter 2.

Mentoring In Greek mythology, Mentor was the wise and faithful advisor to Odysseus. Today, the mentor is a friend, role model, an able advisor and the person who supports in many different ways. Within these functions, the mentor generally takes on the roles as carried out by the assessor, participating actively in formative assessments, but does *not* conduct summative assessments.

Much has been written about mentors and mentorship in the nursing literature (Jokelainen et al 2011, Spouse 2003, 1996, Gray & Smith 2000, Andrews & Wallis 1999). It is well documented that effective supervision, support and facilitation of learning require the mentor to possess certain qualities and skills. Andrews & Wallis (1999:204) report that the literature contains a 'comprehensive catalogue of personal attributes and skills required for effective mentoring'. Students have certain expectations of their mentors and find certain characteristics and behaviours in mentors helpful (Lefevre 2005, Papp et al 2003, Jackson & Mannix 2001, Neary 1997a,b, Spouse 1996, Darling 1984). A common theme is the significance of the personal and professional attributes of the mentor such as approachability, good interpersonal skills, self-confidence, someone who respects and shows interest in students and a competent and enthusiastic practitioner. According to Neary (2000:21), the mentor who can contribute to the clinical environment so that it is an educational environment is the person who is:

- prepared to allocate both time and energy to the role
- up to date with professional practice and is innovative
- competent in the core skills of coaching, counselling, facilitating, giving feedback and networking
- interested and willing to help others
- willing and able to learn
- able to demonstrate the many characteristics advocated by Darling (1984).

These characteristics are described in full below to enable you to assess yourself.

Characteristics of a mentor In her research into the characteristics that students perceive as valuable and helpful in a mentor, Darling (1984) has identified the following:

- a *model* the student can look up to, respect and admire
- an *envisioner* who gives a picture of what could be done, is enthusiastic about opportunities and possibilities and interest is sparked
- an *energizer* who is enthusiastic and dynamic and kindles the student's interest
- an *investor* who makes time for the student; spots potential and capabilities; trusts, 'lets go' and delegates responsibility
- a *supporter* who listens, is warm, caring and encouraging and is available in times of need
- a *standard-prodder* who is very clear about what level of achievement is required and pushes and prods the student to achieve higher standards
- a *teacher-coach* who guides on problem solving and setting priorities, helps in the development of new skills and inspires personal and professional development
- a *feedback giver* who can offer both positive and constructive feedback and help the student explore things that go wrong
- an *eye opener* who motivates interest in new developments and research, facilitates reasoning and understanding and directs the student into seeing the bigger picture

- a *door opener* who provides opportunities for trying out new ideas and suggests and identifies resources for learning
- an *idea bouncer* who not only discusses and debates issues and ideas, but also clarifies and stimulates new thoughts
- a *problem solver* who is tolerant of shortcomings and skilfully uses both the strengths and weaknesses of the student to enable further development to take place
- an *educational counsellor* who is trusted, understands the student's needs to achieve, and supports and guides towards success
- a *challenger* who questions opinions and beliefs, forces the student to examine choices critically while empowering the student towards fulfilment of her/his potential.

Morton-Cooper & Palmer (2000) pointed out that mentors do not have the magic abilities or power to fashion great individuals. They do, though, enable individuals to discover and use their own talents, encouraging and nurturing their unique contributions and to assist them in becoming successful in their own right. Mentors have their own educational experiences, knowledge base, level of competence and history of experiences of caring and practice. These variations will influence the ways individuals practise their roles and how they view the work environment. Phillips et al (2000) found that many practitioners were enthusiastic about having students in the clinical areas and looked forward to sharing knowledge and experiences. Such attitudes will clearly influence the learning climate of the area positively. Conversely, there were practitioners who were so caught up with the 'busyness' of the workplace that students were viewed as an additional burden. The reality about clinical areas is that pressures, busyness and workloads are continually increasing; there is simply no time to 'teach'. This is where the individual's beliefs about how learning takes place can influence the learning climate.

Jarvis (1983) and Rogers (1983) believe that teaching is not essential to learning. Many learners acquire knowledge, skills and attitudes independent of any formal teaching. This is not to say that teaching is unimportant but, given certain conditions, most adults engage in much more learning than is often realized and acknowledged. One way that students learn in the clinical setting is by observing their mentors as they work alongside each other. No formal teaching is done here. McLeod et al (1997:54) state that 'students learn most from observing the actions and understanding the reasoning processes of their role models'. The adage 'actions speak louder than words' aptly describes the power of role modelling, as the actions of the practitioner are probably more powerful in influencing the student than what is said, and what is said by the practice educator is probably more powerful than what is said by the teacher in the classroom

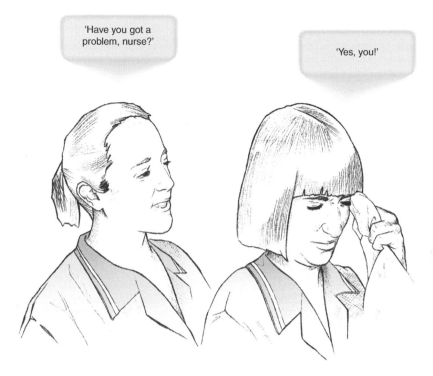

'Have you got a
problem, nurse?'

'Yes, you!'

Figure 8.1 Mentors need good interpersonal skills.

(Stengelhofen 1993). Charters (2000) thinks that this form of facilitating learning has been overlooked or devalued by the very practitioners who employ it. Being a role model is widely recognized as critical in teaching, coaching and shaping as it is the most powerful teaching strategy available to practice educators (McLeod et al 1997). 'Attitudes take time to describe or explain, but are quickly demonstrated by every action and word' (Ogier 1989:36) – attitudes are modelled and learnt by the way the patient/client is spoken to; skills and techniques are demonstrated when care is carried out – all are ways of working and learning at the same time.

By working and talking with the student, the practitioner is teaching as well as getting the work done. Read the following modified extract (Examples 1 and 2) from Ogier (1989:25-26) and then tackle Activity 8.3. The scenarios took place on a busy general surgical ward. Mary is a second year student nurse. Postoperative analgesia was being prepared.

1. Practice educator: 'Mary, can you come here and check this controlled drug with me? Mrs Gavey last had pethidine at 6.00 am, it is now 10.00 am so she can have more.' The practice educator and Mary can be heard preparing syringes, counting the stock and administering the drug to Mrs Gavey. Following documentation, they clear up and go their separate ways.

2. Practice educator: 'Mary, can you check this controlled drug with me? As you heard at the report, Mrs Gavey had a cholecystectomy yesterday afternoon. She last had pethidine 75 mg at 6.00 am, it is now 10.00 am and the physiotherapist is due to see her at about 10.30 am. If we give her more pethidine now, it will be working by the time the physiotherapist comes to help Mrs Gavey with her deep-breathing exercises.' While the practice educator is talking, the injection is being prepared and the sound of syringes being unwrapped and drug cupboards being unlocked can be heard. They administer the drug and sign the documentation, and, while clearing up, the practice educator asks Mary, ''How are you getting on?'

ACTIVITY 8.3

Imagine you are the practice educator. List the information imparted in the interaction described in Example 1, and then do the same for Example 2. What types of interaction took place?

Preparing and giving the drug took the same length of time in each example, but in Example 2 the practice educator was sharing her decision-making process – why the pethidine was being given. Mary also gained an insight into the planning of more effective pain relief. She has learnt through experience, which was triggered by the practice educator's explanation while they worked together. The practice educator also showed interest in how Mary was progressing.

Ask yourself the following questions:

1. How can work be planned so that having students is a help rather than a hindrance?
2. How can students be involved in care so that they are learning while contributing to the work of the team?
3. How can the work be turned into dynamic learning experiences?

Learning opportunities and experiences

Patients and clients and opportunistic teaching and learning

In practice-based health care professions, the best place for learning about care delivery is in the direct context of patient/client care. Burnard & Chapman (1990:48) made this important statement:

> *The basis of clinical learning should be the process of carrying out [care] with patients. The one thing that is always missing in the [academic setting] and always present in the clinical setting is the presence of patients. Encounters with patients, whatever the clinical setting, should always form the basis of learning.*

These learning opportunities are difficult to control as the presence of which patients or clients in the clinical area cannot be prescribed. However, the nature of the conditions, illnesses or problems of patients and clients who require care in any given clinical setting are known. On this basis, the learning opportunities and clinical experiences that can be provided for students in each setting can be determined. Using these learning opportunities, learning contracts and assessment plans (see Ch. 6) can be developed to meet the needs of the student. Although these plans provide the structure to assist the student achieve learning outcomes, the control and predictability of experiences are unlikely to be possible. Each patient or client is different and each has varied needs that require different care and management. The condition of the patient/client could alter, sometimes dramatically. These differences and the unplanned and unpredictable events are learning opportunities that can be capitalized upon.

The way that an unprecedented clinical event is responded to is a learning opportunity in itself. White & Ewan (1991:138) remind us that 'opportunistic teaching is not dependent on the ease of availability of interesting or unusual events but on making opportunities for students to learn'. Opportunistic experiences emerge as the realities of clinical practice unfold. These authors go on to say that the 'ability to see opportunities and use them distinguishes [practice educators] as persons with ingenuity and flair' (White & Ewan 1991:138). For example, during the course of performing 'routine' pressure area care with the student, there are opportunities for involving the student actively in the care of the patient/client by, for example, inviting the student's opinions on the condition of the skin and how the student would manage the situation, pointing out the warning signs of impending pressure sore development, which the student may not have seen, or discussing evidence-based management of pressure areas to prevent pressure sores, the policy of the clinical setting or hospital for the management of patients/clients at risk of developing pressure sores, and so on. If a relative is present who wishes to be involved in the care of the patient/client, involving the relative with care giving will show the student how this is done and the role of family members when a relative requires care. Subsequently, discussions with the student on this aspect of care will reinforce learning.

You may wish to try Activity 8.4 to help you consider the vast range of activities related to direct patient/client care, which are some of the learning opportunities present in your clinical setting.

ACTIVITY 8.4

Make a list of the patients/clients you have looked after during your last three spans of duty. Make a list of their conditions, illnesses and problems that they had presented you with. How did you deal with their range of needs?

Remember that it is not only the direct 'encounters' with patients and clients that are the learning opportunities for students. Other examples of learning opportunities provided by patient/client encounters could be the way you plan and manage your workload, the way you plan care, how you make decisions and how you handle different situations – particularly difficult ones. Chamberlain (1997) found that one strategy by which student midwives used to obtain information was to listen to their midwives' interactions with each other, clients and doctors.

Total patient/client care gives students the opportunity to observe and participate in the provision and delivery of holistic care. Providing opportunities for students to look after the same patients/clients will enable them to learn more about this aspect of care delivery. There is then also the opportunity for students to follow the progress of those patients/clients and their response to care and treatment. Patient/client and staff satisfaction is generally higher with this method of care delivery, which can only contribute to a positive learning climate. Students can also learn, for example, the importance of good team working within a multi-professional team, the range of care-giving activities a patient/client requires, and how to coordinate these, and how to meet the total needs of a patient/client. These are also opportunities for students to realize that an acquisition of technical competence is not enough for professional practice as a health care professional. In the case of nurses, Virginia Henderson (1966) said, very profoundly, that 'nursing is of the head and of the hands and of the heart'. The skills of the practice educator in utilizing the richness of the clinical learning environment will enable the development of a well-rounded health care practitioner as envisioned by that author.

Other clinical activities

Other than the learning opportunities provided by direct patient/client contact, there is generally a huge range of activities in any clinical setting that are learning opportunities for student participation. More often than not, engagement in these activities can generate evidence of competence. Students need to be directed to these activities and assisted to draw up the aims and learning outcomes in order to derive meaningful learning from participating in these activities. You may wish to try Activity 8.5 to help you consider the vast range of other activities that can be learning opportunities for students working in your clinical setting.

ACTIVITY 8.5

Make a list of those activities and events that have taken place during the last 3 days you were on duty. Go on to make another list of those activities and events that you consider to be learning opportunities for students.

White & Ewan (1991) made the observation that students make the surprising but not infrequent comment that they have 'nothing to do' during clinical placements. Pause to consider the undertones of this comment. Students frequently equate real learning with actively 'doing'. When the pace is slower and events less dramatic, students may wonder how such experiences contribute to their preparation for developing competence. Activities that are not directly related to patient/client care may not be viewed as learning opportunities. This is where a list of activities and events with their potential for learning can be useful in directing and guiding students to other sources of learning that contribute to their overall professional development. Some suggestions of activities and events to which students can be directed in most clinical

settings, and which should be considered to be part of the educational environment, are given below. There will be others that will be specific to your own clinical environment.

1. *Learning and gaining insight about the work of the multi-professional team.* The activities for the student could be to:
   a. Observe several different professionals working.
   b. Liaise and communicate with a number of different professionals.
   c. Go on ward rounds.
   d. Attend case conferences and seminars.
   e. Attend staff meetings.
2. *Learning communication skills* within the profession specific team, the multi-professional team and with other carers. The activities for the student could be to:
   a. Liaise and communicate with a number of different team members, professionals in the multi-professional team, including those who provide support services such as pharmacists, and technicians and other carers such as relatives and friends of the patient/client and members of voluntary organizations. In their study of how well prepared newly qualified midwives were for their role, Fraser et al (1997) found that these midwives needed more experience of communicating with and referring to other team members when they were students.
   b. Use the telephone to communicate with a range of people. This activity may appear simple, but can be anxiety provoking for the student who has to speak in public to someone unknown to the student, and the student may fear not having the answers and thus feel foolish.
   c. Participate in ward handovers, ward rounds, case conferences, seminars and staff meetings. The requirement to speak during these events can be anxiety provoking – students need to be encouraged and supported to develop the courage and skills of speaking and voicing their opinions during these events.
   d. Report back to staff on the outcomes of treatment and care given, both verbally and through written reports.
3. *Acquiring administrative and management experience.* Deficits in management and organization skills among newly qualified nurses and midwives in the UK are well documented and cause considerable anxiety and stress. These have been observed since the 1980s in several studies (O'Shea & Kelly 2007, Gerrish 2000, 1990, Vaughan 1980 in Gerrish 2000, Fraser et al 1997). The nurses in Gerrish's studies found the management of self and a team of nurses problematic. They also found prioritizing care especially difficult. A significant number of midwives in Fraser et al's

study found it difficult to manage their time and organize their own workload. The following activities could assist students to develop organization and management skills:

a. Organize the transfer of patients/clients to other units and agencies.

b. Organize the discharge of patients/clients, including hospital transport if required.

c. Order equipment.

d. Manage own workload. Workload should be incremental and commensurate with the student's experience and stage of training. Senior students should be given the responsibility for the care of a group of patients/clients, including making the decisions for their care. The aim is to prepare the student so that transition to the professional role is accomplished at the point of registration.

e. Coordinate the work of the team where appropriate. This activity could include delegating work to the team.

4. *Learning about records and record keeping.* The activities for the student could be to:

a. Find out about the handling and storage of case notes.

b. Retrieve case notes.

c. File patient/client reports.

d. Write in the patient's/client's care records.

e. Extract from and input into computerized record systems.

5. *Learning to use equipment.* The use of equipment should be demonstrated and followed by immediate supervised practice. Opportunities to handle and use the equipment during patient/client care should be provided as soon as possible following demonstration of their use. Repeated practice will help the student acquire dexterity, confidence and consistent performance.

6. *Accessing teaching/learning sessions.* Many clinical areas have these sessions, such as scheduled lectures, seminars, case conferences, demonstration of new equipment by company representatives and teaching ward rounds. Students should be directed to these sessions, as appropriate, and time made available for them to attend these sessions.

When considering the learning opportunities in your clinical setting, it may be useful to remember that 'while students have control over what they want to learn, they have limited control over access to opportunities for learning' (Chamberlain 1997:85). This means that opportunities for learning should be planned so that students can be directed to them and supported while they are learning. This strategy can only contribute to the educational environment in creating an ambience for learning.

Staff commitment to teaching and learning

Support and supervision of learners

Phillips et al (2000) commented that the role of students can be an uncomfortable one – their behaviour and performance are under constant surveillance for what they show about their character and competence. It is widely acknowledged that during clinical placements students experience anxiety and stress for a wide range of reasons. Jimenez et al (2009) reported that nursing students perceived clinical stressors more intensely than academic and other sources of stress. Beginning and third year students are particularly vulnerable. Several studies in the UK (Deary et al 2003, Lindop 1999, Birch 1975) found that third year students experienced greater stress than in the earlier years of the programme. Deary et al also report that, as the programme progressed, there was an increase in psychological morbidity. In a Canadian study, Beck & Srivastava (1991) found that, when compared with the general population, nursing students were at greater risk of having a physical or psychological illness. Sources of anxiety and stress reported in some of the literature include:

- working with dying patients and death (Timmins & Kaliszer 2002, Parkes 1985)
- interpersonal conflict with mentors and other practitioners (Timmins & Kaliszer 2002, Jackson & Mannix 2001, Chamberlain 1997, Parkes 1985)
- insecurity about personal clinical competence and a perceived lack of practical skills (Mahar 1998, Chamberlain 1997, Parkes 1985)
- performing intimate care and caring for someone of the opposite sex (Seed 1995)
- being assessed (Lefevre 2005, Jack 1992) and fear of failure (Jones & Johnston 1997, Williams 1993, Parkes 1985)
- fear of making mistakes (Williams 1993, Kleehammer et al 1990)
- changes in ward allocation (Phillips et al 2000, Jack 1992). Terms such as 'scary', 'frightening', 'terrified', and 'anxious' were used to describe their early days in practice placements (Phillips et al 2000:71).

Many of the above studies also found that stress and anxiety were heightened when staff members were unfriendly, unsupportive and did not make the students feel welcomed. It is important to remember that during clinical placements students are usually removed from their peer support group. Phillips et al's (2000) study showed that the students' chief concern was being made to feel welcome and having time set aside to discuss their learning needs. Students in Jackson & Mannix's (2001) study found the single most helpful behaviour was being recognized as newcomers and shown understanding for their tentativeness and feelings of insecurity. Jackson &

Mannix (2001:274) also found students greatly appreciated any interest shown in them and their learning and liked to be given some degree of responsibility. They quoted one student:

> *I felt useful, because she loaded me with work that I was capable of doing, such as making beds, observations, assisting with hygiene and communicating with the patients. At the end of the day she would ask me questions about the things she had taught me. I found it very rewarding and helpful to my learning.*

It is generally accepted that a degree of anxiety is a healthy basis for growth and development (Lincoln et al 1997). Indeed, we should be perturbed if students had no concerns at all before beginning a placement or throughout a placement. However, there is a curvilinear relationship between anxiety and learning. Decreased learning occurs in the presence of high anxiety (Eysenck 1970, Spielberger 1966 in Kleehammer et al 1990). In the context of clinical learning, Nolan (1998:626) found that 'until students feel accepted learning cannot proceed, as fitting-in takes up most of their time and energy'. Work on humanistic approaches to facilitating learning tells us that adults learn best in an environment that is psychologically comfortable where there is mutual trust and respect for their own worth and that of others (Knowles 1990, Brookfield 1986, Rogers 1983). Powerful feelings such as anxiety, vulnerability, underconfidence, powerlessness, hope and dependence appeared not to interrupt students' learning if support, openness and encouragement were provided as these constructive measures allow mistakes in a trusting and safe learning environment (Lefevre 2005).

The following are some typical questions that students will ask prior to a clinical placement. These questions are based upon and extended from the work of Stengelhofen (1993) and Boud et al (1985).

- What will my role be?
- What will be expected of me?
- How much am I expected to know?
- How much am I expected to do?
- How much help and support will I get?
- What if I am asked to do something I cannot do?
- How will I know how I am doing?
- What are the demands of that setting?
- What will I learn?
- What will the people be like?
- Will they like me? Will I like them? Will I get on with my mentor?

The answers that students seek to these questions could form the basis for the support and supervision that will contribute to the clinical placement being an educational experience for students. You may wish to try Activity 8.6.

ACTIVITY 8.6

Ponder for a few minutes upon the questions above posed by students. What is the reputation of the learning ethos of your clinical area? How do you think a student new to your clinical area might feel?

Information pack Work that has been done into what helps students to learn during clinical placements tells us that making students feel welcome is a prerequisite to creating an atmosphere conducive to learning. Ideally, this 'welcome' should start prior to the commencement of the placement in the form of an information pack sent to the student. Stengelhofen (1993:73) makes an important point:

> *Providing students with a clear picture of the clinical setting and the cases within that setting, as well as identifying the learning outcomes for them, appropriate to the stage of the course, will be a way of reassuring them that they will not be required to do anything or take responsibility beyond what can legitimately be expected.*

An information pack could include, for example:

- a welcome letter; this letter can also contain information to encourage the student to visit the placement prior to starting to meet the practice educator and find out what learning opportunities are available
- maps of the locality and/or the hospital
- facilities such as catering, parking, social and sporting
- staff profile, including members of the multi-professional team
- the allocated practice educator with contact details
- clinical area profile, such as the philosophy, any nursing/midwifery model in use (for nursing and midwifery students), the types of patients/clients seen and treatments offered
- a list of learning opportunities
- a list of learning outcomes
- the roles and responsibilities of students in that clinical setting (this may need to be tailored to individual students depending on their prior experiences and stage of training)
- the shift hours
- guidelines on dress.

When pre-placement information packs are provided, important points can be assimilated by the student prior to commencement of the placement. This helps to reduce information overload during the early stages of the placement. Subsequently, the information is on record for reference. Box 8.1 is an example of a welcome letter extracted from Stengelhofen (1993:68). There are other examples in her text. It is suggested that you draft one to suit your own clinical setting.

Box 8.1 **Example of a welcome letter**

Dear

We hope that you enjoy your placement with us.

The attached information pack is designed to help you understand how our service works, what we have to offer you while you are with us and what we expect from your college. Please read it before your first day. We will go over any queries you may have when we see you, but if you have any urgent questions you can telephone on_____.

Please confirm that you are starting your placement with us on_____. We suggest that you arrive at_____. Before your arrival it would help us in planning your time if you could send us some information about yourself. We would like to know a little about your background, your academic interests, previous clinical experience and your objectives for this placement.

We look forward to meeting you. Involvement in study training is an enjoyable and stimulating, as well as a time-consuming, experience for us. We expect to learn from you as well as with you and we hope that you will be happy with us.

(From Stengelhofen 1993.)

Receiving the student Some hospitals have student support officers who make arrangements to meet all students on the first day of their placement. A programme of orientation for the day introduces the student to the hospital and its various departments, their key functions and personnel. Arrangements are made for the students to be 'collected' by their practice educators or a member of the ward team later in the day, and the students are subsequently orientated to their allocated placement (Hopkins 2000). Hopkins briefed the allocated practice educator who has a particular role in receiving the student and orientating the student to the work setting. When the placement is the first one for a student, practice educators are reminded to take particular care as the student may be highly anxious. There is no doubt that first impressions will influence the student's enjoyment of the placement (Stengelhofen 1993) and may even shape the student's views of the profession (McKenna et al 2010). It is important to make time for the crucial activity of orientation, which is seen to be the 'gateway to a successful placement' (Beskine 2009). This might help students feel that they belong as nursing students say that a sense of 'belongingness' is a prerequisite for clinical learning (Levett-Jones & Lathleen 2008). There should be a plan for the first day. This might include:

- Setting some time aside to welcome the student. It is sensible to start the student on a first shift at a later time than is the routine, preferably after the hustle and bustle of the shift has been dealt with.

- Orientation to health and safety matters (see Ch. 2).
- Orientation to the work place, such as the general layout of the clinical area, working patterns – shift hours, meal breaks.
- Introduction to team members.
- Showing where information sources are kept, such as placement philosophy and policy and procedure manuals.
- Showing communication systems, such as telephones and answering protocols, patient/client buzzer system and emergency call system.
- Spending time to discuss the student's learning needs and previous experiences. Find out at which stage of training the student is. Students' self-esteem is increased if they feel they can share any previously acquired learning with practitioners (Stengelhofen 1993). It should be made clear to students what their roles and responsibilities are and when they should or should not help or participate. Most beginning students breathe a big sigh of relief when they are told that they are not expected to start to give care immediately, and reassured that they will be asked to do only what they are capable of doing.
- Taking prior learning into account, identify learning opportunities available and experiences that are required to enable the achievement of learning outcomes. Jointly develop an action plan for the duration of the placement. It may be necessary to allow students to settle into a placement first and delay this activity.

Providing ongoing support and supervision The practice educator who exhibits the characteristics that students perceive as valuable and helpful (Darling 1984) will most certainly be providing the support and supervision desired by students to help them learn. Ongoing support and supervision should aim to facilitate learning. The development of competence is linked to the effectiveness of support (Lauder et al 2008). Stengelhofen (1993) and White & Ewan (1991) suggest the following activities for the facilitation of learning in the clinical setting:

1. Answer questions – make students feel free to ask questions and to seek help without loss of confidence or self-esteem.
2. Offer suggestions – be careful to foster students' self-confidence. Rogers (1983) suggested that when the student is moving from exploration into understanding, the facilitator responds directly to the content the student is struggling with (e.g. by giving direct answers). When the student starts to focus on actions to be taken during care, the facilitator moves into guiding further development of the student's skills and knowledge. Vygotsky's (1930, in Spouse 1998) theory of the 'zone of proximal development'

(ZPD) states that the potential of a learner to progress to the second stage of development could be capitalized upon by support and guidance from a more experienced other.

3. Allow students to make choices about care to be given – do not limit and constrain the student to your experience.

4. Facilitate development of desired behaviours – the practice educator is reminded that role modelling is one powerful tool for this purpose.

5. Encourage self-monitoring and evaluation – help students to identify where they have reached in their learning and help them to develop the ability to assess their performance accurately and subsequently set realistic learning goals.

6. Provide opportunities and guidelines for students to observe care activities (guidelines for observation are discussed in Chapter 9).

7. Learn from the students – listen to the students and facilitate two-way discussions. Rogers (1983) suggested that facilitators need to be able to respond to the feelings of students as learning experiences are explored together.

8. Give students time to reflect on what is happening and has happened – promote discussion about patient/client care.

9. Give students time to prepare – when assigning work to students, spend time briefing them and allocate time for them to prepare to give care. These points are developed in Chapter 9.

10. Allow students to make mistakes in the confines of patient safety – show confidence in students and give positive reinforcement; reinforce the expectation of success. Allow 'hands on' experience even when you think the task is complex. Manipulate the session to allow students to experience success.

11. Encourage students to think for themselves – structure and sequence questions so that students are led through their own paths of thinking to show how they came to a certain conclusion. Questions should therefore challenge students to trace their own thinking strategies and to explain how they drew inferences or came to certain conclusions.

The following questions may help you evaluate whether students are receiving adequate support and supervision:

1. How do I help students settle into the workplace?
2. What do I do to make their first days more enjoyable?
3. How do I make their placement an educational experience?
4. How do I help students feel confident about their role?
5. Do students in my area feel valued and respected?
6. When students are unhappy at work, do I know the contributory factors?

Continuing professional development (CPD)

When the clinical environment provides a culture where learning and professional development take place, it becomes a positive learning environment where the atmosphere becomes one where there is a commitment to lifelong learning and CPD activities. Staff members are more likely to develop the commitment to seek to learn for themselves and to share their learning with one another. There is encouragement to undertake CPD activities through further formal education through accredited courses and informal in-house training. This kind of environment will assist nurses and midwives who are mentors to pre-registration nursing and midwifery students to fulfil the requirement to develop their own knowledge, skills and competency beyond that of registration through CPD – either formal or experiential learning (NMC 2008a).

'Lifelong learning' is the term used to refer to the planned or unplanned learning that occurs throughout the life, usually the working life, of an individual (Hinchliff 1998). The undertaking of further education is indeed necessary as professionals of health care cannot hope to practise safely and effectively in a context of continuous change without undertaking updating activities. The importance of CPD was recognized by the UKCC and endorsed by the NMC (2008b) in *The Code: Standards of conduct, performance and ethics for nurses and midwives* and the HCPC in its *Standards of Continuing Professional Development* (HCPC 2012). In *The Scope of Professional Practice*, the UKCC (1992) stated:

> *Pre-registration education prepares nurses, midwives and health visitors for safe practice at the point of registration … [It] is therefore a foundation for professional practice … This foundation education alone, however, cannot effectively meet the changing and complex demands of the range of modern health care. Post-registration education equips practitioners with additional and more specialist skills necessary to meet the special needs of patients and clients.*

The statement above is applicable not only to nurses and midwives but to all professionals of health care. It is also as applicable today as it was in 1992.

An important question about mandatory professional development needs to be asked here: Does mandatory professional development serve to inculcate the sense of what Houle (1980:124) termed a 'zest for learning' possessed by an individual, which ultimately controls the amount and kind of education that is undertaken?

Pause to review how CPD can be encouraged in the clinical setting. Are there activities in your clinical area that you think would contribute to the CPD of staff? It is important to utilize learning opportunities in the workplace – not only is such learning directly relevant to practice, but also there can be many constraints on the availability and accessibility of formal courses in a resource-limited system. It is my belief that you and your colleagues, including members of the multi-professional team and unqualified staff members, are the most important teaching and learning resource in your work area. The following questions are intended to help you explore how the 'human resource' for learning can be used to contribute to your clinical setting as one that motivates staff to engage in CPD:

- How can you contribute? How much do you contribute? Remember that your contributions such as developing a teaching/learning pack can be used as evidence of CPD.
- How can your colleagues and members of the multi-professional team contribute? How much do they contribute? Do not forget unqualified staff members – someone may have a personal health experience which they can talk about.
- Are there planned teaching programmes? When this is an established routine, staff will be encouraged to contribute and attend.
- After staff members have been on study days and courses, is there a mechanism for the dissemination of information? This can serve several purposes – it helps the individual learn further through teaching or preparing a paper, and brings what is learned to the clinical area to improve professional practices.
- Are there staff support groups where staff members get together to debrief and reflect? Sharing ideas and experiences in a group is an effective way of developing practice wisdom – wisdom being the distillation of knowledge and experience (Hull 1998).
- Are there activities such as case discussions and conferences and seminars? If you have cared for the patient/client featured in the case you will be able to contribute to the discussion. Subsequently, if what you have learnt is written up, preferably with reference to literature as appropriate, it is again evidence of CPD.

Material resources

Having examined how the human resource can make direct contributions to the learning environment of the clinical setting, go on to consider those non-human resources that can contribute to the learning environment. You may wish to try Activity 8.7.

ACTIVITY 8.7

Have a good 'look' round your clinical setting. Taking a look in the form of walking around may prove to be revealing. What material resources are there to contribute to the learning environment?

The following questions may guide you in your 'walkabout':

- Do you have a resource room/area where text material such as books and journals are housed? If not, is it possible to make space for one? This resource area could also house contributions such as learning packages and posters developed by staff after they have been on study days, conferences and courses.
- If you have a resource room/area, is the area conducive to reading, browsing and study? For example, is text material shelved and filed in some kind of order; is it up to date; is the area generally tidy; is there some fairly comfortable seating; and so on?
- Is there someone who is designated to 'maintain' this area and keep resources up to date? Staff could take it in turns and be given time out to perform this function, such as going to the library to seek out relevant journal articles/ relevant professional material, and do the general 'housekeeping'.
- Is there a file that contains information specifically for students and new staff members? This file could have information about the learning opportunities in your setting, core experiences that students should participate in, names and designations of specialist members of the team and so on.
- Are there places such as notice boards where information, such as flyers about courses, teaching/ learning events and so on, can be displayed? If not, is it possible to find a suitable wall space for a notice/ pin board to be installed? These are generally not too costly.
- Are policy and procedure manuals up to date? Are they in an accessible location?
- Is there a philosophy of care for your area? If there is, where is it displayed? Are staff members aware of the intentions of this philosophy of care?
- Is there a collection of material such as health promotion leaflets and so on from both charitable and government organizations relevant to your clinical area? These are frequently free and provide useful information for both patients/clients and staff.
- If there are audiovisual aids such as DVDs, videos and CDs, are they still up to date? Is the equipment for using these aids in good working order?
- Are there other teaching/learning aids such as models and mannequins? Are they in good order?
- Are information technology facilities available to access electronic sources of information from the Internet, databases or CD-ROM teaching/ learning packages? If these are available, are staff members conversant with the usage of information technology?

QUALITY ASSURANCE

Quality assurance can be viewed simply as comprising all those activities in an organization that help to identify and promote good practice and prevent poor practice (ENB 1993). It is now widely accepted that quality can be achieved and maintained through the use of audit, which has become the most prominent and important mechanism for improving the quality of health and education sector services (Nicklin & Kenworthy 1995). In its publication on educational audit, the ENB (1993:12) went on to say that 'educational audit involves monitoring, measuring and evaluating educational provision'. Thus, the educational audit of clinical placement areas should be in terms of 'the standards of care and service provision and the learning environment, to facilitate their continuing suitability for students' practice experience' (ENB & Department of Health 2001:11). The ENB & Department of Health go on to say that the outcomes of audit and monitoring should lead to the dissemination of good practice and joint action planning between placement providers and higher education institutions to address any areas of concern or those needing enhancement. When attempts are made to judge the quality of the students' experiences, White & Ewan (1991:160) say that 'only the students are capable of judging the value of the experience since they are the ones having the experience'. The ENB & Department of Health (2001) and the NMC (2004) reinforce the importance of actively soliciting student feedback, which should contribute to the ongoing evaluation of the learning environment.

As can be seen from the exploration of the clinical setting as an environment for learning, there are many factors that influence and interact with each other to impact on this learning environment. These factors and the concomitant processes arising consequent to the interaction of these factors should not be left to chance – they need to be worked at to ensure that there are positive influences. Higher education institutions, in partnership with their service colleagues, need to work together to ensure that high-quality practice placements, in a supportive environment, help students achieve the learning outcomes of their educational programme and ensure that they are able to provide the care needed by patients and clients (ENB & Department of Health 2001). The ENB & Department of Health (2001:8) also pointed out that higher education institutions and service providers are 'responsible for the quality of learning opportunities provided for students'.

An essential element of the legislation establishing the NMC and the HCPC as health professions regulators is the role of the quality assurance of the education of aspiring professionals. As guardians of the professional registers and their duty to protect the public, it is essential that regulators are able to judge whether a health care student is fit to join the register once they have completed their pre-registration education and training. Within the wider context of quality assurance, the regulators' activities should be considered in conjunction with the other quality assurance exercises that education providers engage in. At institutional level in England, Wales and Northern Ireland, the Quality Assurance Agency (QAA) carry out 6-yearly institutional audits, focusing on the ability of the higher education institution to manage the quality of its educational provision. In Scotland the Council for Healthcare Regulatory Excellence (CHRE) has a similar function; its enhancement-led institutional reviews are carried out on a four-yearly cycle (CHRE 2009).

The four main areas of quality assurance activity of the NMC and HCPC are:

- new programme approval
- ongoing monitoring of approved programmes
- approving major changes to programmes
- programme re-approval.

Approval is the process of validation and accreditation that leads to decisions about whether a programme is approved so that it can be launched, or is re-approved/re-accredited so that it may continue. Through the systematic process of approval, decisions are made about the ability of the proposed programme to meet, over a period of time, the requirements of regulatory bodies, education providers, health and social care providers, service users and education commissioners.

Ongoing quality monitoring and enhancement is the process by which education providers and external stakeholders satisfy themselves that the quality of educational programmes is being maintained and improved upon. It includes all activity that occurs on an ongoing basis in both the academic and practice based settings – for example, practice placement audit and regular monitoring (normally annually or every 2 years) by the regulatory bodies. The quality assurance approach of the NMC focuses on risks to be controlled in the delivery of programmes (CHRE 2008). These risks are:

- inadequate resources
- inadequate safeguards for monitoring student conduct
- inadequate governance of practice learning
- failure to provide learning opportunities of a suitable quality
- unreliable conformation of achievement
- failure to incorporate essential skill clusters or address required learning outcomes
- failure of internal quality assurance systems to provides assurance against NMC standards.

The quality assurance agency

In the UK, the Quality Assurance Agency (QAA) has made it a requirement that assessment of the quality of practice placement experience is incorporated into every quality assurance process within the quality assurance framework that guides the educational practices of higher education institutions (QAA 2007).

The *Code of Practice* for work-based and placement learning (QAA 2007) outlines the precepts that programmes have to meet in order to provide quality placement experiences for students to meet programme learning outcomes. The following principles to support and monitor placement learning are specified in the code:

- Where work-based or placement learning is part of a programme of study, awarding institutions ensure that their intended learning outcomes are clearly identified, contribute to the overall and coherent aims of their programme and are assessed appropriately.
- Awarding institutions are responsible for the academic standards of their awards and the quality of provision leading to them, and have in place policies and procedures to ensure that their responsibilities, and those of their partners involved in work-based and placement learning, are clearly identified and met.
- Awarding institutions ensure that all partners providing work-based and placement learning opportunities are fully aware of their related and specific responsibilities, and that the learning opportunities provided by them are appropriate.
- Awarding institutions inform students of their specific responsibilities and entitlements relating to their work-based and placement learning.
- Awarding institutions provide students with appropriate and timely information, support and guidance prior to, throughout and following their work-based and placement learning.
- Awarding institutions ensure that work-based and placement learning partners are provided with appropriate and timely information prior to, throughout and following the students' work-based and placement learning.
- Awarding institutions ensure that: their staff involved in work-based and placement learning are appropriately qualified, resourced and competent to fulfil their role(s) where applicable, other educational providers, work-based and placement learning partners have effective measures in place to monitor and assure the proficiency of their staff involved in the support of the relevant work-based and placement learning.
- Awarding institutions have policies and procedures for securing, monitoring, administering and reviewing work-based and placements learning that are effective and reviewed regularly.

One of the emphases made by the QAA is on regular placement audit so that institutions can demonstrate that they can provide quality placement experiences for students. The precepts given by the QAA provide the framework for the educational audit of placements.

Criteria for educational audit

You may wish to try Activity 8.8.

ACTIVITY 8.8

Obtain a copy of the tool for the educational audit of your clinical area. What are the aspects of the clinical environment that are audited? How well do they reflect the clinical environment that is an educational environment?

In 1993 the ENB proposed the use of the following eight aspects, with their associated criteria, for auditing practice placements. Although published in 1993, these aspects are still relevant today as the guiding principles for the audit.

1. Ethos of the placement:
   - general climate
   - channels of communication
   - approachability of staff
   - relationships between the higher education institution and the placement
   - commitment to teaching and learning.
2. Organization of care:
   - philosophy and approach to care
   - the organization of workload so as to promote continuity, e.g. team nursing
   - involvement of students in multi-professional teamwork.
3. Supervision and assessment:
   - effectiveness of supervision and assessment activities by first-level practitioners
   - contribution by academic staff
   - fulfilment of clinical contact hours
   - compliance with regulations in supervision and assessment of students.
4. Teaching programme and assessment:
   - planned programmes
   - opportunities for students to achieve competencies through continuous assessment
   - learning outcomes set at appropriate academic and professional levels
   - patient/client groups support achievement of learning outcomes.
5. Research basis of care planning and delivery:
   - evidence of the application of research in teaching and implementation of care.
6. Academic and professional qualifications of staff.
7. Staff development programmes.
8. Physical environment.

The following three aspects should be added:
9. Teaching/learning resources and strategies:
   - a designated study area
   - a range of teaching/learning resources are provided
   - there is availability of information technology with access to electronic sources of information
   - teaching/learning strategies practised to help students relate theory to practice and reflect on care given.

10. Management of the learning environment. There is a designated learning environment manager who:
   - has overall responsibility for all teaching/learning activities and the learning environment
   - liaises with the clinical link lecturer
   - supports mentors and assessors.
11. The clinical link lecturer. There is a designated clinical link lecturer from the higher education institution who liaises with placement staff to ensure effective implementation of the curriculum by:
   - providing support and guidance for staff and students
   - acting as a resource for educational activities such as compiling a profile of learning opportunities.

In a later publication, the ENB & Department of Health (2001) provide what I see as a useful checklist containing key questions that address the planning, provision and evaluation of practice placement experiences. This checklist is reproduced in Appendix 5.

The process of educational audit

Generally, prior to a clinical area being used as a placement area for pre-registration students, an educational audit of that area is required to ensure that it is able to support student learning. Subsequently, the area is audited annually. Typically this is done by the learning environment manager and the clinical link lecturer. However, it should also be conducted whenever the circumstances of the clinical setting changes, such as a reduction of bed numbers and the type of patients/clients cared for. Nicklin & Kenworthy (1995) suggest that when a clinical area is consistently rated negatively by students, or if there is a high sickness or absence rate amongst students, an educational audit should be carried out for diagnostic purposes.

You may wish to try Activity 8.9.

One higher education institution, in collaboration

ACTIVITY 8.9

How do you, your colleagues and students contribute to the educational audit of your clinical area? How is your clinical link lecturer involved?

with its service colleagues, requires students to complete a questionnaire at the end of each placement. Staff members complete a questionnaire once a year. The responses of students are collated half-yearly, and yearly, with the responses from staff. Responses to questionnaire will contribute only in part to the educational audit. The overall educational audit requires the clinical environment to be monitored and assessed much more comprehensively.

CONCLUSION

What helps students learn and develop into the professionals we desire them to be? Clinical settings provide unique learning experiences and opportunities for students – these must be planned, structured, managed and coordinated (ENB & Department of Health 2001) so that students undergo professional socialization positively and develop the competencies for professional practice that cannot be readily acquired elsewhere. The clinical experience for students should be much more than just learning what to do and how to do it – it should be about the education of students who will one day be our professional peers, colleagues and co-learners. Clinical placements for students should contribute to their education so that they become self-directed learners who will also engage in lifelong learning.

Thoughtful and informed development of a clinical environment so that it is also an educational environment will enhance the learning of students and the professional development of staff. The challenge for practitioners is to create this type of environment. It is important to have a good understanding of the characteristics of an educational clinical environment and those factors that contribute to or detract from it. The educational audit of clinical placements helps to monitor and maintain the quality of placement areas. This mechanism may also be helpful in the acquisition of resources to support the continuing development of a learning environment.

Underpinning the success of any effort to develop a positive learning climate is a commitment by all staff to contribute not only to their own learning but also to that of others – the key to engendering this positive learning climate is the people who work in the setting. Students will tell us what does and what does not help them learn during clinical placements, and their feedback should be used to inform changes that are made.

I would like to end this chapter with a short excerpt from Helen Orton's book titled *Ward Learning Climate*. Although her book was published in 1981, I believe that what she wrote in this excerpt is equally true, if not more so, for today's health care climate (Orton 1981:67).

> ... *patient well-being and student well-being have been shown to be inextricably bound together. In terms of potential improvement for either group it is probably not important whether the motive for change stems from a desire to enrich ward experience for patients or for students. What is now certain is that the encouragement and development of 'good' learning climates would bring improvements for all those involved in ward life and that the benefits could be measured not only in economic terms but also by the increase in human happiness and well-being.*

KEY POINTS FOR REFLECTION

When considering the clinical environment as an educational environment, several groups of factors and the interaction between them need to be taken into account. These factors can be grouped as:

1. The people:

   The leader of the team: the creation of a democratic and non-hierarchical structure promotes teamwork and good communication, as facilitating learning cannot be divorced from competent management and humane leadership.

   The members of the team: each team member contributes to the creation of the learning environment. The clinical setting provides opportunities for students to learn and work as part of a multi-professional team so that each learns to function as an effective team member.

   The students: students bring their own personalities, dispositions, hopes and aspirations, past experiences and backgrounds, and also worries and anxieties to the clinical setting. They should be viewed as valuable student members of the team with specific clinical learning needs while being socialized into the profession.

   The practice educator: to facilitate learning effectively, the practice educator needs good teaching and interpersonal skills as well as being clinically competent and knowledgeable.

2. Learning opportunities and experiences 'provided by':

   Patient/client care: in any clinical setting, encounters with patients/clients should always form the basis of clinical learning.

   Other clinical activities: a list of activities and events with their potential for learning can be useful in directing and guiding students to sources of learning other than participating in direct patient/client care.

3. Staff commitment to teaching and learning:

   Support and supervision of learners: this starts with sending learners an information pack that includes a 'welcome' letter. Be ready to welcome and receive the learner on the first day. Subsequently, provide adequate ongoing support and supervision to enable students to maximize their learning. The following questions may be helpful in guiding the activities of the mentor:

   - How can work be planned so that having students is a help rather than a hindrance?
   - How can students be involved in care so that they are learning while contributing to the work of the team?
   - How can the work be turned into dynamic learning experiences?
   - How do I make their placement an educational experience?
   - How do I help students feel confident about their role?
   - Do students in my area feel valued and respected?

   Continuing professional development (CPD): in order to meet the changing and complex demands of the range of modern health care effectively, practitioners must develop their own knowledge, skills and competence beyond that of registration. CPD can be either formal or informal, e.g. through experiential learning.

4. Material resources: text information needs to be kept up to date and teaching aids need to be in good repair.

   Quality Assurance processes ensure that the quality of educational programmes is being maintained and improved. It includes all activity that occurs on an ongoing basis in both the academic and practice-based settings.

Generally, prior to a clinical area being used as a placement area for pre-registration students, an educational audit of that area is required to ensure that it is able to support student learning. Subsequently, the area is audited formally at least annually so that institutions can demonstrate that they can provide quality placement experiences for students.

REFERENCES

Andrews, M., Wallis, M., 1999. Mentorship in nursing: A literature review. J. Adv. Nurs. 29 (1), 201–207.

Beck, D.L., Srivastava, R., 1991. Perceived level and sources of stress in baccalaureate nursing students. J. Nurs. Educ. 30 (3), 127–133.

Beskine, D., 2009. Mentoring students: Establishing effective working relationships. Nurs. Stand. 23 (30), 35–40.

Birch, J., 1975. To Nurse or Not to Nurse. Royal College of Nursing, London.

Boud, D., Walker, D., 1990. Making the most of experience. Stud. Contin. Educ. 12 (2), 61–80.

Boud, D., Keogh, R., Walker, D., 1985. Promoting reflection in learning. In: Boud, D., Keogh, R., Walker, D. (Eds.), Reflection: Turning Experience into Learning. Kogan Page, London, pp. 18–40.

Bray, L., Nettleton, P., 2007. Assessor or mentor? Role confusion in professional education. Nurse Educ. Today 27, 848–855.

Brookfield, S., 1986. Understanding and Facilitating Adult Learning: A Comprehensive Analysis of Principles and Effective Practices. Open University Press, Milton Keynes.

Burnard, P., Chapman, C.M., 1990. Nurse Education: The Way Forward. Scutari Press, London.

Chamberlain, M., 1997. Challenges of clinical learning for student midwives. Midwifery 13, 85–91.

Charters, A., 2000. Encouraging student centred learning in a clinical environment. Emerg. Nurse 7 (10), 25–29.

Council for Healthcare Regulatory Excellence (CHRE), 2009 Quality Assurance of Undergraduate Education by the Healthcare Professional Regulators, Unique ID: 16/2008. Online. Available: <http://www.chre.org.uk/_img/pics/library/pdf_1286379841.pdf> (accessed March 2012).

Darling, L.A., 1984. What do nurses want in a mentor? J. Nurs. Adm. 14 (10), 42–44.

Deary, I.J., Watson, R., Hogston, R., 2003. A longitudinal cohort study of burnout and attrition in nursing students. J. Adv. Nurs. 43 (1), 71–81.

Dunn, S.V., Burnett, P., 1995. The development of a clinical learning environment scale. J. Adv. Nurs. 22, 1166–1173.

Dunn, S.V., Hansford, B., 1997. Undergraduate nursing students' perceptions of their clinical learning environment. J. Adv. Nurs. 25, 1299–1306.

ENB, 1993. Guidelines for Educational Audit. English National Board for Nursing, Midwifery and Health Visiting, London.

ENB, Department of Health, 2001. Placements in Focus. The English National Board for Nursing, Midwifery and Health Visiting and The Department of Health, London.

Eraut, M., Alderton, J., Boylan, A., et al., 1995. An Evaluation of the Contribution of the Biological and Social Sciences to Pre-registration Nursing and Midwifery Programmes. The English National Board for Nursing, Midwifery and Health Visiting and The Department of Health, London.

Eysenck, M.W., 1970. Anxiety, learning and memory: A reconceptualisation. J. Res. Pers. 13, 365–385.

Fraser, D., 1994. Evaluation of the Non-Midwifery Placements in a Pre-Registration Midwifery Education Programme. University of Nottingham, Nottingham.

Fraser, D., Murphy, R., Worth-Butler, M., 1997. An Outcome Evaluation of the Effectiveness of Pre-registration Midwifery Programmes of Education. The English National Board for Nursing, Midwifery and Health Visiting, London.

Fretwell, J.E., 1982. Ward Teaching and Learning: Sister and the Learning Environment. Royal College of Nursing, London. RCN Research Series.

Gerrish, K., 1990. Fumbling along. Nurs. Times 86, 35–37.

Gerrish, K., 2000. Still fumbling along? A comparative study of the newly qualified nurse's perception of the transition from student to qualified nurse. J. Adv. Nurs. 32 (2), 473–480.

Gilmore, A., 1999. Report of the Analysis of the Literature Evaluating Pre-registration Nursing and Midwifery Educators in the United Kingdom. United Kingdom Central Council for Nursing, Midwifery and Health Visiting, London.

Gray, M.A., Smith, L.N., 2000. The qualities of an effective mentor from the student nurse's perspective: Findings from a longitudinal qualitative study. J. Adv. Nurs. 32 (6), 1542–1549.

Health and Care Professions Council, 2012. Standards of Continuing Professional Development. HPC, London, Online. Available: <http://www.hpc-uk.org/aboutregistration/standards/cpd/index.asp> (accessed February 2012).

Henderson, V., 1966. The Nature of Nursing. Macmillan, New York.

Hinchliff, S., 1998. Lifelong learning in context. In: Quinn, F.M. (Ed.), Continuing Professional Development in Nursing. Stanley Thornes, Cheltenham, pp. 34–58.

Holland, K., 2002. Inter-professional education and practice: The role of the teacher/facilitator (editorial). Nurse. Educ. Pract. 2, 221–222.

Holloway, D., 1985. Accountability in further education: teachers' perceptions. J. Further High. Educ. 9 (2), 31–45.

Hopkins, S., 2000. Support for students. Nurs. Manag. 7 (7), 36–37.

Houle, C., 1980. Continuing Learning in the Professions. Jossey-Bass, San Francisco.

Hull, C., 1998. Open learning and professional development. In: Quinn, F.M. (Ed.), Continuing Professional Development in Nursing. Stanley Thornes, Cheltenham, pp. 182–204.

Jack, B., 1992. Ward changes and stress in student nurses. Nurs. Times 88 (10), 51.

Jacka, K., Lewin, D., 1987. The Clinical Learning of Student Nurses. Nursing Educational Research Unit, Kings College, University of London, London. NERU Report No. 6.

Jackson, D., Mannix, J., 2001. Clinical nurses as teachers: insights from students of nursing in their first semester of study. J. Clin. Nurs. 10, 270–277.

Jarvis, P., 1983. Adult and Continuing Education: Theory and Practice. Croom Helm, Beckenham.

Jimenez, C., Navia-Osorio, P.M., Diaz, C.V., 2009. Stress and health in novice and experienced nursing students. J. Adv. Nurs. 66 (2), 442–455.

Jokelainen, M., Turunen, H., Tossavainen, K., et al., 2011. A systematic review of mentoring nursing students in clinical placements. J. Clin. Nurs. 20, 2854–2867.

Jones, M.C., Johnston, D.W., 1997. Distress, stress and coping in first-year student nurses. J. Adv. Nurs. 28, 475–482.

Kadushin, A., 1992. Supervision in Social Work. Columbia University Press, New York.

Kleehammer, K., Hart, A.L., Keck, J.F., 1990. Nursing students' perceptions of anxiety producing situations in the clinical setting. J. Nurs. Educ. 29 (40), 183–187.

Knowles, M., 1990. The Adult Learner: A Neglected Species, fourth ed. Gulf Publishing, Houston.

Kotzabassaki, S., Panou, M., Dimou, F., et al., 1997. Nursing students' and faculty perceptions of the characteristics of 'best' and 'worst' clinical teachers: A replication study. J. Adv. Nurs. 26, 817–824.

Lait, J., Suter, E., Arthur, N., et al., 2011. Interprofessional mentoring: enhancing students' clinical learning. Nurse Educ. Prac. 11, 211–215.

Lauder, W., Watson, R., Topping, K., et al., 2008. An evaluation of fitness for practice curricula: self-efficacy, support and self-reported competence in preregistration student nurses and midwives. J. Clin. Nurs. 17, 1858–1867.

Lefevre, M., 2005. Facilitating practice learning and assessment: The influence of relationship. Soc. Work Educ. 24 (5), 565–583.

Levett-Jones, T., Lathleen, J., 2008. Belongingness: A prerequisite for nursing students' clinical learning. Nurse Educ. Prac. 8 (2), 103–111.

Lincoln, M., Carmody, D., Maloney, D., 1997. Professional development of students and clinical educators. In: McAllister, L., Lincoln, M., McLeod, S. (Eds.), Facilitating Learning in Clinical Settings. Stanley Thornes, Cheltenham, pp. 65–98.

Lindop, E., 1999. A comparative study of stress between pre- and post-Project 2000 students. J. Adv. Nurs. 29 (4), 967–973.

Mahar, G., 1998. Stress and coping: junior baccalaureate nursing students in clinical settings. Nurs. Forum 33 (1), 11–19.

McAllister, L., 1997. An adult learning framework for clinical education. In: McAllister, L., Lincoln, M., McLeod, S. (Eds.), Facilitating Learning in Clinical Settings. Stanley Thornes, Cheltenham, pp. 1–26.

McKenna, L., McCall, L., Wray, N., 2010. Clinical placements and nursing students' career planning: a qualitative exploration. Int. J. Nurs. Pract. 16, 176–182.

McLeod, S., Romanini, J., Cohn, E., et al., 1997. Models and roles in clinical education. In: McAllister, L., Lincoln, M., McLeod, S. (Eds.), Facilitating Learning in Clinical Settings. Stanley Thornes, Cheltenham, pp. 27–64.

Marton, F., Hounsell, D., Entwistle, N., 1984. The Experience of Learning. Scottish Academic Press, Edinburgh.

Melia, K., 1987. Working and Learning. Tavistock, London.

Morton-Cooper, A., Palmer, A., 2000. Mentoring, Preceptorship, Clinical Supervision: A Guide to Clinical Support and Supervision, second ed. Blackwell Science, Oxford.

Neary, M., 1997a. Defining the role of assessors, mentors and supervisors: part I. Nurs. Stand. 11 (42), 34–39.

Neary, M., 1997b. Defining the role of assessors, mentors and supervisors: part II. Nurs. Stand. 11 (43), 34–38.

Neary, M., 2000. Teaching, Assessing and Evaluation for Clinical Competence. Stanley Thornes, Cheltenham.

Nicklin, P.J., Kenworthy, N., 1995. Teaching and Assessing in Clinical Practice, second ed. Baillière Tindall, London.

Nolan, C., 1998. Clinical education: a system under pressure. Aust. Nurs. J. 3 (9), 20–24.

Nursing and Midwifery Council, 2004. Q.A. Fact Sheet C/2004UK. Nursing and Midwifery Council, London. Online. Available: <http://www.nmc-uk.org> (accessed February 2012).

Nursing and Midwifery Council, 2008a. Standards to Support Learning and Assessment in Practice, second ed. NMC, London, Online. Available: http://www.nmc-uk.org/Publications/Standards (accessed August 2011).

Nursing and Midwifery Council, 2008b. The Code: Standards of Conduct, Performance and Ethics for Nurses and Midwives. NMC, London, Online. Available: <http://www.nmc-uk.org/Publications/Standards/> (accessed February 2012).

Ogier, M., 1989. Working and Learning. Scutari Press, London.

Ogier, M.E., 1982. An Ideal Sister? A Study of the Leadership Style and Verbal Interactions of Ward Sister with Nurse Learners in General Hospitals. Royal College of Nursing, London. RCN Research Series.

Orton, H.D., 1981. Ward Learning Climate. Royal College of Nursing, London.

O'Shea, M., Kelly, B., 2007. The lived experiences of newly qualified nurses on clinical placement during the first six months following registration in the Republic of Ireland. J. Clin. Nurs. 16, 1534–1542.

Papp, I., Markkanen, M., von Bonsdorff, M., 2003. Clinical environment as a learning environment: Student nurses' perceptions concerning clinical learning experiences. Nurse Educ. Today 23, 262–268.

Parlett, M.R., Dearden, G.J., 1977. Experiences of teaching and learning. In: Parlett, M.R., Dearden, G.J. (Eds.), Introduction to Illuminative Evaluation: Studies in Higher Education. Pacific Soundings Press, Cardiff-by-the-Sea, California, pp. 143–146.

Parlett, M.R., Hamilton, D.F., 1977. Evaluation as illumination. In: Parlett, M.R., Dearden, G.J. (Eds.), Introduction to Illuminative Evaluation: Studies in Higher Education. Pacific Soundings Press, Cardiff-by-the-Sea, California, pp. 9–29.

Parkes, R., 1985. Stressful episodes reported by first year student nurses: a descriptive account. Soc. Sci. Med. 20 (9), 945–953.

Pembrey, S., 1980. The Ward Sister – Key to Nursing. A Study of the Organisation of Individualised Nursing. Royal College of Nursing, London. RCN Research Series.

Phillips, T., Schostak, J., Tyler, J., 2000. Practice and Assessment in Nursing and Midwifery: Doing it for Real. The English National Board for Nursing, Midwifery and Health Visiting, London.

Quality Assurance Agency, 2007. Code of Practice for the Assurance of Academic Quality and Standards in Higher Education: Work Based and Placement Learning, second ed. QAA, Gloucester, Online. Available: <http://www.qaa.ac.uk/Publications/InformationAndGuidance/Documents/COP9PlacementLearning.pdf> (accessed February 2012).

Rogers, C., 1983. Freedom to Learn for the 80's. Charles E. Merrill, Columbus, Ohio.

Saarikoski, M., Leino-Kilpi, H., 2002. The learning environment and supervision by staff nurses: Developing the instrument. Int. J. Nurs. Stud. 39, 259–267.

Seed, A., 1995. Crossing the boundary – experiences of neophyte nurses. J. Adv. Nurs. 21, 1136–1143.

Spielberger, C.D. (Ed.), 1966. Anxiety and Behaviour. Academic Press, New York.

Spouse, J., 1996. The effective mentor: A model for student-centred learning in clinical practice. Nurs. Times Res. 1 (2), 120–133.

Spouse, J., 1998. Scaffolding student learning in clinical practice. Nurse Educ. Today 18, 259–266.

Spouse, J., 2003. Professional Learning in Nursing. Blackwell Science, Oxford.

Stengelhofen, J., 1993. Teaching Students in Clinical Settings. Chapman & Hall, London.

Taylor, I., 1997. Developing Learning in Professional Education: Partnerships for Practice. The Society for Research into Higher Education and Open University Press, Buckingham.

Timmins, F., Kaliszer, M., 2002. Aspects of nurse education programmes that frequently cause stress in nursing students – fact-finding sample survey. Nurse Educ. Today 22, 203–211.

UKCC, 1986. Project 2000: A New Preparation for Practice. United Kingdom Central Council for Nursing, Midwifery and Health Visiting, London.

UKCC, 1992. The Scope of Professional Practice. United Kingdom Central Council for Nursing, Midwifery and Health Visiting, London.

White, E., Riley, E., Davies, S., Twinn, S., 1994. A Detailed Study of the Relationship between Teaching, Support, Supervision and Role Modelling in Clinical Areas within the Context of P2000 Courses. The English National Board for Nursing, Midwifery and Health Visiting, London.

White, R., Ewan, C., 1991. Clinical Teaching in Nursing. Chapman & Hall, London.

Williams, R.P., 1993. The concerns of beginning nursing students. Nurs. Health Care 14 (4), 178–184.

Chapter | 9 |

Learning through clinical practice: unearthing meaning from experience

INTRODUCTION

There are some who see the initial preparation of health care practitioners as providing would-be professionals with a set of prescribed theory, rules, routines and behaviours in a pre-packaged and pre-determined curriculum. The argument for preparing practitioners in this manner is that it reduces the risks of professionals failing to provide a reliable service. This so called 'technical–rational' view of professionalism has received much criticism from writers such as Schön (1987, 1983) who stated that such simple offerings do not prepare practitioners to meet the real situations of practice, as this model makes assumptions that practice is a relatively simple interaction in which the practitioner gives and patients and clients receive. Schön emphasized that practice is messy, unpredictable, unexpected and requires the ability to improvise – this ability is often diminished by training and routines.

One important 'hallmark' of the health care professional is generally acknowledged to be the need to be aware of, and to deal with, complex human issues as part of practice (Fish & Twinn 1997). These essential human interactions between professionals and patients/clients make the detailed knowledge and skills needed in each interaction unpredictable. Fish & Twinn (1997:38-39) take this point further:

> *Professional practice involves complex decision-making and elements of professional judgement and practical wisdom guided by moral principles but that these [cannot] be set down in absolute routines.*

A professional needs to be able to exercise professional judgement and select or even create knowledge necessary to the unique situation. Practitioners need to be prepared so that they are able to engage in these processes not only through their initial pre-registration preparation but also through continuing post-registration education. The technical–rational model of professional preparation, and its consequent influences on how the practitioner practises, does not equip the practitioner fully to deal with what Schön (1983:3) termed the 'swampy lowlands' of practice – those aspects of professional work that cause the greatest human concern and yet defy the use and application of rules and routines. Furthermore, professional knowledge and practices change constantly; this requires the practitioner to be motivated in order to refine and update knowledge and practices so that professional expertise and thus 'practice wisdom' (Hull 1998) is continually developing. What is therefore also needed is a model for preparing for professional practice that does not rely slavishly on the use and application of rules, schedules and prescriptions.

The model for learning from experience

This model should be holistic in nature. A holistic model for the initial preparation, and the continuing professional development of health care practitioners, should have clinical experiences as one of its key foci. A *model for learning from experience* is proposed and explored. This model is used as the framework to consider experience-based learning and how students can be assisted to interact with the clinical environment in order to learn through practice and unearth meaning from experiences. The model has four phases. Each phase of the model focuses on several factors and skills/strategies that influence how the learner engages with the experience. The phases, factors and skills/strategies are:

1. *The preparatory phase.* The preparatory phase focuses on:
   - the student as a learner
   - developing noticing skills
   - developing intervening skills.
2. *The experiencing phase.* During this phase the student 'reflects-in-action'. Several teaching/learning strategies will assist and influence how the learner engages with, and reflects during, the experience:
   - sharing, explaining and 'pointing out'
   - questioning and challenging
   - allowing to experiment
   - giving feedback on performance.
3. *The processing phase.* The experience is systematically reflected on during this phase. There are three key stages in reflecting on experience:
   - description of the experience
   - processing through critical analysis
   - synthesizing and evaluating.
4. Outcomes and action:
   - linking learning to action.

EXPERIENCE-BASED LEARNING

In 1926, Lindeman made the point that experience is the richest resource for adults' learning and put forward the case for the core methodology of adult education to be the analysis of experience. Despite Lindeman's counsel, the dismal picture was that more than half a century later student nurses were still learning clinical practice 'by doing' only (Alexander 1982a,b). A study by Phillips et al (2000) suggests that the 'analysis of experience' called for by Lindeman in 1926 is still predominantly absent in the learning of student nurses and student midwives during their clinical placements. Work on experience-based learning (Boud et al 1993, Boud & Walker 1990, Kolb 1984, Dewey 1938) tells us that learning from clinical experience is not the simple 'learning by doing' as has been accepted for too long. What students do, see, hear and smell during clinical placements can often remain

at a superficial level unless they are stimulated to analyse critically their observations and to question the meaning of their experiences and their implications for future learning. They also need to be stimulated to apply theory to practice. Thirty years ago, Alexander (1982a,b) made it clear that student nurses need help in learning how to learn from their everyday work with patients, to apply theory to practice and to use facts learned in the classroom in a variety of clinical experiences with individual patients. The implications of all this for the education of health care professionals is that students need to learn to relate theoretical material to a variety of clinical problems from the earliest days of training.

For students, learning during clinical practice is a complex activity. The student has to contend and learn to deal with the complex, unstable and uncertain worlds of practice (Schön 1987). At the same time, the student needs to be able to synthesize theoretical content from various fields, become familiar with the patients/clients and their needs and problems, learn to analyse those needs and problems and, during the course of needs analysis and problem solving, attempt to apply theories learnt and experiences gained previously. Subsequently, the student has to learn to evaluate the effectiveness of care given and make the appropriate changes that may be required. Learning through clinical experiences is far more diverse and pervasive than is conceived. Effective facilitation of learning in the clinical setting and the supervision and assessment of clinical practice are challenging. The most complex skills such as the ability to translate theory into practice are likely to take longest to develop (Moriaty et al 2010). If students are to learn to 'think', the thought patterns required by the practitioner need to be determined as successful clinical practice requires the highest level of intellectual functioning – namely that of application, synthesis and evaluation (Stengelhofen 1993).

Boud et al (1985:7) ask the following questions about experience-based learning:

- What is it that turns experience into learning?
- What specifically enables learners to gain the maximum benefit from the situations they find themselves in?
- How can they apply their experiences to new contexts?
- Why can some learners appear to benefit more than others?

In practice-based professions like nursing, midwifery and other health care professions, it is particularly pertinent that attempts are made to answer these questions so that students can be best assisted to extract maximum learning and achieve personal and professional development as a result of their experiences during clinical placements.

In order to explore the 'model for learning from experience' in detail, each phase is considered in turn, focusing on those issues that, in my view, are important in ensuring that the process of learning through experience is an effective one. First, I consider some of the characteristics of the nature of experience for learning.

The nature of experience for learning

It is perhaps appropriate to start by considering what the word 'experience' could mean in the context of learning and the role of experience in learning. In trying to describe the nature of experience for learning, I am mindful of the difficulty of the task. Within the clinical context, is it what a student has observed, encountered or undergone or is it what a student has done? Or is it all of these? Dewey (1925, in Boud et al 1993:6) considered that experience is not simply an event that happens, but rather than this event has meaning, pointing out that 'events are present and operative *anyway*; what concerns us is their meaning'.

Following on from Dewey's ideas of experience, Boud et al (1993:6-7) consider meaning to be an essential part of experience. They suggest that:

> *Experience is a meaningful encounter. It is not just an observation, a passive undergoing of something, but an active engagement with the environment…*

They go on to point out that experience is not singular or limited by time and place, as much experience is 'multifaceted, multi-layered and so inextricably connected with other experiences that it is impossible to locate temporally or spatially'. Indeed, in 1938, Dewey pointed out that educational experiences have continuity and integrate with one another so that 'every experience should do something to prepare a person for later experiences of a deeper and more expansive quality. That is the very meaning of growth, continuity, reconstruction of experience' (Dewey 1938:47). Work on the cognitive learning theory (see, for example, Ausubel 1968) also tells us that learning always relates in some way to what has gone on before. Boud & Walker (1990) refer to the 'personal foundation of experience' of a learner, which is the accumulation of previous experiences. Contributory sources to this personal foundation of experience may be the social and cultural environment of the learner, prior clinical placements and experiences. The social, cultural and professional norms and mores assimilated contribute to the formation of the perceptual lenses through which the learner views, and acts, in the world of work. The response of the learner to new experiences is determined significantly by these past experiences, as presuppositions and assumptions have been developed – the past creates expectations, which influence the present. The present context can serve to reinforce or counterbalance this.

What students bring to the clinical area – their expectations, knowledge, attitudes and emotions – will influence their construction and interpretation of what they experience. The way one learner reacts in a situation will not be the same as another. Boud et al (1993) believe that, in general, if an event is not related in some way to what the student brings to it, whether or not they are conscious of what this is, then it is not likely to be a productive opportunity. Even when starting a first clinical placement in a hospital, students will bring memories, feelings and knowledge of hospitals, whether or not they have been in one. It will be a rarity to have a clean slate on which to begin – unless new experience and ideas link to previous experience to form 'new wholes' (Ausubel 1968), they will exist as abstractions, isolated and without meaning (Boud et al 1993). Planning clinical experiences is therefore important: they should provide continuity rather than being separate and discrete. Furthermore, students should be assisted to make links and connections between experiences to provide new meanings and enable them to 'see' new whole pictures. This encourages a deep approach to learning (Marton & Säljö 1984) in which students seek an understanding of the meaning of what they are learning, relate it to previous material and interact actively with the material at hand.

Most people would agree with Boud et al (1985:7) when they state that 'experience alone is not the key to learning'. Dewey (1938:15) was critical of how experiences were offered to students. He asked this question:

> *How many acquired special skills by means of automatic drill so that their power of judgment and capacity to act intelligently in new situations was limited?*

Students were then rendered callous to ideas and lost the impetus to learn. Does this still happen in the education of health care professionals today? Boud et al (1993) believe that experience cannot be considered in isolation from learning – experience is the central consideration of all learning. Although experience is the foundation of, and the stimulus for, learning, it does not necessarily lead to learning unless there is active engagement with it. Aitchison & Graham (1989, in Critocos 1993:161) state that:

> *Experience has to be arrested, examined, analysed, considered and negated in order to shift it to knowledge.*

Working with experience in the manner suggested by Aitchison & Graham is the key to learning from experience. For learning to take place, the experience need not be recent. We may return to the same experience again and again and draw different meanings from each 'visit'. Boud et al (1993:9) believe that 'learning occurs over time and meaning may take years to become apparent … learning from it can grow, the meaning can be transformed, and

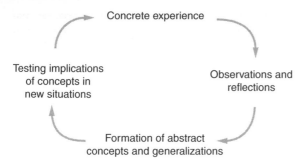

Figure 9.1 The Lewinian–Kolb experiential learning model. (From Kolb, DA. Experiential Learning: Experience as the Source of Learning and Development. ©1984. Adapted with permission of Pearson Education, Inc., Upper Saddle River, NJ.)

the effects of it can be altered'. The meaning of experience is not a given: it is subject to interpretation. Only the person who experiences can ultimately give meaning to the experience. It is the learner's interaction with the learning milieu that creates the particular learning experience (Boud & Walker 1990). No matter what external prompts there might be – mentors, interesting opportunities, resources – learning can occur only if the learner chooses to engage in, and with, the experience.

The emphasis in experiential learning is thus on the process of learning. It proceeds from the assumption that ideas are not fixed and immutable elements of thought, but rather are continuously derived from, and tested out, through experience (Kolb 1984). Kolb's well-known model of this learning process is termed an 'experiential learning model' to emphasize the important part that experience plays in the learning process. Learning is conceived of as a four-stage cycle, as shown in Figure 9.1. The here-and-now personal experience is real and concrete, and forms the focal point for learning 'giving life, texture and subjective personal meaning to abstract concepts' (Kolb 1984:21). The core of the model is the translation of experiences into concepts through reflective activities. These concepts are subsequently used to guide and inform new experiences.

THE 'MODEL FOR LEARNING FROM EXPERIENCE'

Each phase of the 'model for learning from experience' (Chapter 9) will now be considered in detail.

The preparatory phase

Advanced preparation helps address some of the challenges that students will encounter. The quality of the preparation before the experience also potentially determines the learning extracted during the experience and from later reflection and exploration. The preparatory phase at the start of a clinical placement would normally consist of a number of elements:

- An outline of the aims of the placement and a broad structure of what is to take place. These should be agreed jointly between the practice educator and the student after the first meeting/interview has taken place, as discussed in Chapter 6.
- An introduction to staff, resources and learning opportunities that are available to help the student during the placement. Suggestions on how these may be used to help the student learn are discussed in Chapter 8. Those resources and learning opportunities that are specifically required to enable students to achieve their learning intent should be identified.
- Students should have the opportunity to seek clarification.

Subsequent preparation for experience focuses on *the student as a learner* and on helping the student develop *noticing and intervening skills*, as these are two of the prerequisite skills required for learning through clinical experience.

Focusing on the student as a learner

As discussed in an earlier section, what the learner brings to the clinical setting has an important influence on what is experienced and how it is experienced: these factors, including the individuality of the student, should be taken into account during the preparatory phase. The other important element to consider is 'learning intent' (Boud & Walker 1990:64). Intent can be regarded as a personal determination – there is a clear reason for being there, which prompts learners to take steps to achieve their goals. The learning outcomes of a formal educational programme may influence the learning intent. Boud et al (1985) believe that intent to learn for a particular purpose can assist in overcoming many obstacles and inhibitions. Intent can be determined only by direct reference to the learner. For example, during a particular placement the student's intent may be to develop communication skills with very ill patients and their relatives. This intent will influence how the student is likely to experience these types of care situations – it acts to focus and intensify, or play down, perceptions in relationship to these experiences. 'The intent can act as a filter, or magnifier' (Boud & Walker 1990:64); these authors give the example of the photographer who, when using a zoom lens, will see certain things more clearly but in the process of doing so eliminates other things from the frame.

Students may arrive at a clinical placement with little conscious learning intent or even commitment to being there. Unless the mentor can assist the student to form an intent during the preparatory phase, opportunities for learning will not be well utilized owing to a lack of focus;

this is likely to result in superficial learning. Mentors can play an important role in helping students to clarify their intent and guide and direct students to the appropriate learning opportunities in the clinical setting. Mentors should be careful that they do not impose their own intents on the student. A discrepancy in intent between the mentor and student may lead to unproductive experiences and considerable frustration for both parties (Boud & Walker 1990).

Typically, during the preparatory phase there will be a high level of anxiety. Based on the well-documented evidence of student anxiety and stress in clinical settings (see Ch. 8), time should be spent in assisting students to identify and voice their concerns so that ways may be found to reduce their stress and anxiety and increase their confidence. Knowledge that they will not be alone and will not be expected to do more than they are able to will provide reassurance and make students feel less vulnerable. Boud et al (1993) believe that support, trust and confidence in students can help to overcome past negative influences and allow them to start to act and think differently. Similarly, conditions of threat or lack of confidence in the student are usually antithetical to any new motivation the student may have and serve to reinforce any negative images the student may already hold.

During the preparatory phase, when students start to focus on their learning intent they start to explore what is required of them, how they can contribute, what their role might be, what the demands of the setting are, what they can learn and how they can use their own resources such as knowledge, skills and what they have learnt from prior clinical experiences.

Focusing on noticing and intervening skills to help students learn through clinical experience

Asking the following questions may prompt both mentor and student to focus on how best to prepare for learning through particular experiences:

- Why has this particular experience – e.g. the care of a certain patient, a visit to another department – been arranged?
- What can be learnt through this experience?
- How can learning from previous experiences be linked to this experience?
- How can students be assisted to plan thoughtfully so that they '[act] deliberately, [observe] the consequences of actions systematically and [reflect] critically on the situational constraints and practical potential of the strategic action being considered' (Carr & Kemmis 1986:40)?
- How can students be assisted to engage in the clinical experience so that it means 'living through actual situations in such a way that it informs [them] of the perceptions and understandings of [other similar] subsequent situations' (Benner & Wrubel 1982:28)?

Answers to these questions are of course not straightforward, as each clinical situation is different. However, if 'coaching' (Schön 1987:20) of the students starts during the preparatory phase, they can be assisted to extract maximal learning through their experiences. Boud & Walker (1990) believe that there are two aspects of experience–based learning that are necessary to enhance the working of the processes for learning through experience. The first aspect is *noticing*, by which the student becomes aware of the event or particular things within it. The second aspect is *intervening*, in which the student takes an initiative and is active in the event. I see noticing and intervening as two prerequisite skills for learning through experience.

Developing noticing skills

Boud & Walker (1990:68) define noticing as 'an act of becoming aware of what is happening in and around oneself. It is active and seeking and involves a continuing effort to be aware of what is taking place in oneself and in the learning experience. As well as paying attention to the happenings around the care-giving situation – the experience – it is equally important that students pay attention to what is happening in themselves. They need to be aware in three areas:

- how they are acting
- what they are thinking
- how they are feeling.

Being aware of *how they are acting* and *what they are thinking* can alert students to what might be influencing them in the event. Being aware of *how they are feeling* will make students more aware of their emotional responses to the event in order for these to be attended to. Attending to feelings involves being sensitive to the situation: seeking to detect the nuances and the affective climate, as well as what is overt. Neglect of emotions can lead to a build-up of 'stress and a numbing of awareness which can inhibit the ability to act and distort learning' (Boud & Walker 1990:69). Stuart (2000) gave the example of midwives being in constant contact with women in pain during labour without acknowledging their own feelings and thoughts. This may eventually lead them to become less sensitive to the needs of women during this time.

Noticing provides students with the basis for becoming more fully involved in a care-giving situation and enables them to 'reflect-in-action' (Schön 1983) as they become more aware of the processes of how decisions are made to inform actions taken. It is essential to the initiation of the reflective processes during the third phase of the 'model of experience' so that sufficient information is retained for retrospective analysis and interpretation of practice after the event. Noticing seems to be a skill that has to be present to cause the experience to be the basis for learning (Stuart 2001). Stuart (2001) found that students in her study who did not know 'how' and 'what' to notice were unable to enter into experiences and subsequent reflective interactions with their experiences. As two frustrated student midwives said:

I think it is very routine … what they did, I learnt in the first week … It's just like in the morning she [the community midwife] goes round and does the visits, and in the afternoon she does the clinics, and the clinics are all the same, and then going to houses is pretty much the same … (p. 178).

I think on community all your days are very much the same … so, no, basically I have nothing to talk about … (p. 180).

As can be seen from the excerpt above, virtually every care event has the same meaning for these students. These students did not know how to notice. The starting point for the learning process in order to unearth meaning through experience is *noticing* – paying close systematic attention to detail, noticing exactly what occurred, including any thoughts, feelings, actions and reactions. Developing the skills of noticing will help students utilize their 'observer' status to benefit – how this status can be used for learning is poorly understood and has robbed students of valuable learning opportunities (May et al 1997). This has contributed to the unpopularity of the observer status (Neary

2000). Paying attention to those aspects suggested in Box 9.1 will assist in the development of noticing skills.

Learners can be directed to use these aspects in a general way, which will lead them to notice things that might have gone unnoticed otherwise. Alternatively, the mentor can indicate specific aspects to be noticed to help the learner achieve particular learning intents. For example, if a student wishes to learn how to assess the needs of clients at home following major orthopaedic surgery, the student could be directed to notice specific aspects about individual clients visited. The following example is based upon and extended from the work of Stengelhofen (1993).

The setting We are visiting Mrs Jones for the first time today since her discharge from the general hospital 3 days ago following internal fixation of her fractured neck of femur, which she sustained after a fall 6 weeks ago. She is 84 and lives on her own in a terraced house.

Aspects for noticing are:

1. Start observing when we reach the house:
    - How long does she take to answer the door?
    - Note the use of any walking aids – is she using them correctly?
2. During discussion with her:
    - How does she appear to be coping?
    - Is she anxious/confident/confused?

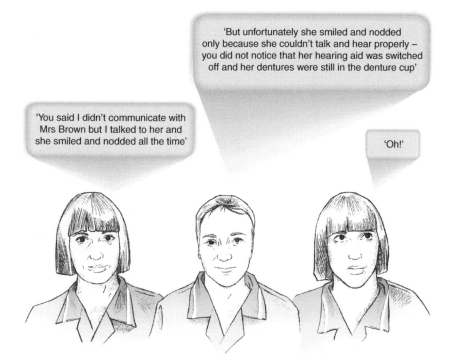

Figure 9.2 Students have to learn *how* and *what* to notice.

Box 9.1 **Aspects to be considered for the development of noticing skills**

NOTICING while engaging in an experience:

- The context of the episode, such as the history of the patient/client; time of day; location; and team members involved
- Other factors in the environment, such as sights, smells and sounds
- What were the patient/client's needs/problems?
- What care was given?
- How were the patient/client, family and significant others involved?
- Personal thoughts during, and after, the episode
- Personal feelings during, and after, the episode
- Personal concerns at the time
- What was noticed about yourself and others, such as the verbal and body language; what you said; what others said; how you behaved; how the patient/client behaved/said; how the practitioner(s) behaved; the approach used by the practitioner(s)?
- What was the immediate aftermath of the event?

3. What does she think are her major concerns/difficulties?
4. What do you think are her major concerns/difficulties? What do you think could be causing these concerns/difficulties?
5. Observe her functional activities. Can she manage important manoeuvres such as using the stairs, sit-to-stand and vice versa, independently?
6. How does she get her food supply? Can she manage activities of living such as washing, dressing, preparing a meal, cleaning the house, independently?
7. What are your thoughts and feelings about someone like Mrs Jones living on her own?

Students should be encouraged to keep written records of what they have noticed, as these serve as valuable 'memory joggers' for later critical reflection.

Developing intervening skills

Intervening is when the learner takes an initiative and is active in the event (Boud & Walker 1990). This can be any verbal or physical action taken by the learner within the learning situation. Learning through experience is an active process that involves the learner not only in noticing but also in taking initiatives to extend and test their knowledge. Looking on is no substitute for active involvement, as the learner who intervenes is adopting an active approach to the experience and is therefore likely to make more of the potential for learning from the event.

The learner's personal foundation of experience will influence interventions taken – it can either be limiting or act as a trigger for further actions. Boud & Walker (1990) believe that the greatest barriers to intervention are past failure and feelings of inadequacy or embarrassment, which inhibit clear thinking. These negative self-images can paralyse learners so that they are unable to perform or they act so maladroitly that learning opportunities are lost. On the other hand, past success and feelings of confidence and willingness to 'give it a go' can carry the learner through initial periods of discomfort. During the preparatory phase, the best way to help learners to intervene is to attend to those feelings that are blocking their ability to act (see, for example, Rogers 1996, for strategies for unblocking blocks to learning).

Learners need to learn the skills to be players. They need to know how and when to intervene and the nature and content of the interventions. Many clinical situations require the exercise of technical skills. Knowing how to perform these, such as doing a bed bath, changing an intravenous infusion, removing a urinary catheter, can act as great confidence boosters as the learner can intervene directly. Learning how and what and when to intervene is learning how to cope with the experience, as one major concern of students is knowing 'how to cope in clinical' (White & Ewan 1991:108). Typical care events could be analysed and suitable responses rehearsed. The use of role plays, case studies or audio or video recordings of typical events, followed by rehearsal of intervention strategies, will enable learners to practise appropriate intervention sequences. This will help them overcome anxieties and uncertainties and develop a degree of confidence before entering unknown situations. Prior to the experience (e.g. before going to the patient/client) it may be possible to predict what common chain of events may arise and a range of strategies can be developed and discussed with the learner. The learner could be asked searching questions such as 'Knowing what you know about Mr Johns, what problems do you foresee? … What care do you think he needs? … What actions would you take?'. The mentor may suggest particular interventions that the learner could implement or ways in which the learner's own ideas could be put into practice.

Because of the uncontrollable and unpredictable milieu surrounding clinical situations, not all the possibilities available in practice can be anticipated. Boud & Walker (1991) believe that it is neither possible nor desirable to cover every eventuality – part of learning from experience is dealing with the unexpected when it arises. There should, however, be sufficient preparation to ensure that learners can act effectively and that they are able to remain conscious of what they want to learn.

The experiencing phase

During the experiencing phase, the key role of the mentor is to facilitate reflection and interventions of the learner within the situation. The learner needs to be assisted to make judgements about when and where to take the initiative and what should be the nature and content of the intervention. Boud & Walker (1990) believe that the most significant influence on the actions of the learner during the situation is the reflective process that run through it as this active working with the data of the situation by the learner influences actions taken. Reflection within the situation can also lead to a recognition of the feelings and thoughts that accompany intervention, which can significantly influence the quantity and quality of learning extracted from experiences. This, in turn, will influence the learner's ability to transfer learning from this event to other events. As Dewey (1938:51) pointed out:

> We always live at the time we live and not at some other time, and only by extracting at each present time the full meaning of each present experience are we prepared for doing the same thing in the future [a]ll this means that attentive care must be devoted to the conditions which give each present experience a worthwhile meaning.

It appears that the 'taking on board of what is going on' while 'performing' needs to be accompanied by the 'thinking' and the 'feeling'. As discussed earlier in this chapter, work on experiential learning theory (Kolb 1984:34) suggests that 'learning involves transactions between the person and the environment'. In their 'model of experience', Boud & Walker (1990) also point out that learners' engagement with an experience, and their level of reflection during it are influenced by their personal foundations of experience, learning intent, noticing and intervening skills and the learning milieu. During the preparatory phase, the learner's personal foundation of experience and learning intent would have been explored so that the learner is as 'ready to learn' (Knowles et al 1998) as possible. Although the learner has been prepared to notice and intervene, these learning processes need to be actively facilitated. The mentor also needs to take into account the milieu in which the event is taking place at the time of the experience. The richness of the clinical environment is a facilitating factor for learning, but there are many demands that compete for the learner's attention, such as the patient/client condition and even distress, and their need for care and attention, and other disturbing events in the immediate vicinity. At the same time, the mentor may be expecting the learner to listen to an explanation or suggestion for intervention.

How can meaningful learning during the 'experiencing phase' be facilitated so that learners' 'power of judgement and capacity to act intelligently in new situations' (Dewey 1938:15) are developed further? The guiding principles of Schön's three models of coaching for learning may be helpful.

The guiding principles of Schön's three models of coaching for learning during the experiencing phase

Schön's three models of coaching have three distinct yet overlapping styles. The coaching role, which mentors might choose to adopt, may call on the use of the style of only one or all three models, depending on the level of experience of the student and the complexity of the event. These three models – *joint experimentation, follow me* and *hall of mirrors* – are now described.

Joint experimentation Joint experimentation can succeed only when learners already know what they want to do in order to intervene. The learner must be willing to step into the intervention and 'have a go' with the unfamiliar. The mentor's skill here lies in helping the learner formulate the interventions to be achieved and leading the learner to search for and decide on a suitable way of achieving the intervention. As different interventions are explored together, the mentor works at 'creating and sustaining a process of collaborative inquiry' (Schön 1987:296). The mentor must resist the temptation to tell the learner how to intervene or intervene on behalf of the learner, but may generate a variety of interventions and leave the learner free to choose and produce new possibilities for action. Joint experimentation is inappropriate when learners are unable to intervene or when the mentor wants them to grasp a new way of seeing and doing things.

Follow me When the mentor wants to offer a new way of seeing and doing things, the *follow me* approach is most useful. The mentor provides detailed descriptions of interventions while they are being performed, being careful to give rationales for the interventions. Schön emphatically stated that the 'relations between a whole performance and its parts, between the whole and *aspects* of the whole, are crucial' (Schön 1987:296) and should therefore be emphasized. During this 'analysis in action' the mentor draws on a repertoire of 'media, languages, and methods of description' (Schön 1987:297), as the ultimate aim is to present images that will 'click' with the learner. While observing the mentor, the learner will be attempting to remember the actions and explanations, and subsequently trying to derive meaningful learning through personal interventions. As the learner attempts to imitate the mentor, there is great potential for ambiguity and confusion. Guidance and feedback from the mentor are important, as the learner will be 'testing by further words and actions how the meanings she (sic) has constructed are like or unlike his (sic) [mentor]' (Schön 1987:297).

Hall of mirrors In this model of coaching, there is willing cooperation between the mentor and learner as they try to grasp their own and each other's understandings of the clinical situation. As learners seek to exemplify their proposed interventions in practice, they are assisted to see their interventions from several perspectives. To achieve this, the mentor and learner continually shift perspective – this may be carrying out the intervention proposed by the learner or having a dialogue about it or mutually redesigning the intervention. The mentor's skill lies in having the courage to allow the student to experiment and take 'risks'. Schön believed that 'to the extent that he (sic) can do so authentically, he models for his student a new way of seeing error and "failure" as opportunities for learning' (Schön 1987:297).

Using Schön's (1987) three models of coaching to provide the underlying principles for learning during the experiencing phase, several strategies are suggested for use during this phase. These are shown in the framework in Figure 9.3. The strategies in the framework may be seen as 'coaching strategies'. As indicated in Figure 9.3, the central activity, which underpins these coaching strategies, is 'talk during practice'. This is an essential activity between mentor and learner for meaningful learning to take place during the 'experiencing phase'. Each of the coaching strategies will now be discussed.

Sharing, explaining and pointing out

When mentors work alongside learners, opportunities are provided to engage learners in 'situated negotiation of their practice' (Phillips et al 2000:111). Informal on-the-job conversations take place that allow the sharing of ideas and understanding about care, which are then put into practice. These mutual exchanges not only value each other's ideas and understandings but also enable the learner's understandings of practice to be clarified. Phillips et al (2000:111) give the example of a mentor and her student working together as they made a heavily sedated terminally ill patient as comfortable as possible. As they work, the mentor and student discuss how best to

position the patient. The student could see areas of tissue damage which the mentor could not from her position. The position that was planned to be used was modified using the information from the student's evaluation. The mentor in this instance shared how she solved the problem and made the decision by 'thinking aloud' thus:

> *Oh well, if you can see that and that's actually happening now, we really can't put her over on her side – well, not completely. If I take her through a bit more this way – I'll not come round to see. It means disturbing her more. So what if we just gently lift her through to me? What if I work your side next time we move her? That way I can get a look at it myself without disturbing her too much.*

It can be seen in the above event how the opinion of the student is valued, which can only increase her confidence. As the mentor talked through the rationale for the choice of new better position for the patient, she was also sharing and pointing out other aspects of care that this patient required, such as not being unduly disturbed and the necessity to be gentle. For this student the event would probably have meant much more than merely changing the position of the patient. Through this experience the student may have learnt to 'read' some of the needs that such patients require, thus deriving meaningful learning from what may appear to be the routine task of repositioning a patient.

Most students, even senior ones, need to be alerted to 'signals' from patients and clients. They need to develop skills in interpreting the presenting signs and symptoms of patients and clients so that the physical condition and illness stages can be noted. They also need to become skilled in noting the emotional responses such as fear, distress, withdrawal and other overt indications. White & Ewan (1991) point out that inexperienced practitioners

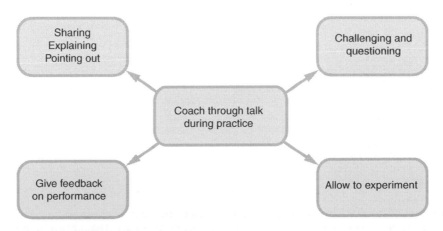

Figure 9.3 The coaching strategies during the experiencing phase.

such as students are concerned that their performance should be accurate. They focus on following guidelines and rules. Consequently, they have difficulty in managing the competing demands of the situation. The more subtle cues of response and reactions within a clinical event are often missed. Opportunities for learning through these experiences are thus lost to them. As mentors work alongside students, opportunities are provided for pointing out the messages and signals that patients and clients are overtly or covertly giving – teaching them how to handle the 'sensitive moments [which] can be the most difficult aspects of practice to handle' (Open University 2001:55). Based on such information, explanations can then be given on how care is tailored to meet the needs of the patient/client at the time. Learning through a clinical event is incomplete if a student focuses only on the 'content' of the particular activity – to unearth the real meaning of the experience the student also needs to be aware of its 'extension into the framework of the patient's situation and surroundings' (White & Ewan 1991:132) so that there is awareness of the context of the whole situation for the patient and the carer.

Sharing, explaining and pointing out can be in the form of overt physical guidance of actions such as placing your hand on the student's at times to transfer the amount of pressure to be used in massage, or placing your hand on the student's to transfer the movements and manoeuvres which need to be made to deliver a baby, or listening with the 'student' to body sounds through monitors, or seeing with the 'student' fine discriminations of change in the patient's colour, or smelling with the 'student' to note the odour characteristic of some body fluid or discharges. White & Ewan describe these ways as 'giving away skills – your skills' and guidance is provided by leading 'behind' the student (White & Ewan 1991:135).

Drawing from the work by Vykotsky (1930, in Spouse 1998) on the zone of proximal development (see also pp. 106, 114, 158), Spouse explored how students' learning during clinical practice can be improved. One of the conclusions she came to was that students who are cognitively ready to move to the next stage could be assisted to reach this potential through support and guidance from a more experienced other. Development is best facilitated if the mentor's speech guides the student to a level beyond that currently in use or practised. Having an accurate assessment of a learner's level of capability is crucial in assisting a learner to develop a higher level of competence.

Questioning and 'challenging'

The mentor is advised not to give all the answers, which deprives the student of the opportunity of carrying out some of the problem-solving and decision-making activities (Stengelhofen 1993). These cognitive processes foster deep learning, and thus help the student extract more meaningful learning through experiences

(McAllister 1997). White & Ewan (1991) state that asking students stimulating and challenging questions helps them to uncover the hidden meaning of their clinical experiences and points them to the 'hidden curriculum' of clinical learning, which may be missed by some students altogether as they are primarily concerned with the task to be completed. Students say they need the mentor to think of things that might never occur to them (Windsor 1987). Skilful questioning and the challenging of thinking help 'awaken' students to the otherwise unrecognized insights and discoveries. Also, we 'need to be challenged so that we do not fool ourselves with our own distorted assumptions or fail to consider new information which is outside our present range of experience' (Boud et al 1993:15).

Some suggestions on how to use questioning and 'challenging' are made below. These are based upon and extended from the work of Tilley et al (2007), Stengelhofen (1993) and White & Ewan (1991):

- Ask the student to explain and justify why a certain course of action has been chosen.
- Ask the student why you are proceeding in a certain way – for example, 'Why do you think I am doing this?'
- Ask the student what actions should be taken in certain situations – for example, 'What assessment should you be thinking of making?', 'What actions do you need to take and why?', 'How would you make Mr Johns more comfortable?', 'What do you intend to do about Mr Johns' request to see his daughter?'
- Place the student in your shoes – for example, 'I have to make a decision as to whether to treat now or leave. What are some of the considerations that might be going through my head?' (Stengelhofen 1993:97).
- Invite the student to come forward with a diagnosis of what the problem may be and how that problem is best managed – for example, 'Have a look at Mr Johns then tell me what you think the major problem is and what we can do about it, then you can tell me how we can fix it' (White & Ewan 1991:141).
- Invite the student's opinions about a situation – for example, 'I would like you to take a look at the patient you looked after yesterday. I think there are some changes … see what you think' (White & Ewan 1991:141), or 'What are the real issues here?', or 'Do you think Mr Johns' request is reasonable? … Why do you say it is unreasonable?'
- The following questions will help the student synthesize data and identify a problem – for example, 'What is the problem?', 'What complications could occur?', 'What clinical data would lead you to believe that this complication will occur?', 'What clinical data would indicate that the patient needs immediate intervention and why?', 'What data are we going to give the doctor or social worker or [another professional in the multi-professional team]?'

Questioning and challenging can be threatening for some students – any threat felt needs to be responded to. Mentors have to be careful not to undermine students' self-confidence. This may be avoided by manipulating situations and questions to allow students to experience success. Be generous with positive reinforcement.

As the student's learning is actively facilitated by questioning and challenging, the mentor needs to be able to facilitate further learning according to the responses of the student as he/she explores a learning experience (White & Ewan 1991). As the student moves from tentative exploration into understanding, the mentor should respond to the content the student is struggling with. When the student's focus is on action, the mentor moves into guiding further development of the student's knowledge and actions.

Allow to experiment

According to Townsend (1990:67) the mentor as facilitator will:

> ... *provide a secure environment in which everyone can experiment, take risks, increase their acceptance for uncertainty and develop mutual trust and commitment. Facilitators are creative, flexible, motivated and involved in mutual goal setting and achievement.*

When being allowed to experiment, the student assumes control of clinical care. As in the joint experimentation coaching strategy put forward by Schön (1987), the mentor supports by helping the student formulate the care to be given by prompting the student in searching for, and deciding upon, the most suitable option of care – the final decision rests with the student.

There is prior agreement that the mentor will intervene only if necessary (e.g. when the situation becomes too complex or there could be detrimental consequences for the patient). There is also agreement for the form of support to be given during care delivery; support may be in the form of verbal affirmation of correct performance or non-verbal by the use of body language or just being the 'silent supporting presence' – 'just standing by' – offering neither approval nor disapproval (White & Ewan 1991). Boud et al (1993:15) made the point that, as learners, we need 'appropriate support, trust and challenge from others. This can enable us to continue our tasks when they seem too much for us or when we get blocked ... '.

If the mentor is present during care giving, the temptation to take over and assume control must be resisted. Mutual trust must exist, with both the mentor and student accepting any uncertainties. Trust in the student's ability is necessary to enable the student to progress and develop clinical competence. Boud et al (1993:15) found that some of the most powerful factors influencing learning from experience are those relating to confidence and self-esteem, saying that 'unless learners believe themselves capable, they will be continually handicapped in what they do'. Many students have said that it is a 'nice feeling' to know that they are trusted. The mentor has to **'let go'** so that the student can have opportunities to experiment and assume control with confidence. This level of responsibility requires the student to be able to make clinical decisions with the guidance of the mentor. When thus engaged in the thinking and the decision-making processes associated with clinical practice, termed 'clinical reasoning' (Higgs 1997), the student must necessarily use knowledge and higher order cognitive skills to make clinical decisions. Skilful facilitation of clinical reasoning will help students 'see and read' the depth and breadth of clinical events so that much more meaning can be derived through clinical experiences. The reader is referred to the work of Higgs for a discussion of strategies available to facilitate clinical reasoning.

Being allowed to experiment should also include being entrusted with responsibility (e.g. responsibility for planning and managing care for a single or a group of patients/clients). The delegation of responsibility for this aspect of care is necessary to assist senior students to develop the skills of prioritizing, decision-making and time management (Gerrish 2000, Fraser et al 1997). In their study of the effectiveness of pre-registration midwifery programmes, Fraser et al found that many of the new midwives experienced a fall in confidence at registration. They concluded that this could perhaps have been reduced if more had been expected of them prior to registration.

Give feedback on performance

Giving feedback to students during the performance of clinical activities presents invaluable opportunities to enhance learning and meaning derived from care activities. Whereas it is important to time feedback so that errors of care delivery are avoided, it is also important to allow the student enough scope to use individual skill and flair during performance. This requires the mentor to have a degree of trust in the student while being a sensitive observer.

Giving immediate feedback on particularly commendable performances or pointing to where desired improvement could occur will help students extract more learning from clinical events. Remarking on the appropriateness of specific initiatives, or praising a demonstration of exceptional caring, or indicating to the student a grasp of principles underlying an action or a behaviour, not only reinforces the student's experience of success (White & Ewan 1991) but may also motivate the student to reflect on the actions taken and care given. As the student thinks through these, awareness of the feelings and thoughts associated with a particular action may develop – further learning and meaning may be extracted from the experiences if the student works on these feelings and thoughts to enhance future actions.

If the judgement of the client or patient is also solicited, this source of feedback may act as a direct indicator as to whether care given was appropriate and performed to enhance comfort – this additional information further helps the student to evaluate care skills and rethink clinical decisions and actions if necessary. Some more learning may take place, which can only allow the student to derive more meaning from a particular clinical experience.

The processing phase

Looking back at the preparatory and experiencing phases, it can be seen that learners have to cope with a considerable amount of new information. Situations force them into active involvement whether they like it or not. They face, and have to deal with, many personal demands. Reflection before and during the experience helps the learner deal with the vast array of inputs and feelings and thoughts generated. Boud et al (1985:26) point out that if 'we are exposed to one new event after another without a break we are unlikely to be able to make the most of any of the events separately'. In the *Four Quartets*, T. S. Eliot spoke of those who 'had the experience but missed the meaning'. Following the experience, it is equally vital, if not more so, to process the experience further through reflection, as reflecting after the event is 'one of the most helpful means of drawing learning from experience' (Boud & Walker 1990:72). What is also significant is that reflection is not an end in itself – the outcome is that knowledge is created through the transformation of experience (Kolb 1984) so that we are 'ready for new experience' (Boud et al 1985:34).

The processing phase is a complex one in which both feelings and cognition are closely interrelated and interactive (Boud et al 1985). Learning is influenced by the socio-emotional context in which it occurs. The role of others in the present, such as support, trust and confidence in the learner, can help overcome negative feelings and allow the learner to act and think differently from the past (Stuart 2001, Boud et al 1993). The climate of the processing phase can act to reinforce or counterbalance both negative and positive experiences – it therefore needs to be planned and managed so that learners may be assisted to extract some more meaning and learning from their experiences. Students are likely to raise many questions and problems that have arisen from their experiences. Generally, it is not possible to 'process' every experience. It may be possible to identify a focus for reflection that addresses several clinical events (e.g. the care of patients who required pressure area care, or discussing the cessation of smoking with clients). An alternative is to select discrete experiences identified by the student as significant clinical experiences.

When conducting the session, it is important to remember that this is not another typical group discussion or individual encounter, nor is it a simple reporting back of clinical events, nor an invitation to students to 'rehash' what they did and to receive comment on how well or badly they performed and what to do about it. Particular care has to be taken to prevent a session from turning into a 'moan session' where no learning takes place and feelings of frustration are heightened (Stuart 2001). Students' presentations of their observations, actions and behaviours, feelings and thoughts in their own words need to be acknowledged and actively worked through with the mentor as facilitator. An interactive non-threatening style of questioning and facilitation will assist the student in drawing out the meaning of what has been experienced. As both mentor and student pose questions and attempt to solve problems that have arisen directly from the experience, previously unchallenged assumptions about theory and practice are likely to be explored (Bedford et al 1993, White & Ewan 1991). Learning through reflection needs to be actively facilitated for many learners (Stuart 2001). The reason may be that certain cognitive skills, which are developed to different stages in different people, are required in order to engage in reflection to learn through this process. Atkins & Murphy (1993) identified these skills as having the abilities to describe, critically analyse, synthesize and evaluate:

- *Description* involves the ability to recollect and replay the experience in its totality. A close attention to detail, noticing exactly what occurred and one's reactions, without making judgements, is required (Boud et al 1985). These authors suggest that this description should be written or verbalized to others.
- *Critical analysis* involves examining the components of a situation, identifying existing knowledge, challenging assumptions and imagining and exploring alternatives (Brookfield 1987, Bloom et al 1956).
- *Synthesis* is the integration of new knowledge with previous knowledge, to form a 'new whole' (Bloom et al 1956). The new knowledge can then be used in creative ways to solve problems and to predict likely consequences of actions.
- *Evaluation*, according to Bloom et al, is the making of judgements about the value of something, for a given purpose. It involves the use of criteria. Mezirow (1981) argues that both synthesis and evaluation are crucial to the development of a new perspective.

These four cognitive skills will now be related to learning through the reflective process during the processing phase. The use of three stages incorporating these cognitive skills is proposed here:

- description of the experience
- processing through critical analysis
- synthesizing and evaluating.

Reflection on experience is treated in this format to aid exposition. It is not intended to imply that the stages must take place consecutively. Each stage may be visited and revisited. Reflective exercises within activity boxes are suggested to help the student extract more learning from care giving experiences – these are offered as a guide and not meant to be a prescription.

Description of the experience

Boud et al (1985) believe that one of the most useful activities for initiating reflection is to recollect what has taken place in as much detail as possible by:

- replaying and describing the event as it happened chronologically; this replay of the event in the mind's eye may be done verbally or committed to paper
- paying close attention to the details of the event
- noticing exactly what occurred
- noticing one's reactions to it in all its elements; of particular importance is an observation of the feelings evoked during the experience.

As far as possible, the description should be clear of any judgements, as these tend to cloud our recollections and may blind us to some of the features that may need reassessing. As we 'witness' the event again, it becomes available for us to reconsider and examine afresh; we may begin to realize how we were feeling and how these feelings may have prompted our responses, which in turn influenced our actions.

Those aspects to be considered for the development of noticing skills outlined in Box 9.1 could be used here to assist with the recall of the details of the event. In recalling past events the nature of memory poses problems, as we inevitably forget. To capture the details and nuances of the event, recall should be done as soon as possible.

As students recall and describe their 'lived experiences', it is important for mentors to listen attentively and respond appropriately, without offering any interpretation or analyses of their own. Mentors need to be highly aware of the ways in which language is used by the students to describe or interpret their experience. As the event is replayed and recalled, students will become aware of the feelings that were present during the experience. These feelings need to be acknowledged, as emotions and feelings can either be a significant source of learning or they can become barriers at times. An examination of feelings may reveal that emotional reactions had overridden rationality to such an extent that there was an unawareness of how behaviours and perceptions were blurred. For example, during an emergency situation, feelings of panic may have overtaken rational thoughts and actions so that the chain of events that ensued compromised the well-being of the patient. On occasions, resultant negative feelings become barriers and may inhibit the student from entering into further similar experiences. These negative feelings act as learning blocks and, unless they are recognized and addressed, further learning will not proceed. For example, if a student is overcome with

anxiety and fear after encountering an aggressive client or a dying patient, this student is likely to shy away from these situations. There are also occasions when students are hurt and distressed after difficult and painful experiences. Phenix (1964:197) urged educators to take responsibility for 'improving the quality of human meaning at the deepest personal level'. As one student in Stuart's (2001:180) study painfully recounted during the processing phase:

> *She's got it [terminal cancer] and she's going to die soon. She's only 44. I think because I'd never come into a situation like this before it hit me hard. I don't know … I think the imagination goes.*
>
> *I just feel guilty myself … just felt like I should not have been there, just don't know what to do. I don't want to go into a situation like that again.*
>
> *I went with [the community nurse] for three days and each time she had her on the list, I just dreaded going. It was just so horrible.*

It is clear that such feelings must be acknowledged, explored and attended to so that undesirable, and even debilitating, influences are removed or the student may remain disabled. Boud et al (1993:15) emphasize that emotions and feelings strongly influence learning, saying that 'denial of feelings is denial of learning'. An increased awareness of emotions will help students to develop the sensitivity required to detect the nuances and the affective tone of the situation so that they can respond sensitively to the needs of the patient/client. In so doing, students will learn to give care as well as *caring* for the patient/client for '… care without caring is empty and meaningless …' (Nordman et al 1998:161). Further, the point when students acquire this form of professional artistry is the point when they have begun to unearth meaning from clinical experiences. Positive feelings should be retained and enhanced so that confidence and self-worth are fostered – these can provide the impetus for students to pursue, or persist with, experiences they may previously have thought to be too difficult or even insurmountable. Unless we believe in ourselves and our capabilities, we can constrain ourselves to such an extent that we ultimately deny ourselves the learning opportunities for further learning and development.

Processing through critical analysis

During this stage, the experience is thought about and mulled over further to examine and seek relationships among the components of the situation and subsequently to see it as a whole picture within the wider context of the care setting and health care. New knowledge and ideas are identified and related to that which is already known, with the aim of integrating the two sources of knowledge to form a 'new whole'. This 'new whole knowledge' can then be used in creative ways to solve problems and predict likely consequences of future actions. Aspects to be considered to assist processing through critical analysis are suggested in Box 9.2. It is necessary to refer to the information provided from the description of the experience.

As students respond to the issues raised by asking the questions in Box 9.2, their responses and explanations could be prompted at times with further questions to probe more deeply and to expand on 'glib' responses. In addition, they could be asked to reconsider the validity and reliability of their knowledge base and clinical data they have used as the basis for the decisions they have made and the care given. It is important to connect the ideas and feelings that arose during the experience and those that arise during the processing phase with existing knowledge and attitudes. Cognitive theorists such as Ausubel (1968) regard this linking of new information with those relevant elements in our existing cognitive structure as one of the central features of the learning process.

This cognitive process has to be facilitated if we want to encourage learners to develop a deep approach to learning (Marton & Säljö 1984), an approach characterized by active interaction with the material at hand as the student searches for further meaning from the experience. This results in an integration of formal learning with personal experience and making links between components of knowledge. For example, the student referred to above in Stuart's study (2001) may be assisted to explore her knowledge about the care

and support of young clients with terminal cancer and the support services available. The student may then evaluate how such care can influence the quality of life of these clients and start to realize that, although it is indeed sad that young people do die of cancer, a quality of life can still be achieved. She has to make connections between the needs of the client, the services available to support the client and her role in meeting the needs of this client and family. This student realized that the client had not had time to come to terms with her illness (Stuart 2001:182):

These defence mechanisms [referring to the stages of the grieving process] we have – she found out at Christmas that she had cancer and she was given a month to live and it's just come so quickly that I don't think she'd been able to go through these defence mechanisms; she hadn't been able to know that she's got it; she hadn't been able to come to terms that she got it. I think all her feelings are muddled up.

Knowledge and understanding of the stages of the grieving process will assist the student in helping the client work through the grief of having terminal cancer. The student needs to make connections between the formal theory of the grieving process and how this client may be best assisted. The student also needs to make links between what her needs are to enable her to carry out the care required and how she can meet those needs. For example, she may have to learn to come to terms with feelings of guilt and pity for these clients, which are present in her existing cognitive and affective structures. The student may realize that she can be a more effective carer if she has an attitude of empathy rather than pity.

The student's feelings of guilt and pity may be a reflection of her assumption that clients with terminal cancer cannot have a quality of life – if this is the case that assumption can be challenged. This challenging may start to take place as the student realizes that, with care and support, these clients can be enabled to experience a quality of life. As the student learns of the strategies she can use to help these clients, and how these strategies may need to be adapted to meet the needs of individual clients, she is beginning to imagine and explore the alternatives for client-centred care.

Synthesizing and evaluating

As students draw conclusions and develop insights into the material they are processing – material from both formal theory and their personal experiences – they develop a set of ideas and perspectives about the management of the clinical situations they were involved with. They have, in effect, developed their own theory of practice through

---

Box 9.2 Aspects to be considered for processing through critical analysis

Consider the following aspects about the experience:

- The rationale of the care given
- The effects on the patient/client/family of the care given
- What aspect(s) of the episode had the most impact on you and why?
- What, if anything, you found demanding
- What you did that was appropriate/inappropriate and the reasons for making the judgement
- What others did that was appropriate/inappropriate and the reasons for making that judgement
- Decisions/choices made by yourself and others and whether these were the 'right' ones; what are the reasons for making that judgement?
- In a similar situation, what were your thoughts, feelings and behaviours?
- Is there a pattern?

personal experiences. Students can demonstrate the knowledge, understanding and values that have informed their actions. A new set of ideas, concepts and/or 'mindscape' (Bedford et al 1993) may emerge, 'enabling them to appreciate the inherent contradictions within professional caring without incapacitating them to the extent that they are unable to act because of their awareness of those dilemmas' (Bedford et al 1993:141). This will lead to altered ways of giving care. Aspects to be considered to assist further processing through synthesis and evaluation are suggested in Box 9.3.

Boud et al (1985) suggest using the process of validation to test for consistency between the new appreciations and existing knowledge and beliefs, and between these and parallel data drawn from others such as those of the mentor and the literature. The literature may be searched for written material that will shed further light on the various facets of the experience, such as data to support the care given. If there are any contradictions, the situation may need to be reappraised. These authors further suggest that, even if our new perception is not consistent with that held by others, it does not imply that we should reject it. Our idea may be breaking new ground or we may wish to hold a certain position regardless of conventional wisdom.

Outcomes and action

The aim of reflecting-on-experience during the processing phase is to make us ready for new experience. However, the benefits gained from reflection could be merely an exercise in abstract thinking if any resultant learning is not linked to action. Students will ask questions such as: 'What do the ideas and concepts mean to me? … How can I make use of what I have learned?' This is an ideal time for assisting students to specify what actions they plan to take so that they can consider the changes in practice and behaviours they want to incorporate into future clinical experiences. The changes may be quite small or they may be large.

In some instances, before changes can be made to practice, students may require to accept the new understanding and approaches into their own value systems. Changing their view of self is involved, as well as the values associated with self as practitioner. As students gain a better understanding of self and their professional practices, their confidence is likely to increase. They are then empowered to try out their new ideas in practice. As they do so, their practices are likely to be reshaped and they then enter into new experiences.

FRAMEWORK TO REVIEW LEARNING THROUGH PROCESSING OF EXPERIENCE

Proposed here is a framework (Table 9.1) to review learning that has arisen as a result of processing experiences. The treatment of learning in this format is to assist the learner and mentor in deciding the quality of learning achieved and what further learning needs to take place. It is not intended to imply that learning through the processing of experiences can be compartmentalized; nor can such learning be quantified (e.g. through the use of grading).

EXPERIENTIAL LEARNING AND CONTINUING PROFESSIONAL DEVELOPMENT

Professional knowledge and practices change constantly and require the practitioner to be motivated in order to refine and update knowledge and practices so that professional expertise, and thus practice wisdom (Hull 1998), is continually developing. Furthermore, it is essential to ensure that practitioners can maintain autonomous practice where they are capable of making their own decisions about their actions and the moral bases of those actions (Fish & Twinn 1997). The ability to exercise professional judgement is essential – professional judgement is seen as a complex skill requiring abilities to notice and analyse the patient's/client's problem, deciding what has to be done and evaluating the effectiveness of actions taken. Such ways of managing professional work cannot be laid down as absolute rules of practice and are termed 'professional artistry' by Schön (1987), which is seen to be

---

> ### Box 9.3 **Aspects to be considered for processing through synthesizing and evaluating**
>
> Students should ask themselves the following questions:
>
> - What made me think, feel and act that way?
> - Could I have acted differently?
> - Did I have any choice?
> - Did I do anything that was different?
> - Why was the care given successful/unsuccessful?
> - Was the care given an accurate reflection of personal and professional philosophies?
> - Were there any conflicts between personal beliefs and values and the care that was given?
> - What conclusions can I draw? What ideas, concepts and generalizations can I form?
> - How do I know that my conclusions are valid?

well beyond technical efficiency and the use of routine craft skills. The professional artistry view relies on frameworks and rules of thumb rather than rules. The practitioner is not less accountable, but is in fact more accountable, as moral accountability for all conduct is exercised (Fish & Twinn 1997). A holistic model for the continuing professional development of health care practitioners, as is the case for pre-registration education, will also have clinical experiences as one of its key points.

Using the 'model for learning from experience' explored so far in this chapter to structure the learning process will help the practitioner use clinical experiences as the key focus for continuing professional development. Although practice is of primary importance, its underlying theory is not set to one side. There is a close interrelationship between theory and practice – no professional action is devoid of theory, for theory involves beliefs, values, ideas and assumptions. Everything we do is thus influenced by theory. What may be absent is awareness of such theories. Many believe that unearthing the meaning of experiences comes after, or at best during, the action. This means that developing expertise (Benner 1984) in professional practice must begin with action.

Table 9.1 A framework to review learning through processing of experience

Stages of processing	Requires further development			Well developed
Description of situation including personal and others' thoughts and feelings	Relevance of description not demonstrated Lacks coherence, organization and clarity	Situation described, but lacks focus and omits sufficient detail	Recognizes and recollects key features of situations, including context, feeling and thoughts	High level of perception evident Subtle nuances in the situation noticed
Critical analysis of situation in relationship to personal and others' involvement	Minimal awareness	Begins to explore thoughts, feelings and behaviour of self and others triggered by the situation	Constructive exploration of thoughts, feelings and behaviour	Demonstrates insight into situation Shows an objective appreciation of how and why self and others felt, thought and behaved as they did in the situation, and how they affected the situation Sees the heart of the matter
Synthesizing and evaluating	Relevant underpinning values not identified. No evidence of forming ideas nor drawing any conclusions	Identifies some values relevant to the situation Limited range of ideas formed Assumptions underlying practice are not explored Conclusions lack depth	Identifies the values, ideas and concepts relevant to the situation Explores some assumptions underlying practice and draws some meaningful conclusions	Critically analyses values, ideas and concepts and their relationship to practice Sees the wider professional implications Constructively challenges own and others' assumptions
Evidence of learning/ outcomes of reflection	No evidence of implications for own practice/ learning	Identifies some implications for own practice/learning Some explicit evidence of learning	Evidence of learning explicit Identifies implications for practice, and begins to specify how own practice can develop	Integrates 'new' knowledge with previous knowledge to reach new/ different perspectives Specifies where and how own practice will develop Relates innovative practice development to the wider professional context

Often the most useful theorizing for action takes place *during* the activity and the most useful theory develops *after* the activity, if the activity has been carefully reconsidered during the processing phase (Schön 1987, 1983). The experience is the vehicle for enabling practitioners to consider what is involved in learning during and after professional activities, and how this learning can be used to develop professional practice.

The principles of learning from each phase of the model, in particular the experiencing and processing phases, will help the practitioner to derive more meaning and learning as professional activities are planned, entered into and reflected upon during and after completion of care. Practitioners enter into a continuum of learning, as this model shows; professional activity cannot be separated into the component parts of theory and practice. Using the principles of learning from the model for learning from experience, you may wish to ask yourself the following questions as you go about developing your expertise through continuing professional development activities:

- What is the nature of learning through professional activities? For example, is it a practical problem-solving activity involving people? Is it refining and defining practical wisdom? Is it developing theory? Is it questioning and challenging established practices?
- What sorts of professional/clinical activities should be used for refining and developing professional practice? Should they be every aspect of your working life? Should they be some aspect of practice that catches your attention? Should they be incidents that are outright critical events, such as emergency situations? Should they be aspects of practice that have simply gone unexamined and unchallenged and are now accepted practices?
- What can you say about yourself as a learner seeking to develop your professional practices? Are you able to get on with it by yourself? Do you find it helpful to bounce ideas off your colleagues? Do your colleagues bounce their ideas off you?
- When was the last time you examined how you practised in a constructive way with others? Bedford et al (1993) believe that as you enter into dialogues with others about your practice, not only do you make your understanding accessible to each other, but also you help to develop both the theory and the practice out of each other. If these dialogic debates are of sufficient depth and breadth, you will be able to explore and understand further the moral dimensions and the ambiguity, complexity and uncertainty of the practice settings.

Within their mandate for continuing professional development, the NMC and the HCPC require their practitioners to keep a record of continuing professional development activities by maintaining personal professional profiles (HCPC 2012, NMC 2011). The profile is to be created by documenting learning activities which are relevant to their practice and the ways in which they have informed and influenced practice. It is suggested here that the learning activities in Table 9.1 and those in the section on the processing phase can be utilized to assist practitioners to maintain their portfolio.

CONCLUSION

Dewey (1938) stated that all genuine education comes about through experience. Certainly, in practice-based professions such as the health care professions, clinical experience should be the basis for learning. To extract learning from experience, we need to create meaning from our experiences as we interact with, and react to, them. We cannot allow any experience to be taken for granted; once we do so, actions become routine and habitual, we stop noticing and enter into a rut.

In this chapter, I have attempted to portray some of the complexities of learning through clinical practice that can hinder meaningful learning from experience. Learning from experience is not a simple rational process – not only do we need to know *what* and *how* to do, but also we need to know *what* and *how* to think. Impacting on, and influencing, these psychomotor and cognitive processes are our feelings, values and beliefs. We therefore also need to exercise our affective self, which very frequently dominates our experience and may become either a positive or negative influence for learning. Forces around us also have their influences on how we engage with and extract meaning from an experience, such as the facilitative presence of others and our surroundings. Schön (1987) stated that learning conditions that are not easily met are an awareness of each other's experience, the ability to describe it and a willingness to make it discussable.

Usher (1993) reminds us that experience always says less than it wishes to say: there are many readings of it, it is never exhausted and total clarity may never be reached. Nevertheless, I hope that the discussion in this chapter has provided a range of perspectives to assist the learner and mentor during clinical practice to unearth meaning from clinical experiences.

If professionals are to develop skills in learning through their experience so as to develop the professional artistry in order to deal with the complex human issues of practice – entering into complex decision making and elements of professional judgement and practical wisdom guided by moral principles – they need to be taught, and encouraged to do so, during their pre-registration training.

KEY POINTS FOR REFLECTION

A model of preparation for professional practice that does not rely slavishly on the use and application of rules, schedules and prescriptions is more likely to equip practitioners to be able to deal with the complexities of clinical practice.

The *model for learning from experience* considers experience-based learning and has clinical experiences as one of its key foci. This emphasizes experiential learning, which proceeds from the assumption that ideas are not fixed, and immutable elements of thought but rather are continuously derived from, and tested out, through experience.

The underpinning principle of the model is that, although experience is the foundation of and the stimulus for learning, it does not necessarily lead to learning unless there is active engagement with it. This model has four phases:

1. **The preparatory phase.** The following questions may assist preparation:
   - Why has this particular experience been arranged?
   - What can be learnt through this experience?
   - How can learning from previous experiences be linked to this experience?
   - How can students be assisted to plan thoughtfully?
   - How can students be assisted to engage in the clinical experience?

   The preparatory phase focuses on:

   The student as a learner: consider 'learning intent', prior learning and the accumulation of previous experiences. The response of the learner to new experiences is determined significantly by these past experiences and their learning intent, as presuppositions and assumptions have been developed – the past creates expectations, which influence the present. The present context can serve to reinforce or counterbalance this.

   Developing noticing skills: noticing provides students with the basis for becoming more fully involved in a care-giving situation and enables them to 'reflect-in-action' (Schön 1983) as they become more aware of the processes of how decisions are made to inform actions taken. As well as paying attention to what is happening around the experience, it is equally important to pay attention to what is happening in themselves. Students need to be aware in three areas:
   how they are acting
   what they are thinking
   how they are feeling.

   Developing intervening skills: intervening is when the learner takes an initiative and is active in the event. This can be any verbal or physical action taken by the learner within the learning situation. Learners need to know how and when to intervene and the nature and content of the interventions.

2. **The experiencing phase.** During this phase the 'taking on board of what is going on' while 'performing' has to be accompanied by the 'thinking' and the 'feeling'. One key aim is to facilitate development of learners' 'power of judgement and capacity to act intelligently in new situations' (Dewey 1938:15). Learners are assisted to 'reflect-in-action'. Several teaching/learning strategies influence how the learner engages with, and reflects during, the experience:

   Sharing, explaining and 'pointing out': students who are cognitively ready to move to the next stage of development can be assisted to reach this potential through support and guidance from a more experienced other. Development is best facilitated if the mentor's speech guides the student to a level beyond that currently in use or practised. Having an accurate assessment of a learner's level of capability is crucial in assisting a learner to develop a higher level of competence. Consider engaging learners in 'situated negotiation of their practice': informal on-the-job conversations take place, which allow the sharing of ideas and understanding about care. Sharing, explaining and pointing out can also be in the form of overt physical guidance of actions.

   Questioning and challenging: skilful questioning and the challenging of thinking help students to uncover the hidden meaning of their clinical experiences. Ask students to explain and justify why a certain course of action has been chosen; explain why you are proceeding in a certain way; come up with decisions and actions that should be taken in certain situations; place the student in your shoes; invite the student to come forward with a diagnosis of what the problem may be and how that problem is best managed; invite the student's opinions about a situation.

   Allowing to experiment: the student assumes control of clinical care. Support by helping the student formulate the care to be given by prompting the student in searching for, and deciding upon, the most suitable option of care – the final decision rests with the student. Trust in the student's ability is necessary to enable the student to progress and develop clinical competence. Learn to 'let go'.

   Giving feedback on performance: immediate feedback on particularly commendable performances or pointing to where desired improvement could occur will help students extract more learning from clinical events. Balance timely feedback to avoid errors of care delivery against giving the student enough scope to use individual skill and flair during performance.

3. **The processing phase.** The experience is systematically reflected on and actively facilitated during this phase, as reflecting after the event is one of the most helpful

means of drawing learning from experience. There are three key stages in reflecting on experience:

Description of the experience: recollect and replay the experience in its totality, paying close attention to detail, noticing exactly what occurred and one's reactions, without making judgements.

Processing through critical analysis: the experience is thought about and mulled over further; assist to make links and connections among the components of the situation, and between other similar situations, and subsequently to see it as a whole picture; new knowledge and ideas are identified and related to that which is already known.

Synthesizing and evaluating: new experience and ideas/concepts formed are linked to previous experience to form 'new wholes'; through the process of validation, test for consistency between the new appreciations and existing knowledge and beliefs and between these and parallel data drawn from others and the literature.

4. **Outcomes and action:** learning is linked to action; assist students to specify actions they plan to take so that they can consider the changes in practice and behaviours they want to incorporate into future clinical experiences.

REFERENCES

Aitchison, J., Graham, P., 1989. Potato crisp pedagogy. In: Criticos, C. (Ed.), Experiential Learning in Formal and Non-Formal Education. Media Resource Centre, University of Natal, Durban, pp. 1–13.

Alexander, M.F., 1982a. Integrating theory and practice in nursing – part I. Nurs. Times., Occas. Pap. 78 (17), 65–68.

Alexander, M.F., 1982b. Integrating theory and practice in nursing – part II. Nurs. Times., Occas. Pap. 78 (18), 69–71.

Atkins, S., Murphy, K., 1993. Reflection: a review of the literature. J. Adv. Nurs. 18, 1188–1192.

Ausubel, D.P., 1968. Educational Psychology: A Cognitive View. Holt, Reinhart & Winston, New York.

Bedford, H., Phillips, T., Robinson, J., et al., 1993. Assessment of Competencies in Nursing and Midwifery Education and Training. The English National Board for Nursing, Midwifery and Health Visiting, London.

Benner, P., 1984. From Novice to Expert: Excellence and Power in Clinical Nursing Practice. Addison-Wesley, Menlo Park, California.

Benner, P., Wrubel, J., 1982. Skilled clinical knowledge: the value of perceptual awareness, part 2. J. Nurs. Admin. 12 (6), 28–33.

Bloom, B.S., Engelhart, M.D., Furst, E.J., et al., 1956. Taxonomy of Educational Objectives, Handbook 1: Cognitive Domain. Longman, London.

Boud, D., Walker, D., 1990. Making the most of experience. Stud. Contin. Educ. 12 (2), 61–80.

Boud, D., Walker, D., 1991. Experience and Learning: Reflection at Work. Deakin University, Geelong, Australia.

Boud, D., Walker, D., 1993. Barriers to reflection on experience. In: Boud, D., Cohen, R., Walker, D. (Eds.), Using Experience for Learning. The Society for Research into Higher Education and Open University Press, Buckingham, pp. 73–86.

Boud, D., Cohen, R., Walker, D., 1993. Understanding learning from experience. In: Boud, D., Cohen, R., Walker, D. (Eds.), Using Experience for Learning. The Society for Research into Higher Education and Open University Press, Buckingham, pp. 3–20.

Boud, D., Keogh, R., Walker, D., 1985. What is reflection in learning?. In: Boud, D., Keogh, R., Walker, D. (Eds.), Reflection: Turning Experience into Learning. Kogan Page, London, pp. 7–39.

Brookfield, S., 1987. Developing Critical Thinkers. Open University Press, Milton Keynes.

Carr, W., Kemmis, S., 1986. Becoming Critical: Education Knowledge and Action Research. The Falmer Press, London.

Criticos, C., 1993. Experiential learning and social transformation for a post-apartheid learning future. In: Boud, D., Cohen, R., Walker, D. (Eds.), Using Experience for Learning. The Society for Research into Higher

Education and Open University Press, Buckingham, pp. 157–168.

Dewey, J., 1925. The Later Works, 1925-1953, Volume I: 1925. Southern Illinois University Press, Carbondale.

Dewey, J., 1938. Experience and Education. Macmillan, New York.

Fish, D., Twinn, S., 1997. Quality Clinical Supervision. Butterworth-Heinemann, Oxford.

Fraser, D., Murphy, R., Worth-Butler, M., 1997. An Outcome Evaluation of the Effectiveness of Pre-registration Midwifery Programmes of Education. The English National Board for Nursing, Midwifery and Health Visiting, London.

Gerrish, K., 2000. Still fumbling along? A comparative study of the newly qualified nurse's perception of the transition from student to qualified nurse. J. Adv. Nurs. 32 (2), 473–480.

Health and Care Professions Council, 2012. Standards of Continuing Professional Development. HPC, London, Online. Available: <http://www.hpc-uk.org/aboutregistration/standards/cpd/index.asp> (accessed February 2012).

Higgs, J., 1997. Learning to make clinical decisions. In: McAllister, L., Lincoln, M., McLeod, S. (Eds.), Facilitating Learning in Clinical Settings. Stanley Thornes, Cheltenham, pp. 130–153.

Hull, C., 1998. Open learning and professional development. In: Quinn, F.M. (Ed.), Continuing Professional Development in Nursing. Stanley Thornes, Cheltenham, pp. 182–204.

Knowles, M.S., Elwood III, F.H., Swanson, R.A., 1998. The Adult Learner, fifth ed. Gulf Publishing, Houston.

Kolb, D.A., 1984. Experiential Learning: Experience as the Source of Learning, Development. Prentice-Hall, Englewood Cliffs, New Jersey.

Lindeman, E.C., 1926. The Meaning of Adult Education. New Republic, New York.

McAllister, L., 1997. An adult learning framework for clinical education. In: McAllister, L., Lincoln, M., McLeod, S. (Eds.), Facilitating Learning in Clinical Settings. Stanley Thornes, Cheltenham, pp. 1–26.

Marton, F., Säljö, R., 1984. Approaches to learning. In: Marton, F., Hounsell, D., Entwistle, N. (Eds.), The Experience of Learning. Scottish Academic Press, Edinburgh, pp. 36–55.

May, N., Veitch, L., McIntosh, J., et al., 1997. Evaluation of Nurse and Midwife Education in Scotland: 1992 Programmes. The National Board for Nursing, Midwifery and Health Visiting for Scotland, Edinburgh.

Mezirow, J., 1981. A critical theory of adult learning in education. Adult. Educ. 32 (1), 3–24.

Moriaty, J., MacIntyre, G., Manthorpe, J., et al., 2010. My expectations remain the same. The student has to be competent to practise: Practice assessor perspectives on the new social work degree qualification in England. Br. J. Soc. Work. 40, 583–601.

Neary, M., 2000. Teaching, Assessing and Evaluation for Clinical Competence. Stanley Thornes, Cheltenham.

Nordman, T., Kasen, A., Eriksson, K., 1998. Reflective practice – a way to the patient's world and caring. In: Johns, C., Freshwater, D. (Eds.), Transforming Nursing Through Reflective Practice Blackwell Science, London, pp. 161–176.

Nursing and Midwifery Council, 2011. The PREP Handbook. Nursing and Midwifery Council, London, Online. Available: <http://www.nmc-uk.org/Documents/Standards/NMC_Prep-handbook_2011.pdf> (accessed March 2012).

Open University, 2001. Assessing Practice in Nursing and Midwifery (K521 WB2). The Open University for the English National Board for Nursing, Midwifery and Health Visiting, Milton Keynes.

Phenix, P.H., 1964. Realms of Meaning. McGraw-Hill, New York.

Phillips, T., Schostak, J., Tyler, J., 2000. Practice and Assessment in Nursing and Midwifery: Doing it for Real. The English National Board for Nursing, Midwifery and Health Visiting, London.

Rogers, A., 1996. Teaching Adults, second ed. Open University Press, Buckingham.

Schön, D.A., 1987. Educating the Reflective Practitioner. Jossey-Bass, San Francisco.

Schön, D.A., 1983. The Reflective Practitioner: How Practitioners Think in Action. Basic Books, New York.

Spouse, J., 1998. Scaffolding student learning in clinical practice. Nurse. Educ. Today. 18, 259–266.

Stengelhofen, J., 1993. Teaching Students in Clinical Settings. Chapman & Hall, London.

Stuart, C.C., 2001. The reflective journeys of a midwifery tutor and her students. Reflective. Pract. 2 (2), 171–184.

Stuart, C.C., 2000. A model for developing skills of reflection. Br. J. Midwifery. 8 (2), 111–117.

Tilley, D.S., Allen, P., Collins, C., et al., 2007. Promoting clinical competence: Using scaffolded instruction for practice-based learning. J. Prof. Nurs. 23 (5), 285–289.

Townsend, J., 1990. Teaching/learning strategies. Nurs. Times. 86 (23), 66–68.

Usher, R., 1993. Experiential learning or learning from experience: Does it make a difference?. In: Boud, D., Cohen, R., Walker, D. (Eds.), Using Experience for Learning. The Society for Research into Higher Education and Open University Press, Buckingham, pp. 169–180.

White, R., Ewan, C., 1991. Clinical Teaching in Nursing. Chapman & Hall, London.

Windsor, A., 1987. Nursing students' perception of clinical experience. J. Nurs. Educ. 26 (4), 150–154.

Appendix 1

Declaration of good health and good character in support of an application for admission to a part of the NMC's professional register

I .... NMC PIN ....

to the best of my knowledge of:

(full name of applicant) ....

whose NMC PIN is ....

believe the above named student's health and character are sufficiently good to enable safe and effective practice and that there is an intention to comply with the *Code of professional conduct: NMC Standards for conduct, performance and ethics*. I also support their application to be entered in the professional register for nurses and midwives.

Signature* .... Date ....

Post held ....

Stamp of education/Training institution

*The individual signing this form must be registered with the NMC and should be the nursing registrant responsible for directing the educational programme. For Midwifery programmes this should be the lead midwife for education. In signing this supporting declaration of good health and good character, the individual should take account of the personal responsibilities and accountability that professional registration confers upon those practitioners registered with the NMC.

(Reproduced with permission of the Nursing and Midwifery Council.)

Appendix 2

Sample unit with its elements and one element of competence with its associated performance criteria

EXTRACT FROM NVQS IN HEALTH AND SOCIAL CARE LEVEL 3 – UNIT HSC35 AND ELEMENT HSC35a (SKILLS FOR HEALTH 2005)

Unit title: Promote choice, well-being and the protection of all individuals

About this unit

For this unit you are expected to protect individuals whilst respecting their diversity, difference, preferences and choice.

Elements of competence

HSC35a Develop supportive relationships that promote choice and independence
HSC35b Respect the diversity and difference of individuals and key people
HSC35c Contribute to the protection of all individuals
Element HSC35a Develop supportive relationships that promote choice and independence

Performance criteria

You need to show that:

1. You respect the dignity and privacy of individuals and key people

2. You treat and value each person as an individual and ensure that the support you give takes account of the their needs and preferences

3. You work with individuals and key people in ways that provide support that is consistent with individuals' beliefs, culture, values and preferences

4. You provide active support to enable individuals to participate in activities and maintain their independence

5. You support others with whom you work, to work in ways that:
   - recognise and respect individuals' beliefs and preferences
   - take account of individuals' preferences in everything they do
   - acknowledge and respect diversity and difference

6. You reflect on, and challenge:
   - your own assumptions, behaviour and ways of working
   - the assumptions of others, their behaviour and ways of working
   - procedures, practices and information that are discriminatory

7. You seek advice when you are having difficulty promoting equality and diversity

SCOPE FOR ELEMENT HSC35a: DEVELOP SUPPORTIVE RELATIONSHIPS THAT PROMOTE CHOICE AND INDEPENDENCE. EXTRACT FROM NVQS IN HEALTH AND SOCIAL CARE LEVEL 3 – UNIT HSC35 AND ELEMENT HSC35a (SKILLS FOR HEALTH 2005)

Scope

Actions that could adversely affect the use of evidence in future investigations

Include: asking inappropriate and/or leading questions; not following organisation and legal procedures; putting undue pressure on individuals.

Communicate

Includes using: the individual's preferred spoken language; the use of signs; symbols; pictures; writing; objects of reference; communication passports; other non-verbal forms of communication; human and technological aids to communication.

Danger

Includes: imminent; in the short term; in the medium term; in the longer term.

Harm and abuse

Includes: neglect; physical, emotional and sexual abuse; bullying; self harm; reckless behaviour.

Key people

Includes: family; friends; carers; others with whom the individual has a supportive relationship.

Risks

Include the possibility of: danger, damage and destruction to the environment and goods; injury and harm to people; self harm; bullying; abuse; reckless behaviour.

Statements that could adversely affect the use of evidence in future investigations

Include: changing information; removing information; adding to information.

KNOWLEDGE AND UNDERSTANDING FOR UNIT HSC35: PROMOTE CHOICE, WELL-BEING AND THE PROTECTION OF ALL INDIVIDUALS. EXTRACT FROM NVQS IN HEALTH AND SOCIAL CARE LEVEL 3 – UNIT HSC35 (SKILLS FOR HEALTH 2005)

Knowledge specification for the whole of this unit

Competent practice is a combination of the application of skills and knowledge informed by values and ethics. This specification details the knowledge and understanding required to carry out competent practice in the performance described in this unit. When using this specification it is important to read the knowledge requirements in relation to expectations and requirements of your job role.

You need to show that you know, understand and can apply in practice:

Values

1. Legal and organisational requirements on equality, diversity, discrimination, rights, confidentiality and sharing of information
2. How to provide active support and place the preferences and best interest of individuals at the centre of everything you do
3. Dilemmas between:
   - individuals' rights and their responsibilities for their own care and protection, the rights and responsibilities of key people and your role and responsibilities for their care and protection
   - individuals' views, preferences and expectations and how these can and are being met
   - your own values and those of the individuals and key people
   - your own professional values and those of others within and outside your organisations
4. How to work in partnership with individuals, key people and those within and outside your organisation to enable the individuals' needs, wishes and preferences to be met
5. Methods that are effective:
   - in promoting equality and diversity
   - when dealing with and challenging discrimination

Legislation and organisational policy and procedures

6. Codes of practice and conduct, and standards and guidance relevant to your own and the roles, responsibilities, accountability and duties of others for valuing and respecting individuals and key people, taking account of their views and preferences and protecting them from danger, harm and abuse

7. Current local, national and European legislation and organisational requirements, procedures and practices for:
   - data protection, including recording, reporting, storage, security and sharing of information
   - health and safety
   - risk assessment and management
   - dealing with comments and complaints
   - the protection of yourself, individuals, key people and others from danger, harm and abuse
   - working with others to provide integrated services

8. Practice and service standards relevant to your work setting and relating to valuing and respecting individuals and key people, taking account of their views and preferences and protecting them from danger, harm and abuse

9. How to access records and information on the needs, views and preferences of individuals and key people

10. The purpose of, and arrangements for your supervision and appraisal

Theory and practice

11. How and where to access information and support that can inform your practice relating to valuing and respecting people, taking account of their views and preferences and protecting them from danger, harm and abuse

12. Theories relevant to the individuals with whom you work, about:
    - human growth and development
    - identity and self-esteem
    - loss and change
    - power and how it can be used and abused

13. The effects of stress and distress

14. Role of relationships and support networks in promoting the well-being of individuals

15. Factors that affect the health, well-being, behaviour, skills, abilities and development of individuals and key people with whom you work

16. Methods of supporting individuals to:
    - express their needs and preferences
    - understand and take responsibility for promoting their own health and care
    - identify how their care needs should be met
    - assess and manage risks to their health and well-being

17. Factors that may lead to danger, harm and abuse

18. How to protect yourself, individuals, key people and others with whom you work from danger, harm and abuse

19. Signs and symptoms of danger, harm and abuse

20. Correct actions to take when you suspect danger, harm and abuse or where it has been disclosed

21. The types of evidence that is valid in investigations and court, actions and statements that could contaminate the use of evidence

22. Methods that are effective in forming, maintaining and ending relationships with individuals and key people

23. Different ways of communicating with individuals, families, carers, groups and communities about choice, well-being and protection

(Reproduced with permission of Skills for Health and Skills for Care and Development from Skills for Health website, http://www.skillsforhealth.org.uk (accessed December 2005). National Occupational Standards are reviewed and updated on a regular basis: see the National Occupational Standards Directory website, http://www.ukstandards.org.uk.)

Appendix 3

Skills checklist

GUIDELINES ON THE USE OF THIS RECORD OF ACHIEVEMENT

This record section is designed to help you direct your learning in relation to your clinical skills development and assist you in keeping a record of your progress. You may find it is useful in providing additional evidence for your professional portfolio.

It lists the core skills addressed within the main text. Clearly the list of skills is not exhaustive; in recognition of this fact, spaces are included for you to add any skills unique to your personal learning experiences.

It is suggested that you initial and date the first column when you have been instructed in or studied the theoretical underpinnings of the skill and initial and date the other columns when:

Level 1 – you have observed the procedure in the practice setting

Level 2 – you have participated in the skill under direct supervision

Level 3 – you have performed the skill on a number of occasions and now require minimal supervision

Level 4 – you can perform the skill safely and competently, giving the rationale for your actions

Level 5 – you have taught the skill to others

It is recommended that initials denoting achievement of Levels 4 and 5 be those of a Registered Nurse Assessor, though this will clearly require local negotiation as this document is not intended to circumvent your locally determined summative assessment(s) of practice.

When performing each skill, remember it is important to not only exhibit the psychomotor element but also the affective and cognitive components (i.e. attitude and knowledge).

Table A3.1 Skills related to the activity of breathing						
Skill	**Instructed/studied**	**1**	**2**	**3**	**4**	**5**
Assess individual's ability to breathe normally						
Monitor and record respiratory rate						
Monitor and record peak flow						
Maintain airway of:						
infant						
child						
adult						
Monitor and record expectorant						

(Continued)

Table A3.1 (continued)						
Skill	**Instructed/studied**	**1**	**2**	**3**	**4**	**5**
Disposal of sputum secretions						
Obtain sputum specimen						
Maintain safe administration of oxygen as prescribed via:						
mask						
nasal cannulae						
humidifier						
Perform rescue breathing (artificial respiration):						
infant/child/adult						

Table A3.2 Skills related to the activity of mobility						
Skill	**Instructed/studied**	**1**	**2**	**3**	**4**	**5**
Assess individual's ability to mobilize safely						
Care of self						
Assess task, individual capacity, load and environment						
Move inanimate objects						
Moving and handling of a range of clients into the following positions:						
upright						
recumbent						
semi-recumbent						
lateral						
semi-prone (recovery)						
prone						
side to side						
Move a range of clients from:						
chair to chair						
bed to chair						
chair to bed						
up the bed						
up in the chair						
cot						
Care for an individual who is falling						
Care for the individual who has fallen						

Table A3.3 Skills related to the activity of personal cleansing and dressing						
Skill	**Instructed/studied**	**1**	**2**	**3**	**4**	**5**
Make a bed/cot that is:						
unoccupied						
occupied						
Changing a sheet on an occupied bed:						
top to bottom						
side to side						
Dispose of linen that is:						
uncontaminated						
contaminated						
Assist individuals requiring a:						
shower						
general bath						
wash						
Assist individuals maintain their oral hygiene:						
cleansing of teeth/dentures/mucous membranes						
use of mouthwashes/dental floss/ interdental sticks						
Administration of eye care						
Facial shaving:						
with a safety razor						
with an electric shaver						
Care of hair:						
washing in bed						
dealing with infestation						
Assist a variety of individuals to dress:						
infant						
child						
adult						

Table A3.4 Related to the activity of maintaining a safe environment						
Skill	**Instructed/studied**	**1**	**2**	**3**	**4**	**5**
Universal precautions – effective:						
hand washing						
use of gloves						
use of plastic aprons						
safe disposal of equipment						
Adheres to Health & Safety at Work Act in relation to:						
disinfection policies						
disposal of infected materials						
dealing with mercury spillage						
dealing with blood and body fluids						
Radiation:						
report untoward occurrences						
Perform a simple dressing using aseptic technique						
Obtain a wound swab						
Monitor pulse:						
radial						
carotid						
apex						
femoral						
Monitor and record blood pressure using:						
a mercury sphygmomanometer						
an aneroid sphygmomanometer						
an electronic device						
Administration of medicines (under direct supervision in keeping with trust policies)						
Storage of medicines						
Respond in the event of an actual or suspected fire						
Respond in the event of a cardiac arrest						
Respond in the event of other emergency (state type)						

Table A3.5 Skills related to the activity of eating and drinking						
Skill	**Instructed/studied**	**1**	**2**	**3**	**4**	**5**
Assess individual's nutritional status						
Assist clients in selecting appropriate meals/fluids						
Monitor and record nutritional intake						
Monitor and record fluid balance						
Assist clients with feeding						
Assist clients with drinking						
Feed dependent clients						
Recognize and report changes in clients' condition						
Provide first aid to a client who is choking						

Table A3.6 Skills related to the activity of communicating						
Skill	**Instructed/studied**	**1**	**2**	**3**	**4**	**5**
Respond appropriately to telephone calls						
Assess the communication needs of clients						
Communicate effectively with clients who have a:						
hearing difficulty						
speaking difficulty						
language difficulty						
comprehension difficulty						
Manage a client exhibiting an aggressive outburst						
Recognize and report changes in clients' condition						
Give and receive reports of clients' condition:						
orally						

Table A3.7 Skills related to the activity of dying						
Skill	**Instructed/studied**	**1**	**2**	**3**	**4**	**5**
Communicate with dying patients						
Communicate with relatives of dying patients						
Communicate with the bereaved						
Perform last offices						

Table A3.8 Skills related to the activity of eliminating

Skill	Instructed/studied	1	2	3	4	5
Assess individual's ability to eliminate effectively						
Assist clients to use:						
bedpan						
urinal						
toilet/commode						
Apply/change a nappy						
Empty a catheter bag						
Monitor and record urinary output						
Monitor and record bowel actions						
Monitor and record vomit/gastric aspirate						
Obtain specimen of urine/faeces/vomit for laboratory examination						
Identify and report changes in clients' condition						

Table A3.9 Skills related to the activity of maintaining body temperature

Skill	Instructed/studied	1	2	3	4	5
Assess an individual's ability to maintain a normal body temperature						
Assist individual's select suitable attire to maintain a normal body temperature						
Monitor and accurately record the temperature of a(n):						
infant						
child						
adult						
Orally						
Axillary						
Aurally						
Using fever strips						
Use appropriate strategies to raise body temperature						
Use appropriate strategies to lower body temperature						
Participate in the assessment of clients' ability to maintain body temperature						

Table A3.10 Skills related to the activity of expressing sexuality

Skill	Instructed/studied	1	2	3	4	5
Maintain privacy and dignity						
Assess individual's ability to express their sexuality:						
child						
adult						
Assist individuals express their sexuality:						
child						
adult						

Table A3.11 Skills related to the activity of working and playing

Skill	Instructed/studied	1	2	3	4	5
Assess individual's ability to work and play						
Assist individuals select appropriate work activities						
Assist individuals select appropriate recreational activities						

Table A3.12 Skills related to the activity of sleep and rest

Skill	Instructed/studied	1	2	3	4	5
Assess individual's needs related to sleep and rest						
Monitor and record individual's sleep and rest patterns						
Assist individuals achieve a balance between activity and rest						

Table A3.13 Additional skills

Skill	Instructed/ studied	1	2	3	4	5

(Reproduced by permission of John Wiley & Sons Ltd, from Hilton, P.A. (Ed.,) 2004. Record of achievement. In: Fundamental Nursing Skills. Whurr Publishers Ltd, London, pp. 306–313.)

Appendix 4

Professional behaviours inventory

1. Reliability in care delivery within expected capability

Achieved	Achieved	Achieved	Not achieved
Exceptionally reliable at all times	Very good level of reliability	Satisfactory level of reliability	Unreliable

2. Attending to client's needs and requests within expected capability

Achieved	Achieved	Achieved	Not achieved
Exceptionally attentive and conscientious at all times	Very attentive and conscientious	Satisfactory level of attention and response paid to clients' needs and requests	Insufficient level of attention and response paid to clients' needs and requests

3. Consistency of efforts to achieve the requisite standard of care

Achieved	Achieved	Achieved	Not achieved
Constantly and consistently makes best efforts in pursuit of excellence	Constantly makes good effort to achieve high standards of care	Makes satisfactory effort to achieve high standards of care	Perfunctory effort made to achieve required standard of care

4a. Relating and working with colleagues and other team members

Achieved	Achieved	Achieved	Not achieved
Outstanding ability to work as a team member	Good ability to work as a team member	Functions satisfactorily as a team member	Uncooperative in the team

4b. Relating and working with colleagues and other team members

Achieved	Achieved	Achieved	Not achieved
Contributes very actively	Contributes well	Makes occasional contributions	Does not contribute to the team

4c. Relating and working with colleagues and other team members

Achieved	Achieved	Achieved	Not achieved
Has outstanding rapport	Has good rapport	Has satisfactory rapport	Unable to establish rapport

5a. Acknowledgement of colleagues' experience and opinions

Achieved	Achieved	Achieved	Not achieved
Polite, listens carefully and highly respectful of colleagues' experience and opinions at all times	Listens carefully and shows a good level of respect for colleagues' experience and opinions most of the time	Satisfactory level of respect for colleagues' experience and opinions most of the time	Poor respect for colleagues' experiences and opinions

5b. Acknowledgement of colleagues' experience and opinions

Achieved	Achieved	Achieved	Not achieved
Manages differences of opinion very well	Manages differences of opinion well	Manages differences of opinion fairly well	Unable to manage differences of opinions

6. Management of personal opinions

Achieved	Achieved	Achieved	Not achieved
Outstanding ability to contain and voice own opinions	Good ability to contain and voice own opinions	Some difficulty in containing and voicing own opinions	Voices own opinions inappropriately

7. Recognition of own limitations within expected capability

Achieved	Achieved	Achieved	Not achieved
Outstanding level of self-awareness and ability to recognize own limitations	Good self-awareness and recognition of own limitations	Satisfactory self-awareness and recognition of own limitations	Limited self-awareness; unaware of own limitations; potentially unsafe

8a. Response to feedback

Achieved	Achieved	Achieved	Not achieved
Responds positively and in a mature manner to constructive feedback at all times; considers it carefully	Responds positively and in a mature manner to constructive feedback most of the time	Has some difficulty in responding appropriately to constructive feedback	Resents criticism, reluctant to accept feedback

8b. Response to feedback

Achieved	Achieved	Achieved	Not achieved
Uses feedback to inform practice at all times	Uses feedback to inform practice most of the time	Uses feedback to inform practice some of the time	Does not change practice through feedback

9a. Verbal and non-verbal interpersonal skills

Achieved	Achieved	Achieved	Not achieved
Verbal communication and interpersonal skills are congruent, clear, effective and appropriate at all times	Verbal communication and interpersonal skills are congruent, clear and appropriate most of the time	Verbal communication and interpersonal skills are satisfactory most of the time	Poor interpersonal skills, frequently gives mixed messages

9b. Verbal and non-verbal interpersonal skills

Achieved	Achieved	Achieved	Not achieved
Non-verbal communication and interpersonal skills are congruent, clear, effective and appropriate at all times	Non-verbal communication and interpersonal skills are congruent, clear and appropriate most of the time	Non-verbal communication and interpersonal skills are satisfactory most of the time	Poor interpersonal skills, frequently gives mixed messages

10a. Communication with women and their partners within expected capability

Achieved	Achieved	Achieved	Not achieved
Exceptionally reassuring and supportive	Makes very good efforts to reassure and support	Satisfactory ability to reassure and support	Does not provide adequate reassurance and supporting care

10b. Communication with women and their partners within expected capability

Achieved	Achieved	Achieved	Not achieved
Very encouraging of their involvement as partners in care	Encouraging of their involvement as partners in care	Satisfactory ability to involve them as partners in care	Discourages their participation as partners

11. Promotion of fair and anti-discriminatory practice

Achieved	Achieved	Achieved	Not achieved
Actively promotes fair and anti-discriminatory practice at all times; always alert to discriminatory practice	Always maintains fair and anti-discriminatory practice; will recognize and act on evidence of discriminatory practice	Does not knowingly permit unfair or discriminatory practice; shows satisfactory awareness of the same	Shows poor awareness of fair and anti-discriminatory practice or promotes discriminatory practice

12. Respect for women and their families

Achieved	Achieved	Achieved	Not achieved
Shows exceptional and consistent level of respect for women and their families	Very respectful of women and their families	Satisfactory level of respect for women and their families	Poor level of respect for women and their families

13. Promotion of rights for women and families

Achieved	Achieved	Achieved	Not achieved
Always actively promotes rights for women and families; always alert to circumstances where rights may be overlooked	Always maintains rights for women and families; will recognise and act on evidence of rights being overlooked	Does not knowingly permit breach of rights for women and families; shows satisfactory awareness of the same	Shows poor awareness of, or disregards, rights for women and families

14. Observation of ethical practice

Achieved	Achieved	Achieved	Not achieved
Extremely effective in identifying ethical aspects of care and raising or handling ethical issues skilfully and collaboratively	Identifies ethical aspects of care well and always raises or handles ethical issues appropriately and collaboratively	Satisfactory awareness of ethical aspects of care, reflected in care given	Poor awareness of ethical aspects of care or handles ethical issues inappropriately

15. Attention to professional appearance and dress code

Achieved	Achieved	Achieved	Not achieved
Always maintains exemplary standard of professional appearance and dress code	Very good standard of professional appearance and dress code	Satisfactory standard of professional appearance and dress code	Careless or unprofessional standard of appearance and dress code

16. Punctuality and timekeeping

Achieved	Achieved	Achieved	Not achieved
Completely dependable; always punctual	Very good level of reliability; usually punctual or communicates appropriately if unavoidably delayed	Satisfactory time-keeping; satisfactory communication if delayed	Unreliable; poor timekeeper and/or poor at communicating when delayed

Appendix 5

Checklists for the clinical learning environment

The checklists below contain key questions that address the guidance for good practice.

Those responsible for practice placements within higher education institutions (HEIs) and service environments should ensure that all these questions have been considered in the planning, provision and evaluation of practice placement experiences.

1. Providing practice placements

- Is there a jointly developed strategy agreed by HEI and service for the selection development and monitoring of practice placements?
- Is the strategy for the selection and monitoring of practice placements shared with other health care education providers?
- Does the strategy for the selection of practice placements enable supply to meet demand?
- Is the identification of practice placements a joint exercise between HEI and service providers?
- Does the strategy require a profile of practice placements?
- Do all placement providers have a profile that determines:
  - maximum number and type of students at any time in a placement
  - the skills required by the student before beginning the practice experience
  - the learning opportunities available and the learning outcomes expected from
  - the placement?
- Have practitioners working in practice areas received preparation for their role in teaching, supporting and supervising students?
- Do the arrangements for practice placements enable students to have equity of opportunity for their learning experiences?

- Do programme planners take account of any special needs students may have?
- Does the totality of the practice experience enable the student to meet all statutory/professional requirements of the programme?
- Do students and mentors/assessors know what is expected of them through specified practice outcomes?
- Are placement areas designed to enable students to experience the full 24 hours a day, 7 days per week nature of health care where necessary?
- Are practice placements introduced at an early stage in the programme so students can see the relevance of related theory?
- Are placements of sufficient length to enable students to achieve the stated learning outcomes?
- Do all students have a period of practice experience to support and consolidate their transition to registered practitioner?
- Does practice experience outside the United Kingdom meet the requirements of the statutory/professional body?
- Are all placement areas audited in line with the requirements of the statutory/professional body as to their continuing suitability for students' practice experience?
- Is the quality of practice placements monitored jointly by service providers and HEIs, and is feedback provided to all participants?
- Is good practice disseminated following audit and monitoring and does joint action planning address areas of concern or needing enhancement?

2. Practice learning environment

- Does the practice area have a stated philosophy of care that is reflected in practice and supports curriculum aims?

- Does the practice provision reflect respect for the rights of health service users and their carers?
- Does the provision of care reflect respect for the privacy, dignity and religious and cultural beliefs and practices of patients and clients?
- Is care provision based on relevant research-based and evidence-based findings where available?
- Does care provision involve different models of care commensurate with current practice and encompassing local and national initiatives?
- Are interpersonal and practice skills fostered through a range of teaching/learning methods?
- Does the practice experience enable students to experience the role of the registered practitioner in a range of contexts?
- Do all placements have an infrastructure to support continuing professional development opportunities for practitioners?
- Do students gain experience as part of a multi-professional team?
- Does the sequencing and balance between university and practice-based study promote the integration of knowledge, attitudes and skills?
- Is a learning resources area available in the practice environment?
- Does student feedback contribute to the ongoing evaluation of the learning environment and the student experience and are all stakeholders aware of the feedback?

3. Student support

- Are students given comprehensive programme information and information about their particular placements?
- Do students receive adequate and appropriate preparation for the practice placements?
- Does this preparation include practice in a skills laboratory?
- Do students receive a comprehensive orientation to each of their placements and is the orientation jointly agreed between mentors/assessors and programme teachers?
- Are students given an initial interview during the first week of the placement, to agree the learning outcomes and ways of achieving them, taking into account their prior knowledge and experience?
- Are students' learning needs, achievements and opportunities reviewed regularly?
- Do students receive agreed written learning outcomes for each placement?
- Do practice placements facilitate progression in terms of the learning experience available?

- Does the experience available among clinical staff support the student's achievement of the learning outcomes of the educational programme at the appropriate level?
- Do students receive consistent supervision and support during all practice placements?
- Is there a named mentor-assessor with qualifications and experience commensurate with the context of care delivery and the requirements of the appropriate professional/statutory bodies, who supervises and guides students in all practice placements?
- Are students supported at the appropriate level in successive practice placements?
- Do practice staff members have dedicated time in educational activities to ensure they are competent in teaching and mentoring/assessing roles?
- Do lecturers have dedicated time in practice to ensure they are competent in the practice environment?
- Are lecturers involved in supporting student learning in practice areas?
- Are students assisted in linking theory and practice and using a research base for practice, by lecturers and practitioners?

4. Assessment of practice

- Are the periods of practice experience used for summative assessment of sufficient length to enable the agreed learning outcomes to be achieved?
- Is there a named mentor/assessor with the appropriate qualifications and experience to assess students in practice placements?
- Are the assessment methods used rigorous, valid and reliable?
- Are there enough mentors/assessors to assess the student's developing competence and to observe the student's achievement of the intended learning outcomes over a suitable period of time?
- Does the student's demonstration of competence involve the achievement of learning outcomes in both theory and practice?
- Is a portfolio of practice experience included in the assessment of the student's fitness for practice?
- Is the student's practice assessed in the context of a multi-professional team?
- Does the assessment strategy reflect progression, integration and coherence?

REFERENCE

ENB & Department of Health, 2001. Placements in Focus. The English National Board for Nursing, Midwifery and Health Visiting and The Department of Health, London.

Index

A

Abbatt, F. 82
Access Northern Ireland 31
Accountability
    clinical practice assessment 22–38
    professionalism and 19–20
    responsibility and 20–22, 21f, 22–27,
        27–38
'Activities of Living' model 56
Administration experience 155–156
Affective domain 55, 110
Aggleton, P. 56
Aggression, student reaction 140–141
Aitchison, J. 171, 171–172
Albarran, J. 139
Alexander, M.F. 170
Allan, H.T. 11–12
Allitt, Beverley 6, 30
Analysis, Bloom's taxonomy 72t
Andrews, M. 151–152
Anger, student reaction 140, 140–141, 141
Anti-discrimination issues
    law 32–33
    practice, promotion 205
Anxiety 113, 141
    assessment 9–10, 102, 105–106, 107
    clinical placements 150, 155,
        156–159, 173, 175
Application, Bloom's taxonomy 72t
Apprenticeship system 151
Armstrong, N. 23
Ashworth, P. 26–27
*Assessing Students: How Shall We Know
    Them?* (Rowntree) 66
Assessment
    clinical practice 10–14
    criteria 127–129
    decisions 135–137

defined 1
educational audit 162
fair *see* Fair assessment
feedback 104
matrix 92–93
nature of 1–2
problems 137–142
purposes 2–10
Assessment methods 67–84
    care records 83
    case studies 83–84
    continuous *see* Continuous
        assessment
    discussion 73–74
    examination of products 70
    formative *see* Formative assessment
    learning diary 74–75
    observation *see* Observation of practice
    overview 63–64
    projects/assignments 84
    questioning 70–73, 72t
    selecting/combining 84–85
    simulation *see* Simulation
    summative *see* Summative assessment
    witnesses *see* Testimony of others
    see also Self-assessment; Triangulation
Assessors 1–2, 2
    assumptions 35, 37
    bias 66, 66, 66
    defined 1
    evidence log 132f, 133f
    feedback 10
    as 'gatekeepers' 6
    mentor-assessor interface 38–39, 66
    reliability, factor in 96–98
    skills 6
Assignments 84
Atkin, Lord 31–32
Atkins, S. 180

Attitudes 93–94, 110, 137, 152–153
Attributes 48
    cooperative 57–58, 57
    performance and 48, 48, 65, 67
    personal (intrinsic) 57–58, 151–152
    professional 151–152
Attrition rates 3, 3t, 4, 4, 4, 4t
Audiovisual aids 160
Audits, educational 161, 162–163, 163
Ausubel, D.P. 103, 182
Autonomy 20–21

B

Bailey, J. 123–124
Bailey, M.E. 108–109
Beaumont, S. 27
Becher, T. 27
Beck, D.L. 156
Bedford, H. 2, 47–48
    assessment 11, 65, 75, 115–116
    dialogue/discussion 73, 73, 129, 185
    documentation 74, 74
    feedback 122
    meetings 105
    performance levels 111
    practice educators 133
    triangulation 63
Behaviour 125
Behavioural skills 12
Bell, M. 56
Benner, P. 49, 50, 69, 126–127, 127
Bergman, R. 20–21
Between-methods triangulation 64, 64
Bias 97, 140
    assessors 66, 66, 66
    observer 68
    peers 77
    practice educators 27